Human Fatigue

Fatigue is a condition spanning the breadth of human functioning in health and disease and is a central concern in sport and exercise. Even so we are yet to fully understand its causes. One reason for this lack of understanding is that we seldom consider fatigue from an evolutionary perspective – as an adaptation that provided reproductive success.

This ground-breaking book outlines the evidence that fatigue is a result of adaptations distinctive to humans. It argues that humans developed adaptations which led to enhanced fatigue resistance compared with other mammals and discusses the implications in the context of exercise, health and performance. Highly illustrated throughout, it covers topics such as defining and measuring fatigue, the emotional aspect of fatigue, how thermoregulation affects the human capacity to resist fatigue, and fatigue in disease.

Human Fatigue is essential reading for all exercise scientists as well as graduate and undergraduate students in the broad field of physiology and exercise physiology.

Francesco E. Marino is Professor of Physiology and Head of the School of Exercise Science, Sport and Health at Charles Sturt University, Australia. He was Visiting Professor at the University of Cape Town in South Africa, the University of Verona in Italy and Harvard University in Cambridge, USA. In 2016 he was awarded the prestigious Memorial Spitfire Fellowship for his work on hydration and human performance in the heat.

Routledge Research in Sport and Exercise Science

The *Routledge Research in Sport and Exercise Science* series is a showcase for cutting-edge research from across the sport and exercise sciences, including physiology, psychology, biomechanics, motor control, physical activity and health, and every core sub-discipline. Featuring the work of established and emerging scientists and practitioners from around the world, and covering the theoretical, investigative and applied dimensions of sport and exercise, this series is an important channel for new and ground-breaking research in the human movement sciences.

Available in this series:

The Science of Judo
Edited by Mike Callan

Modelling and Simulation in Sport and Exercise
Edited by Arnold Baca and Jürgen Perl

The Exercising Female
Science and Application
Edited by Jacky J. Forsyth and Claire-Marie Roberts

Genetics and the Psychology of Motor Performance
Sigal Ben-Zaken, Veronique Richard, Gershon Tenenbaum

Psychological Aspects of Sport-Related Concussions
Edited by Gordon A. Bloom and Jeffrey G. Caron

Human Fatigue
Evolution, Health and Performance
Frank Marino

For more information about this series, please visit www.routledge.com/sport/series/RRSES.

Human Fatigue

Evolution, Health and Performance

Francesco E. Marino

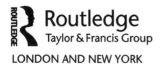

LONDON AND NEW YORK

First published 2019 by Routledge

2 Park Square, Milton Park, Abingdon, Oxon, OX14 4RN
605 Third Avenue, New York, NY 10017

Routledge is an imprint of the Taylor & Francis Group, an informa business

First issued in paperback 2020

British Library Cataloguing-in-Publication Data
A catalogue record for this book is available from the British Library

Library of Congress Cataloging-in-Publication Data
A catalog record for this book has been requested

ISBN: 978-1-138-93973-8 (hbk)
ISBN: 978-0-367-73112-0 (pbk)

Typeset in Goudy
by Apex CoVantage, LLC

For my wonderful wife, Trish, and the three treasures we share, Emma, Alexander and Anabel. Of all the hominins I know, they are indeed the most *infatigable*.

Contents

Preface

There are a number of personal reasons for writing this book. First and foremost is the challenge which comes with trying to put in writing the ideas about human performance and fatigue which I have collected over a period of 25 years as an academic. However, some of those ideas stretch back to my younger days of being an avid footballer (round ball!) and what seemed to be the physical training extremes I endured at the hands of coaches. This book represents my understanding of the concept of fatigue. It is an attempt to harness much of the research which I have been involved with over the past 25 years. Much of this research represents human exercise performance under various conditions, including extreme temperatures.

A second reason is the challenge of writing a book which would be informative and provocative for my fellow exercise scientists and all those that have a love of human performance. This particular challenge was perhaps the most difficult since I had to make assumptions about prerequisite knowledge. A third reason is to share the joy which comes with the appreciation of human performance. A fourth reason, but connected with the third, is that I never had the opportunity to formally study evolutionary biology, except in splashes of curriculum here and there. For this reason, over the course of an academic career I devoured all manner of writings in the field of evolutionary science, which has led me to the conclusion that all observations in exercise science can be explained by evolutionary theory. I even went to the extreme of a sabbatical at Harvard University in the Department of Human Evolutionary Biology. It was during this time that I truly understood how little I understood about evolutionary biology, but it did confirm my view that all things in human performance and disease can potentially be unravelled by evolutionary theory. So, this book is the culmination of this journey. By the way, the journey continues! Thank you, Professor Lieberman!

One of the first studies that I had the privilege to be a part of was on the effect of lowering body temperature for improving exercise performance in the heat, known as precooling. At the time I was captivated by the fact that reducing body temperature by as little as 0.5°C before exercise would result in better times or greater distances. My initial and rudimentary understanding was that body temperature was a limiting factor for exercise – an observation that had general consensus, albeit the mechanism was unknown. Over subsequent years it became apparent that the results from these studies were very much dependent on the exercise protocol that was used – that is, whether the exercise was either self-paced or fixed by the experimenter. This difference meant that experimental results had to be interpreted with some caution and contextualised against the exercise model that was used. It also meant that time to 'fatigue' was highly dependent on the exercise protocol.

A crucial question in the exercise sciences is what determines how fatigue develops during physical performance. This question has been a central tenet of experimental studies in elite, recreationally active, healthy and diseased individuals. The reason for this is that understanding what the exercise 'stopper' might be regardless of health status could mean the difference between winning and losing, improving health or even motivating more people to partake in exercise to gain the benefits of regular physical activity. However, fatigue is not easily defined and requires a nuanced approach to understand how to measure it and what the potential causes might be. The exercise sciences have attacked these questions from many different perspectives so that there are likely to be metabolic, cardiovascular, respiratory, thermoregulatory and neuromuscular answers, all with a specific story to tell and all worthy of investigation. Although much has been learned about these systems and their responses under different conditions in both health and disease, a glaring omission has been why these systems work as they do. The only way to answer this particular question is to go back in time and understand the evolutionary path taken by our biology and that of other animals. It would not be an understatement to suggest that exercise scientists in the main have had little or no formal training in evolutionary biology – including me! Why is this important? As put by (Dobzhansky 1973), the simple answer is that "nothing in biology makes sense except in the light of evolution." For instance, why have mammals adopted a core temperature balance point of 37°C? Why not 25°C or 42°C? What advantages would this particular body temperature have and what were the determining factors for its evolution and eventual adoption? Why the erect posture and bipedal locomotion? Some of these questions have been studied and debated, in some cases for centuries. Definitive answers to these questions will not be found in this book, but potential explanations and propositions are provided that might cause us to think differently about our health and performance capabilities.

The central theme of this book is that evolution played a part in how we as humans, when compared to other mammals, in particular our non-human primates, began on a biological path eventuating in the 'choice' between endurance and power. As such, the contention is that the biological machinery that provides for endurance also improves our fatigue resistance. To make this case, Chapter 1 deals mainly with the basics of evolutionary theory. This includes the concepts of adaptation and exaptation and their relationship to fatigue. Chapter 2 introduces the concepts of safety factors and trade-offs in physiology. Surprisingly this is an area that is under-appreciated in the exercise sciences given that much of the field attempts to explain why some of us are better than others at certain physical feats. Chapter 3 provides physical comparisons between us and our closest living relatives and what this means in terms of structure and function. Understanding fatigue also requires a framework to define and measure it. Therefore, Chapter 4 deals with the framework at the cellular and organismic level and provides examples of how fatigue can be measured. Chapter 5 compares the human morphology to that of Neanderthals and other extinct species. The reason for this comparison is that there are striking similarities and differences between living and extinct species which provide insight into whether endurance was a favoured adaptation and played a part in our survival.

The human brain represents the pinnacle of human evolutionary biology. Chapter 6 discusses the complex nature of the human brain in relation to fatigue and its emotional construct. A striking physiological capacity of humans is our ability to sweat profusely and thermoregulate effectively. Chapter 7 discusses this unique ability, comparing and contrasting that of other mammals that have chosen endurance or power. In Chapter 8 the vexing problem of energy and its relationship to physical activity and health is discussed. The lurking problem of energy-in and energy-out is highlighted in relation to fatigue. Chapter 9 will provide a historical context to the concepts of endurance and power, their measurement and inherent limitations. Finally, Chapter 10 utilises two pathologies (multiple sclerosis and myasthenia gravis) to illustrate the difference between central and peripheral fatigue and how fatigue generally manifests in these illnesses.

A caveat: I am not an expert in all of the areas covered in this book. There are volumes written by scholars about evolutionary biology as a stand-alone topic; this is not an attempt to even remotely replace those writings. It is an attempt to draw the concepts of evolutionary biology closer to human fatigue, performance and health. Throughout the book I have needed to repeat certain concepts for the sake of clarity. My hope is that this book will invite exercise scientists and all those involved or interested in human performance generally to think more broadly about our capabilities. Specifically, that human fatigue is a complex phenomenon and that it cannot be unravelled merely by studying individual systems. Evolution played a major role in achieving the human biology and form so that all of our observations cannot be detached from the tinkering that occurred over some 5 million years. To deny this, and not consider why we might have chosen endurance rather than power, means that we will have missed the opportunity to understand more fully who we are and what our strengths and frailties might be.

Reference

Dobzhansky, T., 1973. Nothing in biology makes sense except in the light of evolution. *The American Biology Teacher*, 35(3), pp. 125–129.

Acknowledgements

When writing a book, it is almost impossible to acknowledge all the individuals who have had a hand in shaping one's thoughts and ideas about a topic. A book is a culmination of many years of thought, discussion, reading, arguments and assistance. I want to apologise upfront if I have missed anyone in this regard. I have done my best to make mention of individuals and groups which have assisted me in my intellectual journey.

As an undergraduate student I attended a conference where Professor Tim Noakes from the University of Cape Town presented on the failure to thermoregulate during distance running. At one point he asked the simple question, "Why do the majority of runners collapse only when they cross the finish line?" I was struck by this obvious yet simple observation, perhaps not because of its scientific merit but rather its philosophical catch. This was surely a paradox worthy of investigation. Having completed a PhD in thermoregulation and performance, I ventured to Cape Town and completed my sabbatical, where I was heavily influenced by the way in which science was practised at this laboratory. For this opportunity I am grateful to Professor Noakes and the staff.

I am also indebted to Professor Mike Lambert, who has been a source of academic integrity and friendship for over 20 years. I am particularly grateful to Professor Daniel Lieberman from the Department of Human Evolutionary Biology at Harvard University. Dan took a chance to host an academic (and family) with an interest in evolutionary biology and gave me time to discuss, critique and develop ideas about human fatigue which might not otherwise have been possible. I want acknowledge Professor Bob Meyenn, the individual who initially gave me a job as an academic and has remained a valued friend. Bob taught me the true value of education and free thinking.

Over a period of about 15 years I have had the privilege to lead a staff dedicated to teaching and learning and to the pursuit of knowledge. I am indebted to my colleagues and the many Honours and PhD students of the School of Exercise Science, Sport & Health who have given me support and inspiration to think differently about all things human.

Finally, I wish to acknowledge my parents, Francesco Snr and Raffaella, who with a limited education understood the power that comes with thinking for oneself.

My wife, Trish, and our beautiful children, Emma, Alexander and Anabel, continue to indulge my many odd behaviours with good cheer. The value of your love and support is beyond any human measure. Thank you.

Chapter 1

Evolution and natural selection in human performance, health and disease

How extremely stupid not to have thought of that.
– T.H. Huxley's reaction after reading Darwin's *The Origin of Species*

Introduction

Any typical textbook dealing with the broad topic of exercise physiology or exercise science will include cursory information on human evolution, if at all. This is perhaps not surprising given that evolutionary theory is generally accepted and that scientists have a working knowledge of the topic. On the surface this is likely to be true, for the basic assumption is that humans, like all other living organisms, evolved over a long period of time – evolutionary time. On this point, we take this to signify millions of years of tinkering that eventually spawned the modern form of *Homo sapiens*. One of the problems with this line of thought is that the evolution of *Homo sapiens* was directional and that we are the outcome. That is, evolution was linear and the only possible result is what we have today. This view is so far from reality and the facts that we have typically become passive in our understanding of evolutionary theory and how it can be applied to understand and solve our modern-day problems. In fact, very few of us would consider evolutionary theory as a means of understanding our biology as applied to human performance and health.

In order to address this fundamental understanding of human physiology as it pertains to performance, health and disease, this chapter introduces some of the most fundamental concepts of evolutionary theory before venturing into the complexities of form and function. This chapter considers the concepts first introduced by Darwin and Huxley, along with the classic studies confirming that evolution is something more than just a theory, but a process which is alive and dynamic. To begin our quest in understanding the place of evolution in biology and in human performance we need only reflect upon the reasoning given by eminent scholars in the field.

In his highly cited 1973 paper titled "Nothing in biology makes sense except in the light of evolution," Theodosius Dobzhansky (1973) outlines the arguments and counter-arguments that are typically used in the debate as to whether evolution is a verifiable theory. Although this paper is usually invoked as a way of asserting that the cornerstone of biology is in fact evolutionary theory, it is worth reiterating the basis of Dobzhansky's argument. In his description of life's remarkable diversity, Dobzhansky also notes that the unity of life is in fact no less remarkable. That is, from the most seemingly rudimentary life, such as a virus, to the most complex organism, the biochemistry is not only similar but also simple. This is not to suggest that DNA and RNA are uncomplicated; on the contrary, it is the universality of the biochemistry that is indicative that all life is intimately connected by preserving the most basic primordial features. The classic theories of Oparin and then Haldane (Miller 1953; Miller et al. 1997) provide the basis from which life likely arose, whereby the Earth's atmosphere, composed largely of nitrogen, ammonia, methane and helium, combined in a primordial soup to form the building blocks of life, the amino acids. The way in which amino acids constitute sequences for given kinds of proteins and that vary within and between species, along with single amino acids arising by genetic mutations, Dobzhansky submits "that all these remarkable findings make sense in the light of evolution; they are nonsense otherwise" (p. 128). However, the essence of Dobzhanky's reasoning is as follows:

> There is, of course, nothing conscious or intentional in the action of natural selection. A biologic species does not say to itself, "Let me try tomorrow (or a million years from now) to grow in a different soil, or use a different food, or subsist on a different body part of a different crab." Only a human being could make such conscious decisions. This is why the species *Homo Sapiens* is the apex of evolution. Natural selection is at one and the same time a blind and creative process. Only a creative but blind process could produce, on the one hand, the tremendous biologic success that is the human species and, on the other, forms of adaptedness as narrow and as constraining as those of the over specialised fungus, beetle, and flies.
>
> (p. 127)

Although there are numerous texts outlining the basic tenets of evolution, the purpose of this section is to provide what might be regarded as the fundamental aspects of evolutionary theory thought to have a direct relationship to understanding human performance and our ability to live healthy lives and avoid disease. To this end, there are two terms used in the foregoing passage taken from Dobzhansky's paper that are fundamental to understanding evolutionary theory. These are *natural selection* and *adaptedness*. In order to apply the principles of both natural selection and adaptedness to any aspect of biology, especially when attempting to understand human health and disease from an evolutionary perspective, we must first consider the context in which they were originally used by Darwin in *The Origin of Species* (Duzdevich 2014). In articulating what Darwin considered to be natural selection, he noted that very slight variations regardless of their causation would in some way benefit the individuals of a particular species in their relationship with other living things and/or their physical environment.

One critical aspect of this would be that these benefits, however small, would be passed on to the offspring. This transmission from parent to offspring will provide a greater chance for reproductive success and, therefore, the preservation of the species. Although the process of natural selection would seem straightforward, Darwin also recognised that this was dependent on the key observation that only a small number of individuals that are born can actually survive. This simply means that every living thing is always striving to increase its numbers. But why? The answer to this is not apparently obvious. Huxley (2010) in his classic work notes that there is a tendency for all organisms to increase in geometrical ratio. That is, in the early stages of existence the offspring are always more numerous than their parents, even though the numbers of a given species tend to remain approximately constant. Thus, if more young are produced than can survive, the only conclusion that can be drawn is that there must be competition for survival (Huxley 2010). It is this competition or *struggle for existence* that will assist in the accumulation of variations as being either favourable and therefore passed on or unfavourable and not passed on because of the failure to reproduce. Natural selection is concerned only with improving the chances of reproducing.

The term *adaptation* or *adaptedness* implies that there is a shaping of a particular feature or features of an organism in order that there is a better fit with its physical environment. However, for adaptation to take place the process relies on the multitude of individual differences which appear in a population. In essence, all species, including humans, are variable. That is to say that individual members of a particular group will vary in a number of their characteristics. Some members of a group will be taller than others, more or less agile, more or less muscular and more or less resistant to disease. In fact, this kind of variation is seen at all levels of the organism – from molecular to gross anatomical features. Let us now look at two typical examples which help illustrate the importance of adaptation. The most widely cited example of rapid adaptation is that of the peppered moth during the Industrial Revolution in England (Cook & Turner 2008). There are two types of peppered moths: the light-bodied and the dark-bodied. Before the Industrial Revolution the dark variety was thought to be rare. However, the light-bodied variety was much more numerous as it was able to blend in with the light-coloured lichens on trees, whereas the black-bodied variety would be easily picked off by birds due to their higher visibility. Within decades of the Industrial Revolution the trees between London and Manchester became darkened as a consequence of soot deposits from coal burning in addition to the lichens dying on the trees as a consequence of the increased sulphur dioxide emissions. The darkened trees now effectively provided less camouflage for the light-coloured moths, whereas the number of dark-coloured moths being picked off by birds was dramatically reduced. The outcome was a rapid increase in the number of dark-coloured moths. To confirm that the population of dark-coloured moths was indeed due to natural selection and rapid adaptation to the environment, it is believed that a series of experiments (Kettlewell 1955, 1959) in which the filming of the predation of birds on moths in both polluted and unpolluted woodlands is an instance where Darwinian evolution was captured in action (Majerus 2008).

The observations on the peppered moth provide some compelling evidence at the macro level for evolution by natural selection. Even more compelling are the experiments conducted on the bacterium E. coli (Lenski & Travisano 1994). These researchers took the opportunity to put to the test evolution by natural selection in fast-forward motion since these bacteria reproduce asexually, so that cloning can create a huge population of identical individuals in a very short time. After taking 12 separate populations of identical bacteria and propagating them in replicate environments for 10,000 generations, they were able to report on two properties of the evolving bacterial population: cell size and mean fitness. These two properties were studied because size is a trait which influences the functional properties of an organism, whereas fitness is the trait which is utilised by the organism to compete for resources. The interesting aspect of this experiment was that the researchers employed natural selection by imposing an environment on the bacterial populations rather than artificial selection. In this way they were able to ascertain whether there were any heritable properties that would enhance reproductive success in that particular environment. A key aspect of this experiment was the chosen environment in which the bacteria were placed. The environment was essentially a glucose broth which was calculated to support a given number of cells. Each day the bacteria were observed to grow until the glucose was depleted, at which time some of the bacteria were transferred to new replicate environments. This continued for 1,500 days until such time that the original bacteria reached 10,000 generations in 12 different populations. The first interesting result is that cell size in the bacterial population increased rapidly for approximately the first 2,000 generations when introduced to the new environment. However, when the environment remained unchanged for several thousand generations, increases in cell size were less than negligible. As suggested by the authors, the trajectories appear to be very similar but reached different plateaus for cell size, leading them to conclude that the populations diverged from the common ancestor and from one another in at least the size of the cells.

To measure the fitness of the bacteria the researchers then resurrected the original (ancestral) frozen bacteria and placed them in direct competition with the more recent generation. The questions they were asking were whether the evolutionary trajectories of fitness were similar to that observed for the cell size or fitness improved at a constant rate throughout the experiment. Beyond the striking similarity between cell size and relative fitness is that adaptation to the environment in all 12 populations was rapid when introduced to the new environment compared to when the environment was constant over several thousand generations. Taken together, the increase in cell size and the change in relative fitness show that significant variation arose in the early stages of the experiment and then persisted until the end of the experiment at 10,000 generations. The fact the mean relative fitness was initially equal to zero in all populations is indicative that mutations arose independently in each population, even though the environments in which the bacteria were placed were identical.

These two examples of the adaptedness of the peppered moth and E. *coli* highlight the three conditions required for evolution by natural selection to occur: (1) there is variation among individuals within a population, (2) the variation is heritable, and (3) the variation is related to the success of individuals in competing for resources.

The preceding discussion considered only the overarching understanding of evolution by natural selection. It did not, for example, consider the workings of genetics in the grand scheme of evolution. The purpose of the preceding discussion was merely to outline the key determinants of evolution and provide the reader with the conceptual framework which will be used throughout the book.

Evolution, disease and human fatigue

In the preceding section, we considered two examples of evolution by natural selection: the peppered moths and the bacterium E. *coli*. One might well ask, what have the peppered moths and E. *coli* to do with evolution by natural selection with respect to human performance, health and disease? The simple answer is that whatever mechanisms were at play in the adaptedness of the peppered moths and the bacteria to their environment would surely also have been at play when we consider our evolutionary path, our resistance to disease and our ability for physical and mental performance in a wide range of human endeavours. It is a safe assumption within the scientific community that there is no dispute that natural selection occurs. However, its significance in explaining human performance in a wide range of activities and situations must be demonstrated by way of evidence. This section will explore factors thought to have led to the unique human traits that distinguish us from our ancestors, both living and past.

When we consider impressive human feats such as the breaking of the four-minute mile, the 100m sprint in under ten seconds, edging ever closer to the two-hour marathon and even the impressive swimming records, one can't help but be amazed at the resilience and beauty of the human in action. We would be forgiven if we thought, just for a moment, that our biology was indeed perfect. In reality, when we consider the uniqueness of humans, we cannot help but also notice that many of our ailments can arguably be related to our imperfect biology. Thus, there is an imperative to understand how and why our biology is the way it is and what limitations it imposes when we interact with our environment. As we have already seen, an organism's survival is dependent to a large degree on its adaptability and whether those advantageous traits are passed on to the next generation. This is the case for humans as well. Therefore, it would be more than helpful to understand how humans evolved and which adaptations are useful and which are not. If we understand this aspect of human evolution, we might then be in a position to not only understand but also predict why we get sick and why our performance is perhaps limited in certain circumstances as well as truly appreciating the wondrous feats we are so accustomed to seeing. By way of illustration, there are some modern-day chronic diseases which we can use to illustrate this point.

There will be little argument that obesity is a prevalent disease for which we seemingly have had no answer, at least within the last 20 years. The latest obesity update from the Organisation for Economic Co-operation and Development (OECD; www.oecd.org/health/obesity-update.htm) indicates that at least 18% of the adult population in OECD countries is obese, constituting about 1%–3% of healthcare expenditure in most countries but up to 5%–10% in the United States. The knock-on effect of the disease is likely to result in the appearance of other chronic diseases, such as Type 2 diabetes mellitus. Although the OECD update and others (Gard 2011) also report the rate of rise in obesity in the last five years has slowed, there is little to indicate that we have dealt with the problem effectively. There is little doubt that significant gains can be made by understanding the physiology on a systemic and molecular level of such a disease, yet little or no attention has been paid to truly understanding why we have been powerless to curb the incidence of the disease. Is there an alternative approach that can be used to solve this problem? How can evolutionary theory by natural selection help us to understand (1) why obesity has increased so rapidly in a relatively short period of human history, and (2) how we can use our knowledge of natural selection to guide us in finding the solution for such a modern-day disease? This, of course, is not to assert that obesity never existed in the past, when it clearly did. Rather, the issue is why this disease has appeared so suddenly and taken hold so rapidly when in 1980 fewer than one in ten people were obese, whereas this is now up to six in ten people in some countries. At the very least this gives us a clue that the disease is almost entirely preventable.

So, the big question it seems is, why does it occur? Why are humans susceptible to this disease and why are some of us more likely than others to fall into its grasp? These questions alone are compelling enough to make us think deeply about our roots and understand the factors of our past that have made us so susceptible to the disease. Perhaps a better question to ponder is, what parts of our biology actually haven't changed since humans appeared, and are these the responsible villains?

Adaptations and health

Returning to the phenomenon of adaptedness, it is perhaps within this construct that the answer to our crisis of chronic ill health lies. In considering this, the most obvious question to ask is, what adaptations took place over millions of years that were useful over a long period of our existence in extremely different environments and provided for reproductive success, but perhaps are now conspiring to cause us grief? There is good reason to believe that the changes in our immediate environment have shifted so much that our physiology has not been able to adapt quickly enough in order to deal with the more accessible availability of energy. There is no doubt that over millions of years of evolution our diets changed, whereby we went from craving and consuming high-energy foods, such as low-hanging ripened fruit, to consuming animal protein (Marlowe 2005); although this was likely sporadic and not abundant, it likely required physical efforts to obtain. In short, we co-evolved with our food so that many of our body's features were actually an adaptation to the environment in which we lived for many thousands of years at a time. However, these features are now less well adapted for the environments we live in today.

The question is why we haven't adapted to the 'new' environment so that diseases which have us in their grip have become so chronic and pervasive that we seem so helpless to do anything to curb their incidence. The simple answer is that the environment has changed more rapidly than what our biology is able to handle. Evolution by natural selection occurs more slowly than we can imagine. To illustrate this, we need only look at the history of sugar consumption and availability. In the year 1700, the per capita consumption of sugar in the United Kingdom was approximately 1.8 kg per person, increasing to 8.1 kg by the year 1800 and then to 45 kg by the year 1950. In the United States this was a staggering 68 kg per person in 1993 (Johnson et al. 2007). In simple terms, the consumption of sugar increased by ~6 kg in the space of 250 years, and then by another 60 kg within the next 43 years. The incidence rates of obesity and diabetes track the increase in sugar consumption, whereby around the 1900s obesity rates were around 3%–6%, but by 1994 they had emerged to be 55%. Type 2 diabetes mellitus emerged as a serious threat to population well-being around 1960, when the incidence rates were 1,000 per 100,000 people, but by 1993 they were around 7,000 per 100,000 (Johnson et al. 2008). In essence, the increase in the consumption of sugar within the recent and miniscule time lapse of 300 years was so rapid compared with the changes that might occur with natural selection at work that whatever our biology was adapted for is now not entirely useful in managing the change in energy availability. As presented, these data imply that the cause of our chronic illnesses, in this case obesity and the comorbidities, can be distilled to one factor: the abundance, availability and consumption of sugar.

If this were so, then the solution would be as simple as removing sugar from our diets. However, this simplistic understanding negates the complexity of the physiology and the process by which it evolved. That is, why would evolution endow us with the propensity to crave and consume highly rich caloric foods, such as sugar, if it was so bad for us? To appreciate the complexity of this question we need only to look to our closest living relatives in captivity, where the situation and environment are vastly different to their normal habitat. We have known for some time that chimpanzees will develop insulin resistance when provided highly processed foods coupled with a lack of physical activity (Rosenblum et al. 1981). Interestingly, captive chimps which had a restricted atherogenic diet but were fed a balanced diet, low in fat, displayed a remarkable abnormal blood lipid profile regardless of whether they were lean or obese (Steinetz et al. 1996). Although the common variable in this scenario is diet, the fact that chimps individually developed different lipid profiles and obesity indicates that individual variability was also at work. These findings highlight the need not to draw simplistic generalised conclusions about our adaptations and our interaction with the environment in identifying the potential solution to our health problems.

Adaptations and fatigue

This book is concerned primarily with understanding human fatigue and how we might manage it in the context of human performance, health and disease. The purpose of the preceding discussion on evolution and adaptation with respect to the chronic disease of obesity and its comorbidity of Type 2 diabetes mellitus was to outline the relationship between what we might have been adapted for and how this might be working against us today. We can apply these same principles in attempting to understand human functioning in other aspects of our lives, including physical performance. How we perform and what things might hamper our performance are fundamental to our existence. We are forever attempting to find new ways of maintaining and improving our health and physical performance. The Olympic motto *Citius – Altius – Fortius* (faster – higher – stronger) perhaps attests to this. In order to achieve this ideal, we need to understand what aspects of our biology and mental capacities hamper our efforts and why humans are the way we are.

The term *fatigue* is derived from the Latin *fatigare*, meaning to 'tire out.' Today, the term has taken on wide usage by describing both biological and inanimate materials for their capacity to withstand failure. In the field of health and human performance, fatigue is used to describe the individual's ability to carry out a task, be it mental or physical. In medicine, fatigue is arguably one of the most ubiquitous conditions spanning the breadth of human health and disease. We have become so used to its inclusion in describing the capacity of people but we do not fully understand its causes. For example, fatigue resulting from physical exertion serves to halt or attenuate the progress of that very exertion. However, mental incapacity due to depression or cancer will serve to diminish physical effort before it ever begins (Curt 2000). According to this difference, both physiological and psychological fatigue can occur either acutely or chronically.

Perhaps one reason for this lack of understanding is that we very seldom consider fatigue from an evolutionary perspective – that is, was fatigue an adaptation that led to reproductive success? Recall that an adaptation is the shaping of a particular feature or features of an organism in order that there is a better fit with its physical environment. Applying this principle to fatigue as a way of understanding its causes is not obvious. For instance, how would fatigue or 'tiring out' be at all advantageous and ensure reproductive success? To answer this question, we must turn back the clock to the earliest human ancestors and make some reasonable assumptions about their environment and how they interacted with it.

The importance of geological time

To understand more completely the story of how our physiology evolved and whether fatigue is an adaptation, it is necessary to get a snapshot of the time it took for humans to evolve. This time scale is only just within our comprehension because we have been able to date the age of the Earth to a reasonable degree. By most accounts the Earth is approximately 4.54 billion years old (Dalrymple 2001; Manhes et al. 1980). The International Commission on Stratigraphy (www.strati graphy.org) regularly updates the chronostratigraphic chart which outlines the age of the Earth in discrete time periods. An *eon* is the largest time, approximating billions of years; *eras* are marked by characteristics rather than time but span hundreds of millions of years; *periods* mark the span of about 100 million years; and several *epochs* are contained within a period and mark the lapse of tens of millions of years. Finally, the smallest of these time frames are *ages*, spanning millions of years.

We have briefly touched on the elements thought to have been needed for life on Earth to get started on its long journey from the primordial soup. For our purpose, however, we will need to fast-forward to the Eocene Epoch, somewhere between 56 million to 34 million years ago. This is an important time period because it is thought that primate evolution took hold during this time. Specifically, it is thought there was a critical split that occurred in primate evolution so that two distinct primate groups emerged: those with wet noses and those with dry noses. We now have strong evidence that this split occurred during the Eocene since the 'in-between' species *Darwinius masillae* (Franzen et al. 2009), commonly known as *Ida* (Tudge 2009), was discovered and is regarded as the most complete primate skeleton dating back ~47 million years. However, the most important aspect of this primate expansion and splitting is not so much that it happened but the likely cause or conditions which drove it.

It is now well accepted that the Cenozoic Era likely started with the Earth being struck by an asteroid, thought to be the most catastrophic event the Earth has ever seen. The size of the asteroid has been estimated to have been about 10 km wide, leaving a crater about 180 km in diameter situated in Chicxulub, Mexico (Schulte et al. 2010). The sizes of the impact and the crater are important as they give us an indication of the release of energy from such a collision, with the most important consequence of this impact likely to be the immediate effect it had on the climate. The estimated energy release is staggering and has been calculated to have been at least 100 million megatons (Alvarez 1983) or ~8 billion times the energy released by the bomb dropped on either Hiroshima or Nagasaki. This enormous release of energy could not have gone without consequences for the environment, with debris sent into the atmosphere resulting in dramatic shifts from cooler to warmer temperatures. This cataclysmic event is now thought to be the major reason for the extinction of the dinosaurs. However, others argue that the population of the remaining creatures would have been too great and they were able to outlive such an event (Prothero 2007,

p. 282). Thus, the terrestrial dinosaurs were either the immediate victims of a cataclysmic event or there was a gradual disappearance. Whatever the catalyst for the mass extinction, the important fact to note is the ensuing change from one dominant creature, the dinosaurs, to another, the mammals. What is known is that during the early Eocene the climate underwent a significant global warming event known as the Eocene Thermal Maximum. This means that the Earth's temperature increased, which provided the conditions in which forests grew and became widespread. This, coupled with the gap left by the dinosaurs' disappearance, allowed the mammals to thrive in a newly expanded ideal world for at least ~7 million years. Long-term cooling, interspersed with shorter, warm stages when forests gave way to more open, drier woodlands, followed this relatively short window of time. The main point to be noted about the Eocene Epoch is that the dramatic change in the climate and by extension the environment, whatever the causes, allowed for particular flora and fauna to dominate the landscape, oceans and the air.

Although there were fluctuations in temperature over the course of the Miocene Epoch from 23 to 5.3 million years ago (MYA), the next major cooling event occurred at the end of the Miocene Epoch, marked by the beginning of the Ice Age (Zachos et al. 2001). The Miocene is characterised by a fossil record replete with evidence of widespread Old World monkeys and apes in East Africa, with migration of primates into Asia and Europe (Dawkins 2005; Stein & Rowe 2000). Thus, we now have two pieces of evidence, the climatic conditions and the fossil record, that can be used to hypothesise about at least one possibility that led to the evolution of humans. We already know that mammals and primates diversified during the preceding Miocene Epoch. It is also apparent that at the end of the Miocene, just when the climate went into the major cooling event, the primate lineage diverged, with *Homo sapiens* and chimpanzees splitting from the last common ancestor (LCA). The reason for the divergence in lineage is not clear; however, the result of the split is what is most important. In summary, there were at least two major climatic events, one at the beginning of the Eocene which led to conditions for the diversification of the mammals and primates, and then, a major cooling event at the end of the Miocene which occurred just when the chimpanzees and *H. sapiens* diverged from the LCA. We will now consider the uniqueness of humans and the possible factors that led to this.

Hominin uniqueness

The term *hominin* refers to the group consisting of modern humans, extinct human species and all our immediate ancestors. This is different to the term *hominid*, which refers to all great apes and their ancestors. This is an important distinction as we consider our evolutionary path since the divergence from our LCA. Before we consider evidence which provides us with some of the clues as to our uniqueness, it is worth recalling that even Darwin reasoned that modern humans evolved in Africa and that we are related to the great apes. Importantly,

Darwin also reasoned that our bipedality was perhaps the initial event that set us on a different evolutionary course from our closest ancestors. (Darwin 1872) wrote in *The Descent of Man and Selection in Relation to Sex*,

> [m]an alone has become a biped; and we can, I think, partly see how he has come to assume his erect attitude, which forms one of his most conspicuous characters. Man could not have attained his present dominant position in the world without the use of his hands, which are so admirably adapted to act in obedience to his will . . . But the hands and arms could hardly have become perfect enough to have manufactured weapons, or to have hurled stones and spears with a true aim, as long as they were habitually used for locomotion and for supporting the whole weight of the body, or, as before remarked, so long as they were especially fitted for climbing trees . . . If it be an advantage to man to stand firmly on his feet and to have his hands and arms free, of which, from his pre-eminent success in the battle of life, there can be no doubt, then I can see no reason why it should not have been advantageous to the progenitors of man to have become more and more erect or bipedal. They would thus have been better able to defend themselves with stones or clubs, to attack their prey, or otherwise to obtain food. The best built individuals would in the long run have succeeded best, and have survived in larger numbers.
>
> (pp. 135–136)

In Darwin's assessment of the uniqueness of man, he noted the freeing of the hands as a key difference, but more importantly the ability to stand and be bipedal had to have been a distinct advantage. The critical consideration is how we took advantage of this uniqueness and what factors conspired to assist us. To understand this, we must consider the timeline of the divergence of chimpanzees and *Homo sapiens* from the LCA. According to our previous analysis this split between *Homo sapiens* and chimpanzees occurred around 5.3 MYA, just as the Earth was moving into major cooling events. Around this time we also had a dramatic expansion in brain size, which according to some scholars (Trinkaus & Holliday 1997) continued for the next 3 million years at close to six times the rate of the previous 4 million years. So, now we have climactic changes, the advent of bipedality and brain expansion conspiring towards an advantage for reproductive success. However, this is not evidence of causation or that other factors were not at play. For instance, others have shown that in addition to paleoclimate variability and fluctuations in temperature, social competition as a selective force for brain expansion cannot be entirely discounted (Bailey & Geary 2009). This suggests that climate may have contributed to population density, but the high variability in cranial volume among the hominid population is likely to be related also to the social interaction and the resulting competition. In fact, current theory suggests that the proclivity for cooperation among our own species was likely a distinct advantage in procuring resources and that this proclivity was perhaps a genetic endowment that other hominin species did not develop (Marean 2015).

To contextualise the conundrum of how we ended up on two feet, various hypotheses have been posited. Each of these has, at one time or another, been attractive and contentious. The reason for contention is that no single hypothesis seems to be able to fully account for the impetus to become bipedal. That is to say, there does not seem to be a unifying theory that can be agreed upon since each proposition leaves some other observation unaccounted for. Thus, it is useful at this point to summarise the various hypotheses to illustrate the pitfalls in deciding which one would be most appropriate. The list is not meant to be exhaustive; rather it is for the purpose of illustration:

1   The *vigilance* hypothesis advanced by Raymond Dart (1926) proposed that early hominids would be at an advantage with the ability to look over tall grasses and spot their prey and avoid predators. However, its popularity as a viable hypothesis waned since many other animals that are not bipedal also display vigilance behaviour – meaning that bipedality is not essential for this to occur.

2   The *aquatic ape* hypothesis by Hardy (1960) claimed that at some point in our evolutionary past bipedalism was useful for wading through water, mainly because our habitat was likely to be on the seacoast. Unfortunately, the explanations for such a necessary posture can also be related to many other reasons, not just an aquatic environment.

3   The *energy efficiency* hypothesis (Rodman 1980) suggested that bipedal locomotion was just as efficient as quadrupedal locomotion. The major point with this hypothesis is that bipedal locomotion is also more efficient than chimpanzee locomotion, suggesting that Homo opted for bipedality since our distant relatives are inefficient walkers. However, the problem here is that early hominids would have likely been energetically inefficient. It seems very unlikely that our early ancestors would have chosen a form of locomotion that might have developed into a more efficient one.

4   The *carrying* hypothesis advanced by Lovejoy (Currey 2003) was attractive as it explained the need to carry food and offspring. The centrepiece of this hypothesis was that the male would gather and acquire food and provision for his mate, while the female would tend to the young. Provisioning would not be possible over longer distances if the hands were not free and bipedal locomotion was not available. However, the problem here is that this hypothesis is constrained by the likelihood that bipedality evolved in forested areas not on the savanna, since the ability to carry must have been available before the need to do so.

5   The *heat* hypothesis proposed by Wheeler (1984) carried some favour, and it does suggest that the Homo capacity for thermoregulation is indeed a distinct advantage over other mammals. Although thermoregulation likely played a part as it provides several advantages, such as less exposure to radiation,

evaporation of sweat and convective heat loss with greater exposure of the torso to the oncoming air, it cannot on its own account for bipedality. The main problem with this hypothesis is that it suffers from the same issue as the carrying hypothesis – namely, that bipedality would have likely evolved in forested areas prior to the transition to the open grasslands (Stanford 2003).

6   The *squat-eating* hypothesis initially suggested by Jolly (1970) and then redis-covered by Kingdon (2003) described the need for hominids to squat and feed off the seeds available to them on the grasslands, while the latter sug-gested that a similar activity took place on the forest floor. No matter where the squatting took place, the key factor in this hypothesis is the need to make morphological adjustments to the joints to make squatting for long periods possible. In other words, Kingdon (2003) suggests that squatting would have led to changes in the anatomy of the pelvis and sacrum and lessened the burden on the arms. In essence, this theory seems to provide for precondi-tions where the morphology was given the opportunity to adapt and make the transition to bipedality. Although this school of thought is attractive, it suffers from the reality that the fossil evidence shows that bipedality evolved over a gradual and long period of time, with different species having more or less advanced bipedal capabilities.

7   The *meat-eating* hypothesis described in the classic text by Stanford (2003) contends that the environmental change of ever-widening food patches, converging with the palate for greater amounts of meat in the diet, was enough to propel our ancestors towards bipedalism. In essence, this hypoth-esis hinges on the ability of early *hominids* to gather and hunt in various ways, which coincidentally accounts for the number of anatomical varia-tions we see in *hominid* species, but the persistent need and search for protein drove the evolution of bipedalism. Although an attractive proposition, this hypothesis does draw on previous ideas that were already in existence, such as the widening food patches due to environmental changes.

The lack of agreement and contentious nature of each of the hypotheses allow us to conclude only that we simply have no absolute understanding for the evolution of bipedalism. Nevertheless, there is a common theme that we can draw upon to make some reasonably solid inferences. At this juncture, it is important to reiter-ate that the cause of bipedality is not what we are attempting to uncover *per se*; rather we are interested in the factors which might have contributed and what these might mean for our understanding of fatigue, human performance, health and disease. It is clear that the climate and the environment in which the first bipeds existed had a major influence on the evolutionary path of humans. Exactly how this might have played out is an educated guessing game, but it is possible to draw some reasonably strong conclusions based on the available evidence. First, if we accept that the major habitat was significantly altered due to climate and temperature changes at the time of the split between chimps and *Homo sapiens* from the LCA, when forest patches were shrinking and savannas expanded, then bipedality must have presented a distinct advantage for at least several reasons. Before considering these reasons in more detail it is useful to contextualise the advantage of being a biped in terms of what problems are overcome compared to being a quadruped, and more importantly compared to a knuckle walker, which our LCA most likely was (Richmond et al. 2002; Lieberman et al. 2009).

Knuckle walking is more energetically costly compared to bipedal locomotion by almost 75% (Sockol et al. 2007). Thus, as the forest patch was beginning to shrink and travelling in open savannas or distances between forest patches to obtain food became more frequent, 75% reduction in energy costs would have been a strong selection pressure for bipedality or at least against knuckle walking. This efficiency hypothesis is also supported by the fact that early hominins had bigger molars and premolars, which are needed for food that requires forceful grinding. This kind of food is in contrast to the foodstuffs that chimpanzees typically acquire in a forest, such as fruits. Thus, the early hominins must have lived in areas other than forest patches and travelled further to acquire the kinds of food that required larger teeth. It is also not possible to consider the change to the environment without also considering the morphology which could have provided a distinct advantage, since morphology is a key aspect that would have led to the optimisation for survival in a given habitat. We shall return subsequently to the question of morphology when considering adaptation and human fatigability.

The second consideration related to the energy cost of locomotion is that metabolic cost itself scales to body mass so that larger-bodied creatures would require more calories per day. Although we have not yet discussed in any detail why brain size increased in hominins, the fact it did would have escalated the energy needs since larger brains consume up to 25% of the metabolic demand of adults (Pontzer et al. 2016; Zauner & Muizelaar 1997). Thus, if the foodstuffs usually available in forests were not available in the savanna, and there were higher energy needs for the upright posture and bipedal locomotion, the next major source of high-energy food would have been animal tissue, such as meat, fat, marrow and all of the other parts of a carcass worth eating.

The third piece of evidence we can consider as advantageous for bipedality is that the open savanna presents a problem of exposure to radiation from the sun. That is, the surface area on which the radiation can act is greatly reduced with the upright posture compared to knuckle walking or quadruped locomotion, where significant surface area would be exposed. In essence, bipedal locomotion would reduce exposure time and surface area in open woodland and the potential for unnecessary heat accumulation. In addition to the reduced surface area for exposure, bipedal locomotion improves the capacity for convective heat loss by exposing the torso to oncoming air movement when running. We shall return to this adaptation in Chapter 8 when we consider the relationship between heat and fatigue. At this juncture it is really only to point out that bipedal locomotion has endowed us with less obvious advantages – in this case a significantly reduced surface area for the sun to act on.

There is one further piece of evidence that we need to consider that likely contributed to the propensity for early hominins to gain an advantage in acquiring high-energy food. It is now thought that the weaponry available to humans was a significant step in our reproductive success, with its 'co-evolution' from simple to more sophisticated projectile armaments. The key point in this evidence is that projectile weapons were not likely part of the hominin arsenal until about 100,000–71,000 years ago (Marean 2015). Therefore, we can conclude only that we must have done without the use of projectile weapons, such as the bow and arrow, for a significant portion of our existence so that harvesting of animal tissue must have occurred by other means – that is, scavenging and hunting.

Unique adaptation and human fatigability

Briefly returning to the question of morphology and its role in the advent of bipedalism, there is certainly plenty of evidence to suggest that humans are well adapted for an erect posture and bipedal locomotion as far as energy consumption and efficiency are concerned. In fact, there are data which show that in terms of resting energy expenditure measured in adult and infant humans when compared to that of dogs when assuming either a supine, lateral or erect posture or during locomotion, adult humans are much less costly compared with quadrupeds (Abitbol 1988). In fact, when assuming naturally erect posture, energy expenditure was almost the same as in the supine position for adult humans, whereas in their natural quadruped stance, dogs had a much higher energy expenditure than in their resting lateral position. However, the most striking finding was that human children when transitioning from crawling to standing had an energy expenditure that was not different with respect to either posture. Although these are interesting data on the comparison of efficiency between bipeds and quadrupeds, Abitbol (1988) suggests that there are at least three key questions that remain unanswered. These are: why is erect posture seemingly more efficient, what is the biomechanical and muscular basis for this efficiency, and what role did natural selection play in this development of efficiency? At present, the answers to these questions remain speculative.

Nevertheless, Hunt (1994) attempted to address these questions based on the extent to which morphology must be refined in order that a particular behaviour is optimised. First, morphology should minimise muscular force necessary to perform a particular behaviour, thereby reducing the energy cost – in this case, an erect posture. Second, optimal morphology should also reduce the joint reaction forces, which in turn reduces joint loading. Third, and perhaps most importantly, is the amount of muscle tissue available for a particular behaviour or movement. From a physiological perspective, the less muscle available the more rapidly fatigue will develop. Thus, when correcting for body mass and comparing the relative cross-sectional area of muscle (cm^2) between human and chimpanzee, we find that humans have a large relative cross-sectional area of skeletal muscle, with the lower limbs of humans making up 38% of the total body mass compared with only 24% for chimps (Zihlman 1992; Thorpe et al. 1999). Taken together, this suggests that morphology played a key role in the adoption of an erect posture.

The relationship between efficiency and morphology is predicated on the assumption that hominins adopted the erect posture because of the drier and more open habitats where bipedal feeding was necessary, either for low-hanging fruit or gathering over longer distances. The adoption of the erect posture and the altered morphology led to adaptations to prevent or resist fatigue and that bipedal posture encouraged bipedal locomotion (Hunt 1994, 2006). Unfortunately, as with other propositions as to the evolution of bipedality, the question as to what role morphology played is theoretical and an educated guess. The only conclusion we can draw from the evidence pertaining to morphology is that bipedal locomotion is less costly when compared to quadrupedal locomotion and that this could have been a key determinant for the adoption of an erect posture and subsequent bipedalism.

The uniqueness of bipedality and the apparent simultaneous events occurring around the same time as it became the preferred method of locomotion have already been discussed. However, this uniqueness was also the ultimate advantage over the other mammals. It is now thought that the capacity for endurance running, made possible by a myriad of other adaptations, such as large bodies, a small gut, enhanced thermoregulation, larger brains and relatively smaller teeth, played key roles in our evolution. The capacity to hunt co-operatively by outrunning or more precisely by running a large animal to exhaustion would have made it far easier to eventually dispatch the animal with a large blow to its head (Bramble & Lieberman 2004). We will consider the evolutionary adaptations that made endurance running possible in later chapters. However, the adaptation of endurance running brings with it an important caveat that we seldom consider in the exercise sciences. That is, in order that we outrun or out-perform a competitor species on the basis of enhanced endurance capability, we must then also be able to resist fatigue, whichever way one wishes to define it. This does not necessarily mean that resistance to fatigue was an adaptation itself, but perhaps a corollary outcome of the capacity for endurance which is arguably a key factor in our evolutionary path. Taking the evolution of endurance running at face value, the capacity to undertake long periods of physical and mental exertion also requires a well-developed capacity to resist fatigue. Therefore, it would not be controversial to surmise that any individual with well-developed resistance to fatigue would have a reproductive advantage.

Much has been written about the advent of endurance running, and some of the elements in its evolution are key in understanding human fatigability. However, this understanding is also heavily dependent on why endurance running would be either a necessity or an advantage resulting in selection for such a characteristic. To evaluate this, two hypotheses have been posited. First, Carrier et al. (1984) reasoned that endurance running was essential to run prey to exhaustion and that this activity provided early hominids a method by which they could increase the protein in their diets. The inclusion of animal protein in the diet is now believed to be one driver for the expansion of brain size (Aiello & Wheeler 1995). A criticism of Carrier et al.'s hypothesis is that the strategy of running down prey "might have been too energetically expensive and low yield for the benefits to have outweighed the costs" (Bramble & Lieberman 2004, p. 351). The interpretation here is that endurance running evolved because it was an effective method to exploit scavenging during a time when the landscape was changing to more open grasslands and the competition for animal protein with other mammals was a necessity (Bramble & Lieberman 2004). Thus, whether endurance running evolved because of the need to pursue prey or whether it was for exploitation through scavenging, the missing piece of this jigsaw puzzle is whether the use of endurance running for persistent hunting required prerequisite skills. In other words, just being able to run long distances without some implied strategy would be limiting in its applicability. It has also been suggested that tracking skills were a requirement for the evolution of persistence hunting, which would then be possible only if endurance running was a developed strategy (Liebenberg 2006). According to this reasoning the advent of endurance running must have developed after or at the very least in conjunction with well-developed tracking skills. This is an important distinction since tracking skills require well-developed cognitive abilities, which by definition would have involved scientific reasoning (Liebenberg 2013). Therefore, the use of endurance running in persistence hunting combined with tracking skills would have increased the likelihood of hunting success and higher protein intake, ultimately contributing to the evolution of a larger brain (Aiello & Wheeler 1995; Liebenberg 2013).

References

Abitbol, M.M., 1988. Effect of posture and locomotion on energy expenditure. *American Journal of Physical Anthropology*, 77(2), pp. 191–199.

Aiello, L.C. & Wheeler, P., 1995. The expensive-tissue hypothesis: the brain and the digestive system in human and primate evolution. *Current Anthropology*, 36(2), pp. 199–221.

Alvarez, L.W., 1983. Experimental evidence that an asteroid impact led to the extinction of many species 65 million years ago. *Proceedings of the National Academy of Sciences of the United States of America*, 80(2), pp. 627–642.

Bailey, D.H. & Geary, D.C., 2009. Hominid brain evolution. *Human Nature*, 20(1), pp. 67–79.

Bramble, D.M. & Lieberman, D.E., 2004. Endurance running and the evolution of *Homo*. *Nature*, 432, pp. 345–352.

Carrier, D.R. et al., 1984. The energetic paradox of human running and hominid evolution [and comments and reply]. *Current Anthropology*, pp. 483–495.

Cook, L.M. & Turner, J.R.G., 2008. Decline of melanism in two British moths: spatial, temporal and inter-specific variation. *Heredity*, 101(6), pp. 483–489.

Currey, J.D., 2003. How well are bones designed to resist fracture? *Journal of Bone and Mineral Research*, 18(4), pp. 591–598.

Curt, G.A., 2000. Impact of fatigue on quality of life in oncology patients. *Seminars in Hematology*, 37, pp. 14–17.

Dalrymple, G.B., 2001. The age of the Earth in the twentieth century: a problem (mostly) solved. *Geological Society, London, Special Publications*, 190(1), pp. 205–221.

Dart, R., 1926. Taung and its significance. *Natural History*, 26, pp. 315–327.

Darwin, C., 1872. *The descent of man and selection in relation to sex*, New York: D. Appleton and Co.

Dawkins, R., 2005. *The ancestor's tale: a pilgrimage to the dawn of evolution*, London: Houghton Mifflin Harcourt.

Dobzhansky, T., 1973. Nothing in Biology makes sense except in the light of Evolution. *The American Biology Teacher*, 35(3), pp. 125–129.

Duzdevich, D., 2014. *Darwin's on the origin of species: a modern rendition*, Bloomington, ID: Indiana University Press.

Franzen, J.L. et al., 2009. Complete primate skeleton from the Middle Eocene of Messel in Germany: morphology and paleobiology J. Hawks, ed. *PLOS ONE*, 4(5), p. e5723.

Gard, M., 2011. *The end of the obesity epidemic*, Oxon: Routledge.

Hardy, A., 1960. Was man more aquatic in the past. *New Scientist*, 7, pp. 642–645.

Hunt, K.D., 1994. The evolution of human bipedality: ecology and functional morphology, *Journal of Human Evolution*, 26, pp. 183–202.

Hunt, K.D., 2006. Bipedalism. In H.J. Brix, ed. *Encyclopedia of anthropology*. London: Sage Publications, pp. 372–378.

Huxley, J., 2010. *Evolution: the modern synthesis: the definitive edition*, Cambridge, MA: MIT Press.

Johnson, R.J. et al., 2007. Potential role of sugar (fructose) in the epidemic of hypertension, obesity and the metabolic syndrome, diabetes, kidney disease, and cardiovascular disease. *American Journal of Clinical Nutrition*, 86(4), pp. 899–906.

Johnson, R.J. et al., 2008. Hypothesis: could excessive Fructose intake and Uric acid cause type 2 diabetes? *Endocrine Reviews*, 30(1), pp. 96–116.

Jolly, C.J., 1970. The seed-eaters: a new model of hominid differentiation based on a baboon analogy. *Man*, 5(1), pp. 5–26.

Kettlewell, H., 1955. Selection experiments on industrial melanism in the Lepidoptera. *Heredity*, 9(3), pp. 323–342.

Kettlewell, H., 1959. New aspects of the genetic control of industrial melanism in the Lepidoptera. *Nature*, 183, pp. 918–921.

Kingdon, J., 2003. *Lowly origin: where, when, and why our ancestors first stood up*, Princeton: Princeton University Press.

Lenski, R.E. & Travisano, M., 1994. Dynamics of adaptation and diversification: a 10,000-generation experiment with bacterial populations. *Proceedings of the National Academy of Sciences of the United States of America*, 91(15), pp. 6808–6814.

Liebenberg, L., 2006. Persistence hunting by modern hunter-gatherers. *Current Anthropology*, 47(6), pp. 1017–1026.

Liebenberg, L., 2013. *The origin of science*, Cape Town: CyberTracker.

Lieberman, D.E., Pilbeam, D.R. & Wrangham, R.W., 2009. The transition from *Australopithicus* to *Homo*. In J.J. Shea & D.E. Lieberman, eds. *Transitions in prehistory essays in honor of Ofer Bar-Yosef*. Cambridge, MA: Paleoanthro.org, pp. 1–22.

Majerus, M.E.N., 2008. Industrial melanism in the Peppered Moth, Biston betularia: an excellent teaching example of Darwinian evolution in action. *Evolution: Education and Outreach*, 2(1), pp. 63–74.

Manhes, G. et al., 1980. Lead isotope study of basic-ultrabasic layered complexes: speculations about the age of the earth and primitive mantle characteristics. *Earth and Planetary Science Letters*, 47(3), pp. 370–382.

Marean, C., 2015. The most invasive species of all. *Scientific American*, 313(2), pp. 23–29.

Marlowe, F.W., 2005. Hunter-gatherers and human evolution. *Evolutionary Anthropology*, 14(2), pp. 54–67.

Miller, S.L., 1953. A production of amino acids under possible primitive Earth conditions. *Science*, 117, pp. 528–529.

Miller, S.L., Schopf, J.W. & Lazcano, A., 1997. Oparin's 'Origin of Life': sixty years later. *Journal of Molecular Evolution*, 44, pp. 351–353.

Pontzer, H. et al., 2016. Metabolic acceleration and the evolution of human brain size and life history. *Nature*, 533(7603), pp. 390–392.

Prothero, D., 2007. *Evolution: what the fossils say and why it matters*, New York: Columbia University Press.

Richmond, B.G., Begun, D.R. & Strait, D.S., 2002. Origin of human bipedalism: the knuckle-walking hypothesis revisited. *American Journal of Physical Anthropology*, 116(S33), pp. 70–105.

Rodman, P.S., 1980. Bioenergetics and the origin of hominid bipedalism. *American Journal of Physical Anthropology*, 52(1), pp. 103–106.

Rosenblum, I.Y., Barbolt, T.A. & Howard, C.F., Jr, 1981. Diabetes mellitus in the chimpanzee (Pan troglodytes). *Journal of Medical Primatology*, 10(2–3), pp. 93–101.

Schulte, P. et al., 2010. The Chicxulub asteroid impact and mass extinction at the Cretaceous-Paleogene boundary. *Science*, 327(5970), pp. 1214–1218.

Sockol, M.D., Raichlen, D.A. & Pontzer, H., 2007. Chimpanzee locomotor energetics and the origin of human bipedalism. *Proceedings of the National Academy of Sciences of the United States of America*, 104(30), pp. 12265–12269.

Stanford, C.B., 2003. *Upright: the evolutionary key to becoming human*, Boston: Houghton Mifflin Company.

Stein, P.L. & Rowe, B.M., 2000. *Physical anthropology*, 7th ed., Boston: McGraw-Hill.

Steinetz, B.G. et al., 1996. Lipoprotein profiles and glucose tolerance in lean and obese chimpanzees. *Journal of Medical Primatology*, 25(1), pp. 17–25.

Thorpe, S.K. et al., 1999. Dimensions and moment arms of the hind- and forelimb muscles of common chimpanzees (Pan troglodytes). *American Journal of Physical Anthropology*, 110(2), pp. 179–199.

Trinkaus, E. & Holliday, T.W., 1997. Body mass and encephalization in Pleistocene Homo. *Nature*, 387(6629), pp. 173–176.

Tudge, C., 2009. *The link: uncovering our earliest ancestor*, London: Little Brown.

Wheeler, P.E., 1984. The evolution of bipedality and loss of functional body hair in hominids. 13(1), pp. 91–98.

Zachos, J. et al., 2001. Trends, rhythms, and aberrations in global climate 65 Ma to present. *Science*, 292(5517), pp. 686–693.

Zauner, A. & Muizelaar, J.P., 1997. Brain metabolism and cerebral blood flow. *Head Injury*, pp. 89–99.

Zihlman, A.L., 1992. Locomotion as a life history character: the contribution of anatomy, *Journal of Human Evolution*, 22(4), pp. 315–325.

Chapter 2

Safety factors, reserve and trade-offs

Fear is the foundation of safety.

– Tertullian (c. 155 – c. 240)

Introduction

In Chapter 1 the general concept of fatigue was introduced, which spans across human performance, health and disease, along with consideration that should be given to understanding the fatigue process from an evolutionary perspective. Specifically, the question as to whether fatigue is an evolutionary adaptation was raised, since an adaptation is the shaping of a particular feature or features of an organism resulting in a better fit with the physical environment. However, to really understand the relationship between an organism's features and the environment, we typically make the assumption that features were designed in such a way that everything about the organism is advantageous and, therefore, all features have a purpose. To illustrate the point that some structures, whether biological or otherwise, are not specifically designed but rather co-opted for use in some other way, renowned evolutionary biologists Gould and Lewontin (1979), in their classic paper, made use of a practical example to illustrate the futility of the assumption that any structure is made for the best purpose. The example these authors provide is illustrated in Figure 2.1, which shows what is commonly referred to in architecture as a spandrel. These are for practical purposes, tapering triangular spaces formed between two rounded arches. Notably, spandrels usually contain a mosaic or some artwork. Nevertheless, the spandrel is a by-product of the necessary architecture (the adjoining arches), but the space occupied by the spandrel itself has no particular use. Since they are a by-product, the artist is not likely to waste the space and hence makes use of them. In other words, spandrels do not simply exist to house the artwork or ornaments; the specific architecture has generated space, so why not make use of that space?

In biological terms, we would not refer to co-opted features as spandrels. Rather, this observation has been termed an *exaptation*: "you can't use a structure until you have it. As a result, most of our so-called 'adaptations' actually start life as

SPANDREL

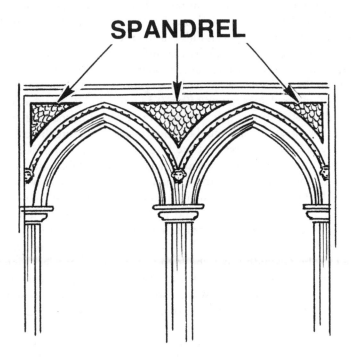

Figure 2.1 According to Gould and Lewontin (1979), spandrels do not exist to house artwork; they are a by-product of the necessary architecture (adjoining arches) which is then made use of.

exaptations: features that are acquired through random changes in genetic codes, to be co-opted only later for specific uses" (Tattersall 2012, p. 44). This is such a critical aspect of our biology as it relates to human performance that we seldom consider what role these exaptations play in physiological and mechanical processes of human movement. With little or no consideration of our exaptations, it is generally thought that all features have natural limitations, so much so that in the exercise sciences we typically make the assumption that there are finite capacities for particular organs and systems, which in turn limit our performance.

Physiological limitation

The question of physiological limitation is a difficult one to study but was considered by a few researchers when attempting to examine the relationship between structure and the functional needs of the organism. This matching phenomenon in biology was originally termed *symmorphosis*, which is predicated on the assumption that structural elements are regulated to satisfy but not exceed the requirements of the functional system (Taylor & Weibel 1981). The underlying premise is that nature is not wasteful but rather economical so that any system is regulated in order that space and energy are maximised. The original studies conducted to verify symmorphosis did so using the respiratory system (Taylor & Weibel 1981; Weibel et al. 1981). These studies attempted to compare the size of the respiratory structures (lungs, mitochondrial volume, capillary number and length within the skeletal muscle) with maximal oxygen consumption (VO_{2max}) in animals of different sizes ranging from 0.5 kg to 240 kg. The overall conclusion from these studies was that animals are designed economically, whereby the oxygen flow at VO_{2max} is limited by the structures that are directly involved so that there are no structures that are in excess of what is needed. However, these authors also revised their initial conclusions somewhat, since they found that the matching of structure with functional capacity was strictly evident only when considering the internal compartments of respiration, such as mitochondrial volume and capillary number and length, but not for the lungs (Weibel et al. 1991). In this instance, the structure of the lungs was far in excess of the requirement for maximal capacity. It was reasoned that this observation may be related to the possibility that the lungs, as the gas exchanger between the body and the external environment, may have other requirements related to stresses that were not measured. What can be concluded from these studies is that there is some matching of structure and functional capacity at some level which could impose a limitation on the system. Where and how this limitation is developed are yet to be elucidated. Interestingly, the concept of symmorphosis has not been advanced since these early studies, likely due to the difficulty in measuring the components of a biological system from the macro to the micro level of organisation.

The basis for physiological limitation in human performance is still a necessary concept to attempt to understand, since much of what we know about human performance is based on what those limitations might actually be. The most obvious physiological limitation that is typically invoked is that of the heart and the circulatory system, for which we have developed at least one simple mathematical prediction which supposedly establishes an upper limit of heart rate by using the simple equation 220 – age. This example is typically given in undergraduate textbooks of exercise physiology, and it comes with the underlying assumption that maximal capacity is seldom, if ever, exceeded. In more simplistic terms, maximal heart rate is likely to be 220 beats per minute no matter who you are. The most curious thing about this simple equation is that no published record of how it was derived actually exists! There is only an estimate based on mean data published in 1971 (Fox et al. 1971). Since this time, this equation has been used almost without question or scrutiny. In fact it is now thought this widely used mathematical model is flawed to the point that it cannot predict maximum heart rate in children or adolescents (Verschuren et al. 2011). Nevertheless, maximal heart rate, however defined, is typically used as a measure of a cardiovascular ceiling or limit. Clearly, it would be futile to suggest that the heart has no limit since the heart cannot beat any faster than the cardiac muscle can contract and relax.

However, it is equally futile to use this limit as a surrogate for establishing a limit on human performance since we rely on a coordinated effort of multiple systems to achieve our performance goal.

The maximum heart rate equation is used here as an illustration of the usual model of limitation in exercise physiology rather than one of regulation. The difference between these two schools of thought can be further illustrated with basic engineering principles. For instance, a bridge that has collapsed is an example of a system that has exceeded its limiting condition (limitation or catastrophe), whereas a bridge that remains intact is a system that is regulated and, therefore, yet to exceed its limiting condition. The system fails the instant the limiting condition is exceeded. Until such an event occurs, the factors which might bring about system failure are essentially unknown. However, engineers would argue that they would likely have a better than average idea as to what those factors might be, given that most of our skyscrapers, bridges and the like remain intact for incredibly long periods of time. Engineers base their mathematical calculations of limitations on what they term *safety factors*.

In this chapter, we will consider the fundamental concepts of safety factors as related to biological "design," along with the potential *reserve* capacities which are an inherent characteristic of organs and their related systems. In addition, we will consider what *trade-offs* might be an outcome of safety factors and what these trade-offs mean in terms of human performance, health and disease.

Safety factors

Since the classic paper by Meltzer (1907), biologists have attempted to determine what rule can be applied to biological systems which would yield the inherent safety factor for a particular organ, system or the entire organism. In an effort to understand what the limitations of any given biological system might be, Meltzer (1907) systematically described what the obvious maximum was for a particular organ and its associated system, noting that it was "self-evident that nature is economical and wastes neither material or energy" (p. 484). However, the caveat for this assumption is that

> organs and complex tissues . . . are built on a plan of great luxury. Some organs possess at least twice as much tissue as even a maximum of normal activity would require. In other organs, especially in those with internal secretion, the margin of safety amounts sometimes to ten or fifteen times the amount of the actual need.
>
> (pp. 488–489)

The question then is, how is a particular safety factor determined? First, a working definition for a safety factor is required. A safety factor is a term used to describe the inherent *capacity* of a system beyond the expected *load* that the system is likely to encounter. In engineering, the safety factor (SF) of any system can be theoretically determined by dividing the capacity (C) by the expected maximum load (L):

$$C / L = SF$$

An example that is usually given to illustrate the workings of this equation is the passenger elevator. The normal safety factor for a passenger elevator is 12. That is, the strength of the cables attached to the elevator is required to have a capacity 12 times for which the expected load of the elevator is required to operate. In practical terms, if the specification sign on the elevator indicates that the maximum load (L) is 27,468 N and it can fit only ten people, then the actual maximum load can be calculated by using the load and the required safety factor:

$$C / 27,468 = 12$$
$$C = 12 \times 27,468 \text{ N}$$
$$C = 329,616 \text{ N or } 33,593 \text{ kg}$$

Thus, the elevator will need to exceed a load of 32,616 N before the cables holding it will fail. In engineering terms this gives us great confidence in the design and operation of structures where the penalty for failure would be significant if not for the safety factors involved. In addition to calculating the maximum load before failure, the basic safety factor equation can be rearranged to predict how much reserve (R) any particular system might have. For instance, if we subtract the load from the capacity, the yield would be the actual reserve:

$$C - L = R$$

Thus, in our example of the passenger elevator, the reserve would be as follows:

$$329,616 \text{ N} - 27,468 \text{ N} = 302,148 \text{ N}$$

At this point we might ask what the relevance of safety factors or reserve might be with respect to fatigue. Fatigue is a term widely used and dependent on context; it nevertheless carries intuitive meaning that conveys a non-specific sense for capacity to undertake the required effort before failure occurs. In biological terms fatigue is used to describe the individual's ability to carry out a task successfully, either physically or mentally. Therefore, it would be of immense practical relevance to be able to use the safety factor rules to further understand fatigue and its causes, since the presumption is that fatigue is a consequence of attaining or avoiding some physiological limiting point. The relationship between fatigue and the reserve is most relevant as it would seem intuitive that when the reserve is compromised, fatigue would set in, in order that the system does not fail.

Safety factors at the macro level of organisation

We will now illustrate the application and determination of the safety factor rule with regards to some biological examples at the macro or systemic level of organisation. An obvious example is the kidney, which in healthy individuals can be donated without any loss or change in normal renal function to the donor, provided that one healthy kidney is retained. On a macro level, this suggests that we have at least twice the capacity of what is normally needed with respect to renal function. In relation to the lungs, studies which have evaluated respiratory capacity following either lobectomy and/or pneumonectomy suggest there is exists a very large reserve. It has been found that exercise capacity as measured by maximal oxygen consumption (VO_{2max}) after lobectomy remains relatively unchanged at 6 months' post-resection, whereas pneumonectomy can result in a 20% decrease, probably due to the reduced area of gas exchange (Bolliger et al. 1996). Interestingly, the perceived exertion is thought to remain unchanged during exercise regardless of either lobectomy or pneumonectomy. These findings also indicate that functional reserve of the lungs is indeed significant. The fact that the removal of a lobe makes little to no difference to exercise capacity confirms that the normal process of respiration can be accomplished with only half of the lung tissue. Bone tissue on the other hand is curiously complex, with the safety factor being less uniform across species. Table 2.1 provides some safety factors related to the compressive resistance of bone in a range of species. These data show that bone safety factors can vary a great deal between terrestrial animals, including *Homo*.

The assumption is that the material strength of bone is similar across species and there would be no difference when bone is scaled for size across large and small animals. By extrapolation this would also mean that as bone increases in size with larger animals and the material strength remains constant, the safety factor for bone would also be similar between small and large animals. When this hypothesis was tested it was found that bending strength does not seem to vary a great deal over the large range of body sizes, leading to the conclusion that large animals have a much lower safety factor than small animals (Biewener 1982).

Table 2.1 The range of safety factors of bones in a range of terrestrial species including *Homo*

Species/structure	Safety factor (compressive force)
Hopping kangaroo/leg bone	3.2
Jumping dog/leg bone	2.8
Running ostrich/leg bone	2.6
Galloping buffalo/leg bone	2.5–5.0
Jumping locust/leg bone	1.2
Man weightlifting/vertebra	1–1.7

Source: Alexander (1981).

It seems somewhat counterintuitive for nature to have endowed large animals with a reduced safety margin compared with their much smaller counterparts. However, it has also been shown that different sized animals during locomotion do not develop a constant peak ground force; rather the peak force decreases as body size increases (Cavagna et al. 1977). These two findings show that the bending strength of bone is not dissimilar between animals of different body size and peak force on the limbs decreases as body size increases. This means that small animals have relatively greater safety factors for bone than do larger animals. Since nature is economical and not wasteful, there must be a usefulness to the greater than expected safety factor in the bones of small animals. Although there is no definitive answer to this safety factor difference with respect to bone tissue, it is thought that bone tissue does not simply react to the normal stresses of constant locomotion; rather it is likely to be under greater stresses from high accelerations and decelerations in smaller animals compared to larger ones, and this might account for the greater safety factor (Biewener 1982). The example of the safety factor of bone used here highlights the fact that safety factors in biological terms are likely to be very complex and directly related to the specific interaction between a given species and its environment.

The safety factors related to human bone are even more complex when considering the bipedality of *Homo*. The general presumption with respect to the human skeletal system is that it is shaped and remodelled by the loads that the various bones are exposed to, which in the end produce the desired safety factors for the individual bones. However, there are at least two basic observations with respect to bone tissue safety factors which are likely to also apply to other species. First, bones actually do fracture and, therefore, safety factors are at times exceeded. Second, there is clearly a delicate balance between resisting fracture and the strength of bone. The main feature of this relationship is that human bones range from poorly adapted for resisting fracture (e.g., the auditory ossicles, femoral neck) to those bones that have high resistance to fracture (skull) (Currey 2003). The intriguing issue about the difference in how safety factors are established between long bones and flat bones, such as the skull, is that the skull is rarely subjected on a day-to-day basis to the external loads which would produce the kind of strength and the subsequent safety factor to resist fracture, as is the case with long bones. The question then is, how does the skull produce the thickness of its bones in order to establish the safety factor? In attempting to answer this intriguing question Lieberman (1996) examined the effect of exercise on the bone thickness of both the tibia and the bones of the skull, specifically the cranial vault in miniature swine and armadillo. After being weaned, the swine were separated into an exercise group, which ran on a treadmill for 30 min each day for 1 month and housed in a large pen, whereas the control swine were confined to a smaller pen but free to roam about. The armadillo were identical twins, with one twin running on a treadmill for 60 min a day for a period of 4 months. As expected, the findings showed that when exercise was compared to normal living, the bone mass of the tibia in both these animals was significantly increased. However, the bone thickness of the cranial vault (frontal, central and mid- sagittal) in the exercised animals was 32.5% and 24.3% thicker (mm) for the swine and armadillo, respectively. These findings indicate that bones of the cranial vault respond to loading during exercise, in addition to the loading from normal mastication and chewing. A further conclusion is that the bones of the skull do not grow to a particular thickness, but they do indeed respond to lower amounts of loading compared to long bones in order to generate the growth required to produce a safety factor which makes them particularly resistant to fracture. This is a critical point as the potential cost of fracture of the cranial vault can indeed be very high. Although these data from animal studies are interesting and point to a positive relationship between physical activity and cranial vault thickness, whether this relationship holds true for *Homo* is also an important point to consider.

From the available fossil record Lieberman (1996) also compares the cranial vault thickness (at bregma and parietal eminence; Figure 2.2) from *Homo erectus* to *Holocene modern humans* and found that cranial vault thickness is possibly associated to some degree with the required level of subsistence. The taxa that are compared suggest that cranial vault thickness is different between post-industrial

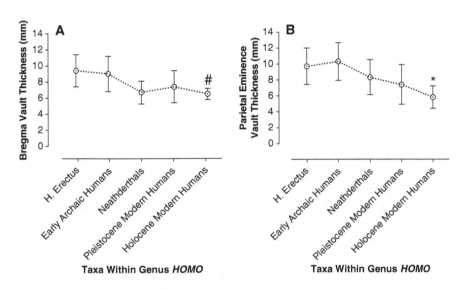

Figure 2.2 The cranial vault thickness at bregma (A) and the parietal eminence (B) of different taxa within the genus *Homo*. The mechanism by which vault thickness is altered is yet to be fully understood. #$P < 0.05$ thickness significantly thinner compared with *H. erectus* and early archaic humans. *$P < 0.05$ thickness is significantly thinner compared with all other humans.

Source: Data are redrawn from Lieberman (1996).

and pre-industrial farming populations. Although the differences between each of the comparisons is minimal, the fact that *Holecene modern humans* have generally significantly thinner vaults compared to *Homo erectus* does suggest at very least that an environmental factor likely influences osteogenesis in these bones. Thus, the safety factor (thickness) associated with the bones of the skull is to some degree dependent on the interaction between the environment and the individual, but the threshold for producing the required safety factor is likely to be lower compared with other bone tissue.

The purpose of the preceding discussion was to highlight the intricate processes that are involved in tissues developing appropriate safety factors. Note that in the discussion about the safety factors of bone, the limiting circumstance is fracture. However, day-to-day living does not typically include fracture of bone tissue; rather it reflects the resistance to fracture — that is, the variations in loading on a day-to-day basis that are meant to deal with the damage inflicted by fatiguing activity. Consequently, loading experienced during fracture must be different to that loading which stimulates the safety factor of individual bones. Although a definitive mechanism has not been identified which determines the safety factor of biological tissue generally, it is nevertheless apparent that low safety factors are observed where loads are likely to be predictable (long bones of the limbs) but safety factors are greater when loads are highly unpredictable (the skull) and the penalty for failure is potentially very high (Alexander 1981).

Safety factors at the micro level of organisation

In the preceding section, we considered some gross examples of safety factors, such as the kidneys, lungs and bone tissue. Although having two of anything implies some type of reserve capacity, how this strategy might translate to the micro level of organisation is not evidently as obvious. We have seen that in some structures, such as the passenger elevator, a safety factor of 12 seems appropriate, but in biological tissue at the macro level this can range from a factor of 3 for some bones in some species to a factor of 1 in other species (Table 2.1). A further consideration in the evolution of a specific safety factor is the penalty of failure; the higher the cost, the higher the safety factor would intuitively be. This explains the higher safety factor for the passenger elevator compared with a freight elevator, to which engineers might assign a safety factor of only 7. Other considerations in arriving at appropriate safety factors are availability of materials, deterioration and replacement costs. In general terms, the higher the cost of materials the lower the safety factor tends to be. In the world of engineering and construction, this decision is usually related to material costs and the economic model that is used at any one time. However, in biology the economic model is always dictated by the laws of nature, or more specifically, reproductive opportunity through natural selection. In this way, a ratio of capacity to load is arrived at, making each biological component economical without reducing the penalty threshold for failure.

To illustrate the evolution of a safety factor at the micro level of organisation, we will first consider one of the earliest descriptions which examined the relationship between pancreatic enzyme outputs and malabsorption (DiMagno et al. 1973). When investigating the functional reserve capacity of the pancreas in patients with pancreatitis versus healthy subjects, malabsorption in these patients did not occur until enzyme output dropped to 10% or less of the normal level. The authors concluded that 90% of the pancreas will need to be destroyed before malabsorption occurs. Specifically, fat digestion can continue until lipase output reaches 10% of normal values. In fact, earlier studies of patients with up to 75% pancreatectomy indicate no significant malabsorption, although exogenous insulin was required (Kalser et al. 1968). These studies clearly show that the pancreas has an enormous reserve for enzyme secretion and well above normal loads, which translates to a safety factor of about 10. The other observation here is that rather than having two of this organ, as with the kidney or lungs, for example, nature has opted for one pancreas but endowed the actual tissue with an enhanced capacity to do its work. This is particularly enlightening when considering the enormous work an organ such as the pancreas does and puts into stark relief what it would take to develop a disease such as Type II diabetes mellitus, given its enormous safety factor. This observation also highlights the reality that biological capacity comes at some cost since the resources available to animals are limited; that is, an excessive amount of resources for one component of a biological system will undoubtedly reduce the resources available for another. Whether the benefit of having two kidneys or two lungs means that we have only one pancreas with an enhanced cellular capacity is difficult, if not impossible, to prove.

An area in which the safety factor has been reasonably well studied at the micro level of organisation is the metabolic capacity of the small intestine. The reasons for studying this system over others lies in the fact this system is intimately connected with our need to acquire, utilise and store energy. Access to and the utilisation of energy are also connected to the general concept of fatigue, whereby low energy availability or lack of access to energy leads to premature fatigue. We shall return to the relationship between energy and fatigue in more detail in Chapter 7. There are some interesting observations reported which show a unique regulatory adaptation of the intestine and its subsequent effects on energy intake and consumption. Located on the epithelial surface of the small intestine are millions of small villi projecting from the mucosa, with a brush border consisting of micro-villi, which protrude into the intestinal chime. The intestinal brush border along with the villi and the folding of the intestine provides an enormous surface area for contact between the intestine and the material passing through it. This is useful in making the cells more efficient, as contact between the cells and the substance to be absorbed or used has to be as economical as possible. It is suggested that this enormous surface area of the small intestine has an absorptive capacity far in excess of the daily intake, whereby several kilograms of carbohydrates, 500 grams of fat and 700 grams of protein in addition to more than

20 litres of water per day can be processed (Guyton & Hall 2006). This maximal processing capacity is clearly a result of the surface area available for absorption and in contrast to the normal intake (load) of energy, which is vastly less, according to dietary guidelines (National Health and Medical Research Council 2013), which place the total intake of macronutrients at around 1.2 kg per day. From an evolutionary perspective, this larger than required capacity must be related to the need to utilise and store fuel at a rate that would enhance our prospects of survival under the most extreme conditions. Humans like many other creatures will consume as much as needed and access whatever storage capacity we might have, especially when we anticipate low supply and scarcity. This point is important when one considers that hormonal regulation of metabolism, particularly insulin secretion, is geared towards energy abundance and the storing of excess energy Guyton and Hall (2006) (pp. 961–962).

At this point it is worthwhile briefly mentioning that fuel storage is a complex phenomenon which does not simply have one directional behaviour – find food, eat, store fuel. This simplistic view negates the obvious observation that in extreme pathology, such as anorexia nervosa, where starvation occurs, the drive for intense and frequent exercise also occurs, which has been a key observation from its earliest description (Gull 1874; Davis et al. 1997). This particular symptom is not simply restricted to the common understanding of physical exercise but is also characterised as hyperactivity and exercise which seems at best aimless (Kron et al. 1978). Thus, if energy depletion leads to fatigue, then anorexia nervosa presents us with a paradox not easily explicable, if lack of fuel storage is thought to reduce our physical capacity to undertake exercise. Fortunately, natural selection can, to some extent, provide some clues as to what might explain this behaviour, which is often thought to be socially and psychologically driven (see Chapter 7). However, for now we will focus on the safety factor relevant to fuel storage.

In attempting to understand why we have evolved such an enormous capacity for intestinal absorption, several studies have undertaken to examine the safety margin associated with uptake of nutrients by the intestinal brush border in particular carbohydrates. Although the process by which absorption takes place is complex and requires an in-depth understanding of specific enzymatic action and processes (see Guyton & Hall 2006), we are more concerned here with the outcomes of this process and what they can tell us about the safety factor for nutrient absorption. Since studies on humans are difficult using the available techniques, much of our understanding comes from animal models. In a classic study (Toloza et al. 1991), mice were transferred from living in a normal ambient temperature of 22°C to a less than optimal temperature of 6°C for a period of 28 days. During this time food intake, digestive efficiency, intestinal morphology and brush-border capacities were measured. The most immediate response observed within 24 hours of being exposed to the cold was a 68% increase in food intake, which was equivalent to 2.5 times the pre-exposure value. Interestingly, the faecal output matched the increased feeding by a similar value. These findings suggest that the intestinal capacity of the experimental mice is at least 2.5 times the normal load. However, the most striking result of this experiment was that within 4 days of being transferred to the cold temperature, the intestine also hypertrophied by 18%, which then resulted in an enhanced transport capacity. The authors noted that the intestinal nutrient uptake, specifically glucose, was typically about 6 mmol/day when the mice were in 22°C, versus a maximal capacity of 19 mmol/day, providing for a safety factor of ~3.1. Given the sharp increase in feeding when transferred to 6°C, the nutrient uptake also rose to 15 mmol/day, which encroached upon the safety factor, leaving virtually no reserve for nutrient uptake for these mice. In response to this low margin of reserve, the mice improved their maximal nutrient uptake by establishing a new capacity of 24 mmol/day. This result is shown in Figure 2.3 as the time course of adaptation for intestinal glucose uptake. The authors noted that complementary organs, such as the liver, kidneys and spleen, also hypertrophied in order that the overall increased metabolic and absorption rates were met.

The changes to the glucose uptake of the intestine and when overfeeding, with a change in the apparent safety factor in response to the ambient temperature challenge, have also been observed in lactating mice (Hammond & Diamond 1992). When already lactating mothers were imposed with an experimentally increased litter size, there was an apparent ceiling on the amount of feeding and

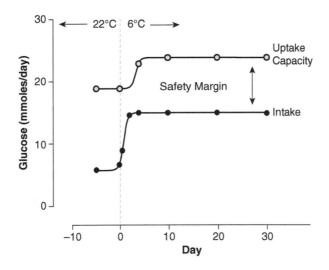

Figure 2.3 The safety margin or reserve for glucose uptake in mice transferred from 22°C to 6°C. The safety margin or safety factor is the difference between the uptake capacity and the dietary intake (load) which changed in response to the extra feeding that occurred due to the shift from moderate (22°C) to cold (6°C) ambient conditions.

Source: Data are redrawn from Toloza et al. (1991).

weaning that could be achieved. In this instance, lactating mothers could manage to wean about double the normal litter size. This was accomplished by four apparent mechanisms: (1) increasing food intake in proportion to the total mass that required nourishing, (2) maintaining digestive efficiency regardless of the increased food intake, (3) increased intestinal glucose uptake while increasing a reserve capacity, and (4) hypertrophy of the gut by a factor of 2.5. Perhaps the most critical aspect of this speedy adaptation is its reversal – atrophy of the intestine when the mother was no longer required to lactate and nourish her young, as shown in Figure 2.4. The other conclusion that can be drawn is simply that biological tissue, in this case the small intestine, must be energetically costly and atrophy ensues if it is not needed, preserving the fundamental tenet that nature does not waste material or energy but aims to preserve a safety factor which is advantageous for reproduction.

Thus far we have discussed the apparent safety factors and reserve capacities of the pancreas and small intestine with some evidence that complementary organs, such as the liver, spleen and kidney, also respond to increased loads, resulting in an improved reserve for the period of time that it is needed (Toloza et al. 1991; Hammond & Diamond 1992). These changes reflect the primitive need for nourishment, energy and the storage of fuel under the specific conditions of temperature and reproduction. How a greater understanding of these reserve capacities might provide clues to solving our chronic health problems needs further work and experimentation.

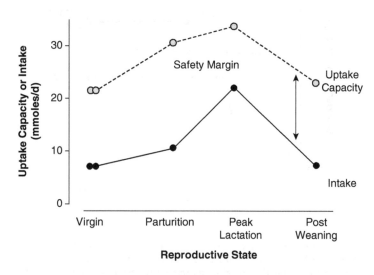

Figure 2.4 The wet mass of the small intestine mucosa from the non-reproductive state through to the post-weaning state in lactating mice.

Source: Data are redrawn from Hammond and Diamond (1992).

Safety factors and skeletal muscle

A system that is directly connected with the typical measurement of fatigue is the musculoskeletal system. We will return to the skeletal muscle and its direct relationship to the observation and measurement of fatigue in Chapters 4 and 5. In this chapter we will briefly explore the safety factor of skeletal muscle and its relationship to performance, fatigue and health. Skeletal muscle is a highly complex organ, being intimately connected with the central nervous system (CNS; neuromuscular), which relies heavily on chemical differences and the generation of electrical impulses. The basic observation is that in healthy humans a failure of neuromuscular transmission is seldom reported even during the most intense muscular effort. There are multiple reasons for this observation, not least of which is the abundance of neurotransmitter substance, which when released at the motor nerve terminal by singular impulses is far in excess of what is needed for excitation of the muscle fibre. This alone implies a significant reserve at least at this point of the chain of transmission. However, since skeletal muscle contraction is a result of a continuum of transmission from the CNS to the actual muscle fibre, there are likely to be multiple safety factors that reside at various points along this continuum.

To appreciate the nature of the skeletal muscle safety factor, it is essential that one is familiar with the basic architecture which gives rise to the chemical and electrical transmission leading to skeletal muscle contraction and subsequent force development. These basic neuromuscular principles are well beyond the scope of this text so the reader is referred to a more comprehensive description (MacIntosh et al. 2006). The following section details some of the important and intricate mechanisms which are critical to the operation of skeletal muscle with respect to its inherent safety factor. Skeletal muscle safety factor can be ascertained and defined in a number of ways, which include but are not limited to the following (Wood & Slater 2001):

1   The fraction of acetylcholine receptors (AChRs) that when blocked prevent action potentials;
2   The ratio of estimated peak amplitude of the end-plate potential to the threshold depolarisation needed to generate the action potential;
3   The estimate of the magnitude of the post-synaptic current that flows in response to a nerve impulse; and
4   The number of chemical transmitter acetylcholine (ACh) quanta released compared to the number required to generate the action potential.

Notwithstanding the possibilities listed earlier, the safety factor which is likely to be most critical is the relationship and interaction of ACh with other elements of the neuromuscular system which determine the capacity for transmission. Along with other chemicals and hormones, the basic compound ACh is stored in the pre-synaptic vesicles, which is then released into the synaptic cleft following an action potential. The amount of ACh released is known as a *quantum*. At the post-synaptic membrane of the muscle fibre are situated AChRs, which are located on the post-synaptic folds, as shown in the electron micrograph in Figure 2.5. There are two architectural elements which are important in understanding the safety factor at this point: the number of AChRs and the post-synaptic folds.

First, we will examine the number of AChRs and what this might determine in terms of action potential and skeletal muscle contraction. Although empirical evidence for the number of AChRs in human skeletal muscle is scant, classic studies on the muscles of the cat and rat provide evidence that the number of AChRs could be one safety factor to consider (Paton & Waud 1967; Chang et al. 1975). These experiments show that by pharmacologically blocking the AChRs, it is possible to estimate the number of AChRs required to generate an action potential. This would be indicative of a safety factor that provides post-synaptic receptors well over and above what would be required for successful chemical transmission. One further curious observation is that the quantity of folding in the post-synaptic membrane (Figure 2.6) is relatively large in humans compared with other species (Slater et al. 1992). This is a critical observation as it is estimated that chemical transmitter ACh quanta is significantly less in humans compared with other species, leaving the safety factor for chemical transmission to be marginally greater than 1 with respect to ACh alone. In order to improve the possibility for transmission, and thus the safety factor, the post-synaptic folding in humans seems to be increased substantially, which amplifies the effect of ACh release. In other words, the comparatively low level of ACh release in humans is balanced with the relatively large post-synaptic folding. Figure 2.5 depicts this relationship for humans and other species.

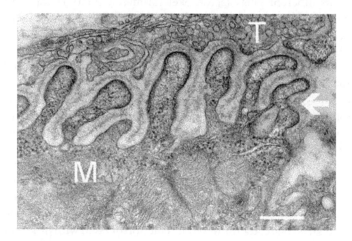

Figure 2.5 Electron micrograph of neuromuscular junction. T is the axon terminal, M is the muscle fibre, and an arrow indicates the junctional folds with basal lamina. The scale is 0.3 μm. From Wikipedia Commons PD.

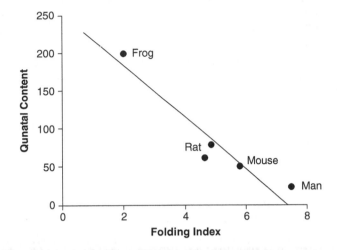

Figure 2.6 The relationship between the post-synaptic folding and the ACh quanta in humans and other species. This relationship shows that a reduction in transmitter substance (quantal content) is balanced by the number of folds (folding index) in the post-synaptic membrane, which is thought to amplify the effect of the transmitter substance ACh.

Source: Data redrawn from Wood and Slater (2001).

Taking the data that are shown in Figure 2.6 at face value leads to the conclusion that different species of vertebrates use different strategies to accomplish neuromuscular transmission by balancing the ACh quanta against the number of post-synaptic folds. This observation is not readily explicable in terms of why different animals would use different strategies to arrive at a given safety factor for neuromuscular transmission. However, we are left with one distinct possibility as outlined earlier – that "nature is economical and wastes neither material or energy" (Meltzer 1907, p. 482). However, one suggestion (Wood & Slater 2001) is that as animals increase in size there would be a need to innervate more skeletal muscle fibres for any given motor unit, limiting the available material in the pre-synaptic space. If this is so, then it makes sense for evolution to have found the economy and compensation in the post-synaptic space. Although attractive, this proposition is by no means definitive.

A further consideration is whether the safety factor changes according to the type of skeletal muscle – Type I (slow-twitch) versus Type II (fast-twitch) fibres, given their well-described and distinctive force-producing properties. For instance, it is apparent that the amount of post-synaptic folding is greater for Type II than it is for Type I fibres (Ellisman et al. 1976; Ogata 1988; Padykula & Gauthier 1970), which is also the case for the voltage gated calcium channels

(Milton et al. 1992; Ruff & Whittlesey 1992). It is also evident there are differences in the properties of sodium channels (Na^+) between fibre types (Ruff & Whittlesey 1992). These are important distinctions as the density of Na^+ channels is thought to contribute to the speed of the muscle action potential – specifically, its resistance to termination. Essentially, the inactivation of the Na^+ channels determines how rapid the action potential is terminated (Ruff & Whittlesey 1992) so that:

1   Fast inactivation of Na^+ channels produces rapid termination of action potentials;
2   Slow inactivation of Na^+ channels produces resistance to termination of action potentials.

This property would allow fast-twitch fibres to fire at high frequencies, while the slow-twitch fibres could have tonic activation. This makes evolutionary sense since the individual safety factor (Ach quanta, post-synaptic folding and voltage gates) should be aligned and be able to predict the functional capacity of the specific skeletal muscle fibre. In the case of Type I fibres, it is known that these fibres are specifically capable of being in a state of continuous action and able to resist fatigue in comparison to their Type II counterparts. We shall return to this physiological difference between muscle fibre types in Chapter 9 when discussing the difference between measuring endurance and power.

Safety factors in health and disease

Any exercise physiology textbook will outline the anatomical and physiological changes to be expected with lifestyle diseases, such as diabetes, obesity, cardiovascular disease and occasionally conditions such as McArdle's syndrome, along with typical muscular dystrophies. The usual description of these conditions is tied to what can be expected of individuals who are afflicted with these diseases when exercising, and whether exercise can ameliorate the condition in some way. In addition, most authors will describe the effects of ageing on exercise capacity and what regular exercise can do to maintain functional capacity and independence. However, few texts explore or consider the effect these pathologies or ageing might have on the individual organ safety factors and what this might mean for our capacity to resist fatigue. In this section, we will deal with how some of these pathologies alter the safety factor of a particular organ or system.

We begin by considering the effects of disease and ageing on bone. There is an assumption that the reader is somewhat familiar with the fundamental processes of bone mineralisation, bone growth, turnover and remodelling during the life span. Central to these processes is that bone not only provides a solid, rigid frame for the body but also, as discussed previously, needs to withstand given loads to avoid fracture and continuous loading associated with daily activity. An important component in determining whether the safety factor of bone is altered as a consequence of disease depends to a large degree on the bone's functional strain to which it has been subjected over a long period of time. For instance, functional loading of bone is predominantly by compressive strain, whereas tensile strain is usually no more than about 80%–85% of compression (Taylor 1986). In addition, bone can be subjected to shearing, bending, torsion and eccentric loading, and although few studies have been conducted in vivo, these kinds of strains are considered to be low in comparison to compression and tension strains. The exposure of various bones to these strains has a great deal of bearing not only on the individual safety factor of bone but also on the probability that it will fail. Thus, the functional strain history and the quality of the bone itself are critical to understanding the effects of health and disease on the safety factor.

One of the most pronounced changes that occur to bone is the increase in the percentage of mineralisation with advancing age. The outcome of this mineralisation is that energy absorption decreases by a factor of three between the ages of 3 and 90, as reported for the cortical bone of the femur (Currey 1979). Effectively, this results in decreased plastic deformation before a fracture occurs. On this basis, the consequence is that the safety factor of bone and more generally the skeleton declines with age because of the quality of the bone material (Biewener 1993). The unavoidable reduction in bone mineral density (osteopenia) and the subsequent development of bone mass loss and the associated microarchitecture (osteoporosis) lead to the increased risk of fracture. However, this is a complex phenomenon that is dependent on so many factors, including genetics, nutrition, gender and the volume of physical activity that one undertakes over the lifespan in addition to the lean and fat mass components (Taaffe et al. 2001). Although it may seem inevitable that the safety factor of the skeleton is reduced over the life span, it is also evident that the decrease in the safety factor can also be retarded given the appropriate conditions. It is well known that exercise, and in particular resistance exercise, can have a positive effect on bone health if the program can be maintained (Lang et al. 2010).

Interestingly, in animal models, mechanical loading of the rat ulna 3 days per week for 5 weeks induced small (<two-fold increases) structural changes which resulted in >100-fold increase in fatigue resistance of the bone (Warden et al. 2004). These findings show the adaptive nature of the skeleton and the effect that appropriate physical activity will have on attenuating the decreased safety factor in bone. It is not inconsequential that physical activity results in the capacity of the skeleton to withstand higher loads since the capacity to resist fatigue is critical in avoiding a catastrophic failure. The opposite of this position is of course that any condition which decreases the safety factor of the skeleton will result in less mobility and potentially fracture.

The safety factor associated with skeletal muscle has already been discussed. However, in what way the safety factor might change as a consequence of deteriorating health is important as it relates to understanding how we might manage or prevent such a change and maintain our quality of life. The most common observation is that commencing at around the age of 30 years there is a progressive loss of skeletal muscle mass (sarcopenia) which is also accompanied by a loss in overall strength (Rutherford 1992). This reduction continues and presents a major health problem since it is associated with reduced mobility, increase in the frequency of falls and loss of independence. Again, and similar to skeletal changes, the loss of muscle is complicated by a number of factors which are not dissimilar to those related to bone loss.

There are two distinct observations which are thought to alter the force-generating capacity of skeletal muscle. First, there is general muscle fibre atrophy, and second, a loss of motor unit number and size (Lexell et al. 1988). However, the skeletal muscle changes are related to the central nervous system alterations with ageing. The loss of motoneurons in the anterior horn of the spinal cord affects the larger, faster motor units more so, which accounts to some extent for the loss of power. Interestingly, the slower motor units tend to survive but these axons sprout towards the fast muscle fibres and innervate them. The reason for this sprouting and re-innervation from slow axons to the fast fibres remains unclear. However, the outcome of this change is that former fast fibres now take on the contractile and biochemical characteristics of slow fibres (Roos 1997). What does this mean for the safety factor of skeletal muscle? Recall that post-synaptic folding is greater for Type II than for Type I fibres and that the density of Na^+ channels is thought to contribute to the speed of the muscle action potential. Thus, the ability to either terminate or resist termination of an action potential is a critical factor in whether we fatigue rapidly or resist fatigue. Since slow-twitch fibres seemingly have low-density Na^+ channels, they are able to resist the termination of action potentials and be in a state of continuous action. Thus, selective denervation of fast motor units and a preference for re-innervation by slow axons suggest that the safety factor is not so much reduced as it is altered to attenuate the reduction in endurance and as a consequence resist fatigue.

Regardless of the mechanism for this selective denervation of fast fibres and re-innervation by slow axons, the observation is a critical one in understanding the human propensity for fatigue resistance. In this example, if the opposite was the case, whereby slow units would be selectively denervated, and then re-innervated by fast axons, the outcome would be improved or maintained power at the expense of endurance and fatigue resistance. Thus, the question remains, why would selection of slow axons over fast axons as we age be an evolutionary advantage? We will explore this question in more detail in Chapter 3 when we consider the differences between us and our closest primate relatives. One interesting observation that is seldom considered is the altered safety factor of neuromuscular transmission as ageing progresses. Few studies have shown that there are gradual changes to the pre- and post-synaptic components of skeletal muscle endplates with ageing (Oda 1984; Wokke et al. 1990). In essence, the paucity of data indicates that there is likely remodelling of the neuromuscular junction as age progresses. In a rat diaphragm model, it was shown that the safety factor of neuromuscular transmission was also relative to the changes in ACh quanta, as shown in Figure 2.7 (Kelly 1978).

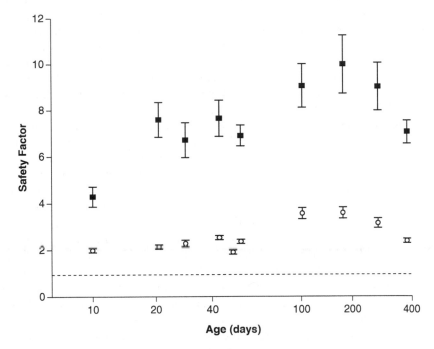

Figure 2.7 The data show the end-plate potential (EPP) when stimulated at 10 Hz (closed boxes) and again during a subsequent plateau phase of the train (open circles). It is evident that the safety factor above 1.0 is sufficient to maintain transmission. However, the safety factor is significantly increased between 11 and 175 days of age and then decreases significantly between 175 and 375 days of age.

Source: Data redrawn from Kelly (1978).

Thus, it is evident that ageing reduces the number of available Type II fibres in preference for their re-innervation by slow axons, in addition to the loss of post-synaptic folding and the associated ACh quanta. This situation in turn reduces the overall safety factor of neuromuscular transmission, but only to a point where transmission itself is still able to be completed with a reserve (Figure 2.7). The studies in this area show that the overall outcome is the decrease in the safety factor of neuromuscular transmission with old age. For now, this observation lends some support to the proposition that fatigue resistance and our ability to harness endurance rather than power must have provided us with an evolutionary advantage, for if the opposite were the case, a preference for Type II fibres and their associated greater post-synaptic folding and ACh quanta, a greater neuromuscular transmission safety factor may have resulted, but the compromise would have been a reduced capacity for fatigue resistance.

Although we have dealt mainly with the ageing process to help describe the expected changes to the safety factor in bone and skeletal muscle, there are many diseases which profoundly alter the structure and functional characteristics of skeletal muscle. These are generally grouped into either myopathies, which are defects in the muscle itself, or neuropathies, which are changes within the nervous system and may lead to secondary changes in the muscle. Generally, myopathies are either atrophic or destructive, but regardless of type, the outcome is a loss of muscle mass. By way of illustration we will deal only with the atrophic myopathies since the destructive myopathies are related to genetic or autoimmune defects and are beyond the scope of this discussion. The interesting observation is that in most cases of atrophic myopathies, the loss of muscle mass is due to the preferential atrophy of II fibres, similar to what is observed with ageing (Ciciliot et al. 2013). However, there are at least two exceptions to this rule in atrophic myopathies. When a limb is immobilised due to a fracture, there is a characteristic loss of Type I fibres, and similarly following spinal cord injury, Type I fibres are converted to Type II fibres, albeit smaller than normal (Burnham et al. 1997). The reasons for this apparent differential switch from Type I to Type II fibres in these two conditions are not entirely clear. Nevertheless, it is now thought that immobilisation results in the expression of increased myosin heavy chain isoforms (the motor protein of muscle) and that maximum shortening velocity of muscle fibres is enhanced (D'Antona 2003). It makes intuitive sense for there to be rapid development of fatigue in this circumstance since it would diminish the capacity to resist fatigue and possibly minimise the likelihood of re-injury. In terms of what this might mean for the safety factor of skeletal muscle, recall that post-synaptic folding is greater for Type II than for Type I fibres and that fast-twitch fibres fire at high frequencies. In addition, the threshold for the activation of fast motor units is much higher. These characteristics are akin to developing force, but given that these fibres fatigue rapidly compared to the more tonically active Type I fibres, the preponderance of Type II fibres in the circumstances of immobilisation and spinal cord injury would maintain the muscle safety factor locally, but reduce the ability to resist fatigue by attenuating endurance.

The preferential switching from Type I to Type II fibres in a diseased state is likely to have some intrinsic advantage. To further illustrate this possibility, it is a common observation that patients with heart failure show progressive signs of muscle wasting (Haehling et al. 2013). However, what is curious about this is that these patients typically show a switch from Type I to Type II muscle fibres (Larsen et al. 2002). This switch of muscle fibre type is likely to be related to the fact that Type I fibres have greater volume of mitochondria and are dependent on the delivery of oxygen for extended periods of muscle activity. Conversely, Type II fibres are less dependent on mitochondria and utilise anaerobic sources for energy. Simply put, the switch from Type I to Type II fibres in heart failure reduces the capacity to resist fatigue and provides a protective mechanism, whereby the individual is unable to produce physical efforts for long periods. In this case, the safety factor of skeletal muscle is perhaps improved by the fibre type switch, but since heart failure is likely to substantially reduce the maximum heart rate achievable (Keteyian et al. 2012), the safety factor of the heart, in this case the heart rate reserve, dictates the ability to resist fatigue, which has been substantially altered.

Evolutionary basis of trade-offs

The basic understanding of trade-offs is most simply explained by the common situation that when confronted with a decision to choose between increasing one factor or characteristic, the result is a decrease in another. In all areas of human endeavour, we are confronted with these familiar choices. For instance, when shopping we might choose to spend money on one particular product, which in turn will leave us short of funds for another, since resources for the majority of us are not unlimited. The most obvious trade-off as far as *Homo* is concerned is the choice to be bipedal rather than quadrupedal, which resulted in a multitude of differences for our species. In the previous section dealing with the concept of the safety factor, the central tenet was that biological systems have finite material, space and energy to provide for the capacity of any one system. Thus, an important aspect of biological capacity is the apparent trade-off that will occur due to limited resources and constraints of space, energy and time, where it would be impossible to increase two traits at the same time (Garland 1988).

Given that we have already introduced the concept of safety factor in skeletal muscle, it remains a good example to illustrate the principle of trade-off with respect to human performance and fatigue. Since we have also established that speed/power and endurance are determined by the skeletal muscle fibre type, improvements in either of these parameters is also likely to be based on a trade-off. In fact, a recognised evolutionary constraint on physical performance is the trade-off between speed and endurance, with its primary basis being the ratio of slow- to fast-twitch muscle fibres in any particular muscle (Garland & Carter 1994). This particular trade-off has been studied in a range of species at different levels of functioning (Bennett et al. 1984; Garland 1988; Van Damme et al. 2002; Vanhooydonck et al. 2001; Wilson et al. 2002; Wilson & James 2004). These studies indicate that at the muscle level there is indeed a negative correlation between maximal power/force generation so that fatigue resistance is a function of the fibre type composition. However, it has been noted that there is a lack of evidence to support an apparent trade-off between speed and endurance at the population level (Wilson & James 2004). For example, an analysis of 600 world-class decathletes showed that individual performances in any pair of disciplines was positively correlated with the entire data set so the expected trade-off between speed and endurance was not detected (Van Damme et al. 2002). However, when these authors restricted their analysis to athletic individuals of comparable ranking, the trade-offs between particular traits were evident so that high-level performance at the power events, such as the 100m sprint, shotput and long jump, was negatively correlated with performance at the 1500m endurance event. These data confirm that high performance in one function may impede performance in another at the individual level.

Although different species are endowed with varying numbers of slow- and fast-twitch muscle fibres, it is the unique adaptability of the muscle fibres which provides evidence that species are adapted either for endurance and fatigue resistance or for power and strength. The popular view is that there is incompatibility between the strength and endurance modes of training (Djamil 1985) so that endurance training does not meaningfully improve muscle force output (Hickson 1980) and strength training has no appreciable effect on maximal oxygen uptake (VO_{2max}) (Hickson et al. 1980), a measure thought to reflect endurance capacity. However, this reasoning merely represents a convenient separation between endurance and power as if they are mutually exclusive. A closer inspection of studies that have examined these relationships reveals there is no sacrifice of endurance by undertaking strength training (Mackinnon et al. 1999) but in fact intense strength training also results in obvious improvement in capacity for higher-intensity cycling and running exercise in trained individuals (Hickson et al. 1988; Hoff et al. 2002). Intense strength training for 3 days/week over 10 weeks improved leg strength by 30% without changes in muscle girth, fibre type or oxidative enzymes (Hickson et al. 1988). Yet, short-duration (4–8 min), high-intensity endurance exercise was improved by up to 13%, whereas long-duration exercise improved by 16% even though VO_{2max} remained unchanged. There is also evidence that combined strength and endurance training will improve both endurance capacity and strength comparably to either strength or endurance training alone in sedentary adults (McCarthy et al. 1995). These findings show that improvements in endurance may not be directly attributable to increases in aerobic capacity *per se* as VO_{2max} is not improved and oxidative enzymes remain unchanged. Rather, an enhanced ability to resist fatigue is more likely to explain these observations.

The observation that strength training can effectively increase endurance, in particular fatigue resistance, without changes in oxidative enzymes, fibre type distribution and VO_{2max} highlights an adaptive paradox. The question then is, what adaptations through resistance training would improve higher-intensity endurance performance and increase the capacity to resist the onset of premature fatigue? The answer must lie in those adaptations which lead to altered neural input to the working muscles, since resistance training increases the tendency of motor units to fire more synchronously, leading to greater efficiency in force production. Carroll et al. (2001) in their review make the point that if more force can be produced after strength training, then fewer motor units need to be recruited so that the amount of cortical activation for any given movement would be reduced. In fact, others have attributed the improved running economy in short-endurance exercise (5 km) following explosive strength training in large part to changes in neuromuscular characteristics and not improvements in aerobic capacity (Paavolainen et al. 1999).

There are at least two aspects of the literature describing the altered endurance capacity and its relationship with fatigue resistance explained by evolutionary theory. First, that improvements in high-intensity endurance are possible with strength training suggests that fitness is characterised by a capacity to attenuate the development of premature fatigue. From an evolutionary perspective, this would also enhance reproductive success as even a small improvement in resisting premature fatigue in a range of ecological contexts could mean the difference between obtaining food and being food. Second, that speed-endurance trade-offs are difficult to detect at the population level merely indicates that nature has more scope and degrees of freedom to manipulate heritable traits (Garland 2014), which is what is expected, since natural selection is primarily an outcome of wide variation of heritable traits. It is also not surprising that speed-endurance trade-offs are most ubiquitous at the individual level and more so at the systemic level of organisation.

References

Alexander, R.M., 1981. Factors of safety in the structure of animals. *Science Progress*, 67(265), pp. 109–130.

Bennett, A.F., Huey, R.B. & John-Alder, H., 1984. Physiological correlates of natural activity and locomotor capacity in two species of lacertid lizards. *Journal of Comparative Physiology B*, 154(2), pp. 113–118.

Biewener, A.A., 1982. Bone strength in small mammals and bipedal birds: do safety factors change with body size? *Journal of Experimental Biology*, 98, pp. 289–301.

Biewener, A.A., 1993. Safety factors in bone strength. *Calcified Tissue International*, 53(Suppl 1), pp. S68–S74.

Bolliger, C.T. et al., 1996. Pulmonary function and exercise capacity after lung resection. *European Respiratory Journal*, 9(3), pp. 415–421.

Burnham, R. et al., 1997. Skeletal muscle fibre type transformation following spinal cord injury. *Spinal Cord*, 35, pp. 86–91.

Carroll, T.J., Riek, S. & Carson, R.G., 2001. Neural adaptations to resistance training. *Sports Medicine*, 31(12), pp. 829–840.

Cavagna, G.A., Heglund, N.C. & Taylor, C.R., 1977. Mechanical work in terrestrial locomotion: two basic mechanisms for minimizing energy expenditure. *American Journal of Physiology*, 233(5), pp. R243–R261.

Chang, C.C., Chuang, S.T. & Huang, M.C., 1975. Effects of chronic treatment with various neuromuscular blocking agents on the number and distribution of acetylcholine receptors in the rat diaphragm. *Journal of Physiology*, 250(1), pp. 161–173.

Ciciliot, S. et al., 2013. Muscle type and fiber type specificity in muscle wasting. *International Journal of Biochemistry and Cell Biology*, 45(10), pp. 2191–2199.

Currey, J.D., 1979. Changes in the impact energy absorption of bone with age. *Journal of Biomechanics*, 12(6), pp. 459–469.

Currey, J.D., 2003. How well are bones designed to resist fracture? *Journal of Bone and Mineral Research*, 18(4), pp. 591–598.

D'Antona, G., 2003. The effect of ageing and immobilization on structure and function of human skeletal muscle fibres. *Journal of Physiology*, 552(2), pp. 499–511.

Davis, C. et al., 1997. The prevalence of high-level exercise in the eating disorders: etiological implications. *Comprehensive Psychiatry*, 38(6), pp. 321–326.

DiMagno, E.P., Go, V.L. & Summerskill, W.H., 1973. Relations between pancreatic enzyme outputs and malabsorption in severe pancreatic insufficiency. *New England Journal of Medicine*, 288(16), pp. 813–815.

Djamil, R., 1985. Incompatibility of endurance- and strength-training modes of exercise. *Journal of Applied Physiology*, 59(5), pp. 1446–1451.

Ellisman, M.H. et al., 1976. Studies of excitable membranes. II: a comparison of specializations at neuromuscular junctions and nonjunctional sarcolemmas of mammalian fast and slow twitch muscle fibers. *Journal of Cell Biology*, 68(3), pp. 752–774.

Fox, S.M., III, Naughton, J.P. & Haskell, W.L., 1971. Physical activity and the prevention of coronary heart disease. *Annals of Clinical Research*, 3(6), pp. 404–432.

Garland, T., Jr, 1988. Genetic basis of activity metabolism. I: inheritance of speed, stamina, and antipredator displays in the garter snake Thamnophis sirtalis. *Evolution*, pp. 335–350.

Garland, T., 2014. Trade-offs. *Current Biology*, 24(2), pp. R60–R61.

Garland, T., Jr, & Carter, P.A., 1994. Evolutionary physiology. *Annual Review of Physiology*, 56(1), pp. 579–621.

Gould, S.J. & Lewontin, R.C., 1979. The spandrels of San Marco and the Panglossian paradigm: a critique of the adaptationist programme. *Proceedings of the Royal Society B: Biological Sciences*, 205(1161), pp. 581–598.

Gull, W.W., 1874. Anorexia nervosa (Apepsia Hysterica, Anorexia Hysterica). *Transactions of the Clinical Society of London*, 7(5), pp. 22–28.

Guyton, A.C. & Hall, J.E., 2006. *Textbook of medical physiology*, 11th ed., Philadelphia, PA: Elsevier Saunders.

Haehling, Von, S., Steinbeck, L. & Doehner, W., 2013. Muscle wasting in heart failure: an overview. *The International Journal Biochemistry & Cell Biology*, 45(10), pp. 2257–2265.

Hammond, K.A. & Diamond, J., 1992. An experimental test for a ceiling on sustained metabolic-rate in lactating mice. *Physiological Zoology*, 65(5), pp. 952–977.

Hickson, R.C., 1980. Interference of strength development by simultaneously training for strength and endurance. *European Journal of Applied Physiology*, 45(2–3), pp. 255–263.

Hickson, R.C., Rosenkoetter, M.A. & Brown, M.M., 1980. Strength training effects on aerobic power and short-term endurance. *Medicine and Science in Sports & Exercise*, 12(5), pp. 336–339.

Hickson, R.C. et al., 1988. Potential for strength and endurance training to amplify endurance performance. *Journal of Applied Physiology*, 65(5), pp. 2285–2290.

Hoff, J., Gran, A. & Helgerud, J., 2002. Maximal strength training improves aerobic endurance performance. *Scandinavian Journal of Medicine & Science in Sports*, 12(5), pp. 288–295.

Kalser, M.H., Leite, C.A. & Warren, W.D., 1968. Fat assimilation after massive distal pancreatectomy. *New England Journal of Medicine*, 279(11), pp. 570–576.

Kelly, S.S., 1978. The effect of age on neuromuscular transmission. *Journal of Physiology*, 274, pp. 51–62.

Keteyian, S.J. et al., 2012. Predicting maximal HR in heart failure patients on β-blockade therapy. *Medicine and Science in Sports & Exercise*, 44(3), pp. 371–376.

Kron, L. et al., 1978. Hyperactivity in anorexia nervosa: a fundamental clinical feature M. Botbol, ed. *Comprehensive Psychiatry*, 19(5), pp. 433–440.

Lang, T. et al., 2010. Sarcopenia: etiology, clinical consequences, intervention, and assessment. *Osteoporosis International*, 21(4), pp. 543–559.

Larsen, A.I. et al., 2002. Effect of exercise training on skeletal muscle fibre characteristics in men with chronic heart failure: correlation between skeletal muscle alterations, cytokines and exercise capacity. *International Journal of Cardiology*, 83(1), pp. 25–32.

Lexell, J., Taylor, C.C. & Sjostrom, M., 1988. What is the cause of the ageing atrophy? *Journal of the Neurological Sciences*, 84(2–3), pp. 275–294.

Lieberman, D.E., 1996. How and why humans grow thin skulls: experimental evidence for systemic cortical robusticity. *American Journal of Physical Anthropology*, 101(2), pp. 217–236.

Mackinnon, L.T., McEniery, M. & Carey, M.F., 1999. The effects of strength training on endurance performance and muscle characteristics. *Medicine and Science in Sports & Exercise*, 31(6), pp. 886–891.

McCarthy, J.P. et al., 1995. Compatibility of adaptive responses with combining strength and endurance training. *Medicine and Science in Sports & Exercise*, 27(3), pp. 429–436.

MacIntosh, B.R., Gardiner, P.F. & McComas, A.J., 2006. Skeletal muscle: form and function, 2nd ed., Champaign, IL: Human Kinetics.

Meltzer, S.J., 1907. The factors of safety in animal structure and animal economy. *Science*, 25(639), pp. 481–498.

Milton, R.L., Lupa, M.T. & Caldwell, J.H., 1992. Fast and slow twitch skeletal muscle fibres differ in their distribution of Na channels near the endplate. *Neuroscience Letters*, 135, pp. 41–44.

National Health and Medical Research Council, 2013. *Australian dietary guidelines*, Canberra, ACT: Department of Health and Aging, Commonwealth of Australia.

Oda, K., 1984. Age changes of motor innervation and acetylcholine receptor distribution on human skeletal muscle fibres. *Journal of the Neurological Sciences*, 66(2–3), pp. 327–338.

Ogata, T., 1988. Structure of motor endplates in the different fiber types of vertebrate skeletal muscles. *Archives of Histology and Cytology*, 51(5), pp. 385–424.

Paavolainen, L. et al., 1999. Explosive-strength training improves 5-km running time by improving running economy and muscle power. *Journal of Applied Physiology*, 86(5), pp. 1527–1533.

Padykula, H.A. & Gauthier, G.F., 1970. The ultrastructure of the neuromuscular junctions of mammalian red, white, and intermediate skeletal muscle fibers. *Journal of Cell Biology*, 46(1), pp. 27–41.

Paton, W.D.M. & Waud, D.R., 1967. The margin of safety of neuromuscular transmission. *Journal of Physiology*, 191(1), pp. 59–90.

Roos, M.R., 1997. Age-related changes in motor unit function. *Muscle & Nerve*, 20, pp. 679–690.

Ruff, R.L. & Whittlesey, D., 1992. Na+ current densities and voltage dependence in human intercostal muscle fibres. *Journal of Physiology*, 458, pp. 85–97.

Rutherford, O.M., 1992. The relationship of muscle and bone loss and activity levels with age in women. *Age and Ageing*, 21(4), pp. 286–293.

Slater, C.R. et al., 1992. Structure and function of neuromuscular junctions in the vastus lateralis of man: A motor point biopsy study of two groups of patients. *Brain*, 115, pp. 451–478.

Taaffe, D.R. et al., 2001. Race and sex effects on the association between muscle strength, soft tissue, and bone mineral density in healthy elders: the Health, Aging, and Body Composition Study. *Journal of Bone and Mineral Research*, 16(7), pp. 1343–1352.

Tattersall, I., 2012. *Masters of the planet: the search for our human origins*, New York: St. Martin's Press.

Taylor, C.R., 1986. Bone strain: a determinant of gait and speed? *Journal of Experimental Biology*, 123, pp. 383–400.

Taylor, C.R. & Weibel, E.R., 1981. Design of the mammalian respiratory system. I: problem and strategy. *Respiration Physiology*, 44(1), pp. 1–10.

Toloza, E.M., Lam, M. & Diamond, J., 1991. Nutrient extraction by cold-exposed mice: a test of digestive safety margins. *American Journal of Physiology*, 261, pp.G608–G620.

Van Damme, R. et al., 2002. Evolutionary biology: performance constraints in decathletes. *Nature*, 415(6873), pp. 755–756.

Vanhooydonck, B., Van Damme, R. & Aerts, P., 2001. Speed and stamina trade-off in Lacertid lizards. *Evolution*, 55(5), pp. 1040–1048.

Verschuren, O., Maltais, D.B. & Takken, T., 2011. The 220-age equation does not predict maximum heart rate in children and adolescents. *Developmental Medicine & Child Neurology*, 53(9), pp. 861–864.

Warden, S.J. et al., 2004. Bone adaptation to a mechanical loading program significantly increases skeletal fatigue resistance. *Journal of Bone and Mineral Research*, 20(5), pp. 809–816.

Weibel, E.R., Taylor, C.R. & Hoppeler, H., 1991. The concept of symmorphosis: a testable hypothesis of structure-function relationship. *Proceedings of the National Academy of Sciences of the United States of America*, 88(22), pp. 10357–10361.

Weibel, E.R. et al., 1981. Design of the mammalian respiratory system. IX: functional and structural limits for oxygen flow. *Respiration Physiology*, 44(1), pp. 151–164.

Wilson, R.S. & James, R.S., 2004. Constraints on muscular performance: trade-offs between power output and fatigue resistance. *Proceedings of the Royal Society B: Biological Sciences*, 271, pp. S222–S225.

Wilson, R.S., James, R.S. & Van Damme, R., 2002. Trade-offs between speed and endurance in the frog Xenopus laevis: a multi-level approach. *Journal of Experimental Biology*, 205(8), pp. 1145–1152.

Wokke, J.H. et al., 1990. Morphological changes in the human end plate with age. *Journal of the Neurological Sciences*, 95(3), pp. 291–310.

Wood, S.J. & Slater, C.R., 2001. Safety factor at the neuromuscular junction. *Progress in Neurobiology*, 64(4), pp. 393–429.

Chapter 3

Not just cousins

I confess freely to you, I could never look long upon a monkey, without very mortifying reflections.

– William Congreve (1670–1729)

Introduction

Chapter 1 introduced and briefly described the fundamental tenets of evolution by natural selection together with hypotheses that have been posited for the path that *Homo* took to bipedality. Although each of these hypotheses has been critiqued at length elsewhere, with a few being dismissed as unlikely candidates for the evolution of bipedalism, there is a more recent consensus that endurance running was at least a major selective pressure (Bramble & Lieberman 2004; Carrier et al. 1984; Aiello & Wheeler 1995; Liebenberg 2013). No matter what the singular or combined factors might have been for the advent of an erect posture and bipedality, we are able to make only educated conjectures based on the fossil evidence and comparisons with other extant primates. Until relatively recently, the notion was held that *Homo* evolved in an uncomplicated linear fashion from quadruped to knuckle walker and then to biped. However, it is now accepted that the human evolutionary tree is anything but uncomplicated and has branches and likely extinct species which we are yet to uncover. Table 3.1 shows a basic lineage of the appearance and disappearance of hominids. This lineage should never be taken as being a linear and progressive path to the evolution of *Homo sapiens*, since it appears that a range of species overlapped and lived side by side for long periods of time. The implication here is that these species survived, took different evolutionary lines and had varying degrees of success before becoming extinct (Bradshaw 1997). Thus, we should not necessarily view our evolution as a tree, but rather more like a bush, with many bipedal species living and overlapping with each other (Wood & Pilbeam 1996; Rightmire 1995).

It is thought that the human lineage split from the chimpanzee about 5–7 MYA from what is termed the last common ancestor (LCA). These dates are based on a number of studies using both the fossil evidence (White et al. 2009) and the genetic (Kumar et al. 2005) comparison of primates to humans. This

Table 3.1 Possible timeline of events that mark the appearance of *Homo*. This list is not a linear progression to the eventual appearance of *Homo sapiens*. The list highlights the overlap when species appeared and disappeared and the real likelihood that hominins lived side by side for long periods.

Species	Million years ago
Ardipithicus ramidus	4.4
Australopithicus anamensis	4.0–4.5
Australopithicus afarensis	3.9–2.9
Homo rudolfensis	2.4–1.8
Homo habilis	2.4–1.5
Homo ergaster	1.9–1.4
Homo erectus	1.9–0.7*
Homo heidelbergensis	0.6–0.2
Neanderthals	0.3–.04#
Homo sapiens	0.20–present

Note: *Considerable debate exists as to this date range, with some experts suggesting this species lived up to 35,000 years ago. However, recent evidence suggests that this may be unlikely (Indriati et al. 2011). #This date range is based on the more recent work of Higham et al. (2014). For a discussion on the overlap of species see Walter (2013).

Source: Revised from Bradshaw (1997).

divergence is depicted as a cladogram against the geological timeline where the LCA of *Homo sapiens*, chimpanzee and gorilla existed (Figure 3.1). The focus of this chapter is not so much what caused the divergence, as this aspect was briefly discussed in Chapter 1; rather it is the outcome that we are most interested in and how this relates to human performance in health and disease. If the current consensus is that endurance was a significant selection pressure (Bramble & Lieberman 2004), it is of significant interest to further understand what benefit endurance might have had for survival. Thus, it is also important to note that part of the journey to bipedality was the drive for nourishment, whereby it is now apparent that meat became a significant part of the hominid diet around 2.6 MYA (Semaw et al. 2003). It follows that in order to obtain meat, early hominins were hunter-gatherers since the projectile weaponry we associate with killing an animal from a distance was not available until about 100,000–71,000 years ago (Marean 2015).

Group cooperation was also likely involved in obtaining meat, but most importantly it necessitated tracking a large animal long distances, alternating between walking and running (Lieberman 2014). If endurance was indeed a key selection pressure, and as shown in Figure 3.1, the transition from being quadruped to biped was likely very gradual over a long period of time and involved diversity in hominin locomotion, not just walking and running (Fleagle 2015).

The difficulty in addressing the evolution of our biology and why we are more adapted for endurance than for power is the fact that our LCA is not available

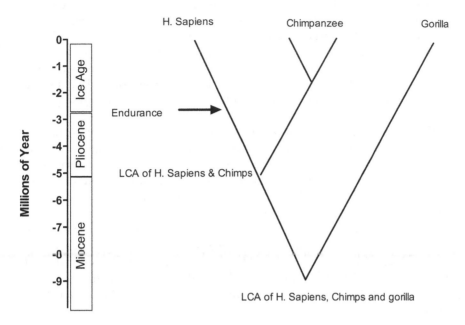

Figure 3.1 A cladogram with the approximate timeline of divergence from the last common ancestor (LCA) of *Homo sapiens*, chimpanzee and gorilla against geological time. Note the approximate date that endurance running was likely already developed by the time evidence of meat eating was discovered and projectile weaponry was likely in use.

Source: Figure adapted from Lieberman (2015).

to us for the purpose of analysis and comparison. The next best comparison is our closest living relative, the chimpanzee. In this chapter, we will examine the major differences between *Homo* and the extant apes, and where appropriate refer to other hominin species in order to develop an insight about our differing capacities and the propensity to undertake long physical exertion, which makes us better equipped to resist fatigue.

The skeleton

In Chapter 2 we examined the concept of safety factor and used some examples pertaining to the skeleton – in particular, the varying degrees by which bones differ in their safety factor to resist fracture, such as the ossicles versus the skull. The complexity by which a safety factor of bone is accomplished was also discussed; however, the overriding principle is that day-to-day living does not result in a fracture, but rather the avoidance of and resistance to fracture. This basically means the skeleton is able to withstand loading which is typically related to fatiguing activity rather than to a one-off force resulting in bone fracture. In addition, recall that the basic observation is that when loads on bone are likely to be predictable – such as for long bones – the safety factor is comparably lower than for bones where unpredictably high loads yield a high penalty. In this section, we will examine the differences in skeletal structure of *Homo*, other relevant species and chimps as a basis for understanding the cost of each in relation to physical performance.

Figure 3.2 shows the typical skeletal comparison of *H. sapiens* with chimpanzee. There are some immediate and obvious differences that are apparent. However, before taking these into consideration with respect to their relationship to physical performance, it is most important that the one skeletal feature that distinguishes *Homo* from other species is given prominence in this discussion. In 1925, Raymond Dart (1925) published what was regarded at the time as his most controversial finding as to the evolution of bipedalism. In this classic paper and later in his book (Dart & Craig 1959) he argued that one of the defining features of the Taung skull was the location of the foramen magnum. Dart estimated it to have a forward relative displacement such that the skull was balanced on a more vertically placed vertebral column compared to a gorilla or chimpanzee, for he wrote,

> the significance of this index, which indicates in a measure the poise of the skull upon the vertebral column, points to the assumption by this fossil group of an attitude appreciably more erect than that of modern anthropoids. The

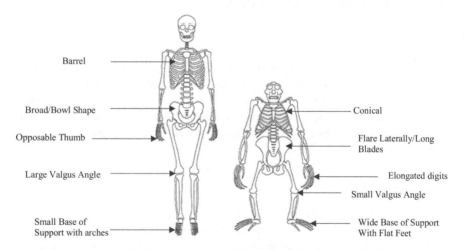

Figure 3.2 A typical comparison of the *H. sapiens* skeleton with an extant chimpanzee. See text for more detailed description.

Source: http://sb.cc.stonybrook.edu/news/_resources/images/1SkeletonsSketchinternet.jpg.

improved poise of the head . . . means that a greater reliance was being placed by this group upon the feet as organs of progression, and that the hands were being freed from their more primitive function of accessory organs of locomotion.

(p. 197)

Although at the time, this conclusion drew much criticism from his contemporaries, it is now regarded as a key characteristic of adapted bipedality.

Returning to the features shown in Figure 3.2, it is evident that the chest and rib cage in humans are barrel-shaped compared with the chimp's, which are rather conical, so that they are much narrower superiorly than inferiorly. The pelvis in humans is broader and bowl-shaped, whereas the chimp's is narrower and longer. Although the femur is shaped similarly, in humans the proximal end is thicker, with the shaft slanted inwards and the proximal end creating a larger valgus angle. This effectively puts the feet closer together under the centre of gravity. In the chimp, this angle is much smaller so that the base of support is wider, which causes the chimp to waddle when attempting to walk bipedally. Notably, the upper limb extends somewhat further in the chimp so that the hands are in proximity of the distal end of the femur. Although not completely visible in Figure 3.2, the chimp's hands have a reduced thumb but elongated digits, which are used more like hooks. Conversely, in humans the thumb is larger and its 'saddle' joint with the wrist enables the thumb to be opposable with the tip of all other digits. Finally, the chimp's feet are rather flat and have no arch, with the large toe pointing out away from the other digits. This allows the foot to be used for grasping. Humans clearly do not possess such a skill to any comparable degree, with our feet having arches and the large toe aligned with the other digits.

The comparative features shown in Figure 3.2 are only those that demonstrate the major skeletal differences which are thought to play a significant part in the capacity for physical performance. There are, of course, many more differences than those provided in Figure 3.2. However, for the main purpose of this book, the differences which are demonstrably important with respect to gross movement and performance are discussed.

The shape of any particular feature is naturally dictated by the kinds of movements and relationships between skeletal features. For instance, the ape rib cage does not provide any major advantage or disadvantage in terms of respiration compared with humans, since this is largely determined by the volume of the thorax. However, the upper and lower limb girdles and their respective functions have produced altered characteristics of the rib cage. In apes, the top of the rib cage is narrow, which allows the scapula to sit on the back and rotate more so in the coronal plane. This particular feature reflects the use of the shoulder and upper limb for arboreal living, grasping and swinging. The inferior portion of the ape rib cage is wide since the blades of the pelvis are tall and flare laterally, whereas the human pelvis is deeper and rounded, making the lower ribs similarly shaped (Figure 3.2). This difference in the shape of the pelvis also brings about a significant difference in the position of the lower limb and hence its capabilities. That is, a long ilium and ischium give the ape longer lever arms for the hamstring muscles for powerful extension of the thigh, while restricting extension in humans but providing greater flexion (Hogervorst et al. 2009; Aiello & Dean 2002) (see Figure 3.3). The critical aspect of this feature is that in humans the ischium, from which the hamstrings arise, is shorter so that the lever arm is able to generate a faster movement, but the trade-off is a loss of power in comparison to the chimpanzee. Finally, since the human pelvis is broader, it naturally places the gluteus maximus muscle posteriorly to the hip joint rather than laterally. Thus, because of its size and location the gluteus maximus in humans is regarded as the most powerful extensor muscle, but its main function is to act as an extensor and to stabilise the torso (Stern 1972). These skeletal characteristics stemming from the shape of the rib cage, which is largely determined by the location and function of the upper and lower girdles, illustrate that the human form is uniquely adapted for an erect posture and bipedal locomotion.

In addition to the unique characteristics of the human pelvic girdle, the human thigh has distinct characteristics which provide for adapted bipedal locomotion. The human femur when in its normal upright position extends downward, where it articulates with the tibia by slanting medially. Figure 3.4 shows what is typically referred to as the carrying or bicondylar angle formed between the line of

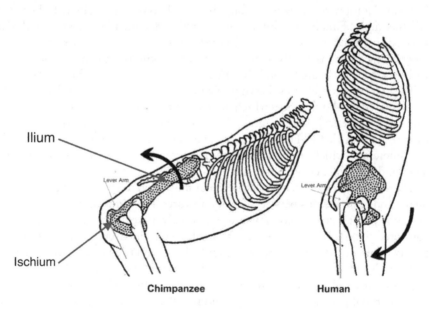

Ilium

Ischium

Lever Arm

Lever Arm

Chimpanzee   Human

Figure 3.3 The lateral view of the chimpanzee and human pelvis in relation to the femur. Note the longer "ischium" in the chimpanzee, which also provides for a longer lever arm compared with that of the human.

Source: Adapted from Aiello and Dean (2002) with permission from Elsevier.

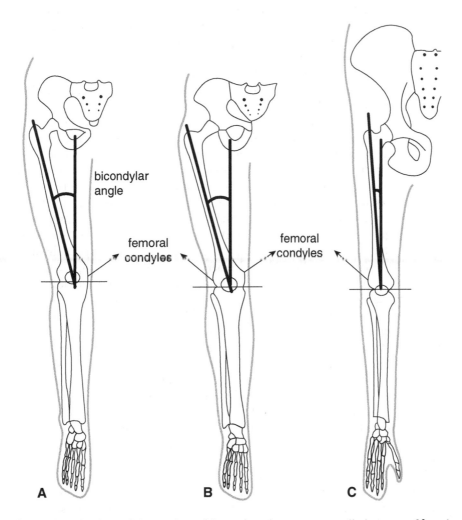

Figure 3.4 The bicondylar angle in (a) modern humans, normally between 8° and 11°, in (b) australopithecines, normally between 14° and 15°, and in (c) chimpanzees, which is normally between 1° and 2°.

Source: Figure is from Shefelbine et al. (2002). Reproduced with permission from Elsevier.

the shaft of the femur and the vertical line created by a line perpendicular to the infra-condylar plane. The important points in this arrangement are that the femoral neck aligns the acetabular joint directly over the knee, which results in the angle compensating for the width of the pelvis. As depicted in Figure 3.4, the large angle is distinctly human. However, the fact that other species, such as the australopithecines, have also been shown to have possessed a large bicondylar angle indicates that other hominins were adapted for a bipedal gait (Shefelbine et al. 2002). The overall outcome of this femoral arrangement with the hip through to the knee joint is that it brings the feet closer together and as a result the need to sway from side to side is alleviated. Chimpanzees, on the other hand, when standing upright maintain a forward leaning posture because of restricted extension and waddle from side to side when walking bipedally because of their wide stance (Figure 3.2).

Beyond the gross features of the shoulder and hip girdles, thigh and leg, researchers have more recently speculated that specific bones of the foot could enhance the proposition that endurance running was indeed an important part in the evolution of *Homo*. Since it has been known for some time that skeletal muscle tendons store elastic energy during loading, producing potential recoil during the stance phase of locomotion, it also stands to reason that the bones these tendons are attached to play a significant role in their mechanical properties (Cavagna et al. 1964). This is particularly the case with the Achilles tendon, which is attached to the calcaneus, and as noted, this tendon is longer in humans than it is in extant apes (Bramble & Lieberman 2004). It is now apparent that the calcaneus may have played a part in the ability of modern humans for endurance running. In a novel study on the comparison of the calcaneus of modern humans with those of early human species and Neanderthals, it was shown that the prime characteristic of this bone, the calcaneal tuber length (CTL; distance from talocalcaneal joint surface to attachment point of Achilles tendon) is ~8% longer in Neanderthals than in humans, with this difference being ~4% compared with early human species. The facts that the Achilles tendon moment arm is positively correlated with the CTL and Neanderthals have a significantly longer CTL indicate that the Achilles tendon in this species was shorter compared with modern humans. Thus, the loading and storage of elastic energy in the Achilles tendon were likely reduced in Neanderthals compared with modern humans.

The potential outcome of this relationship is shown in Figure 3.5, where the CTL increases between modern humans and Neanderthals, with early human species seemingly intermediate for this characteristic (left y-axis, closed symbols). However, when the oxygen consumption (VO_2) during running for humans and the predicted VO_2 for early human species and Neanderthals are plotted (right y-axis, open symbols) against the CTL, it suggests that the cost of running increases as a function of CTL. In other words, the shorter length of the Achilles tendon due to the longer CTL likely reduced the economy for endurance running in Neanderthals. In fact, Raichlen et al. (2011) showed that the relationship between CTL and running economy at 16 km/hr in modern humans is highly significant, and that the CTL explains 80% of the variation in mass-specific energy costs of running at this particular speed. The assumption these authors make is that the running biomechanics of Neanderthals, early human species and *Homo sapiens* are similar, since there is little reason to believe that spring mechanics would have significantly changed.

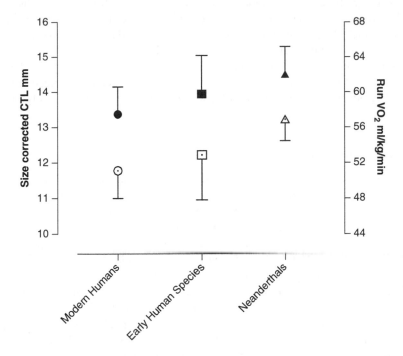

Figure 3.5 The calcaneal tuber length (CTL; distance from talocalcaneal joint surface to attachment point of Achilles tendon) divided by the cube root
of body mass (closed symbols, left y-axis) and estimated oxygen consumption (VO$_2$) (open symbols, right y-axis) during running in modern
humans, fossilised early human species and Neanderthals.

Source: Data redrawn from table 3.1 from Raichlen et al. (2011).

Taking this assumption at face value, Raichlen et al. (2011) suggest their findings should be interpreted with much caution since any data which lie beyond
the regression sample are subject to error. Nevertheless, these data provide an
enticing hypothesis, and if endurance running was indeed a significant factor in
the evolution of *Homo*, it seems predictable that a critical skeletal characteristic,
such as the calcaneus, correlates well with the potential for energy storage and
usage and is favourable to endurance running economy.

However, it is important to note that the use of the calcaneus as an example
does not in any way suggest that this is the only characteristic of the foot that
led to the inevitable improved ability for endurance running, or for that matter
bipedalism. It is now abundantly clear that the skeletal characteristics of the foot
underwent complex changes over long periods when it seems likely that different
hominin species were adapted for both bipedalism and arboreal living (Lieberman 2012).

Although there are many more skeletal characteristics beyond those discussed earlier, these few, ranging from the limb girdles to the rib cage, thigh and foot, are examples of how the skeleton of *Homo* is clearly adapted for bipedalism and favours better endurance running capabilities. More than that, these characteristics underscore that the skeletal adaptations of humans are suggestive of a favourable trade-off for endurance over power, whereby the skeletal arrangements are uniquely adapted for the purpose of endurance running and ultimately fatigue resistance.

The musculature

In Chapter 2, skeletal muscle was discussed in relation to safety factor and the limitations that this imposes on function during physical performance and in disease states. In the preceding section the relationship between skeletal characteristics and muscle was briefly mentioned since it is almost impossible to separate the two when attempting to understand physical performance. In this section, the differences in skeletal muscle between humans and extant apes are discussed with a view to understanding the physical capability of each.

The study of human strength, power and endurance is certainly not lacking, and the data generated in this area stretches from molecular to observational comparisons between different training modalities, gender and race, to name a few. Our understanding of the adaptability of human skeletal muscle is well documented, although much more work is required to further understand certain neurological adaptations in both health and disease.

Unfortunately, comparative experiments in primates are limited since it is not possible to definitively know if an ape has provided a maximal effort under experimental conditions. However, data do exist that show definitively the overwhelming power and strength of extant apes. Early studies attempting to measure the comparative pulling power of chimpanzees showed a distinctive four-fold strength advantage over men when normalised for body mass (Bauman 1926, 1923). In more recent studies, vertical jumping height of bonobos (*Pan paniscus*) was measured between 0.72 and 0.78 m compared to the trained human performance of 0.32 m (Scholz et al. 2006). These findings offer strong evidence that bonobo muscle outperforms human muscle in explosive tasks, speculating that this was likely due to inherent differences in either the contractile material or in the arrangement of the machinery itself.

Table 3.2 summarises some apparent key musculoskeletal differences between humans and chimpanzees that have been shown to account for some of the disparity in mobility, strength and locomotion. It can be seen from these data that chimpanzees have almost twice as much muscle mass in the forelimbs compared to humans. However, humans have significantly more muscle mass in their hind limbs. An important component of skeletal muscle mechanics is the bundle of muscle fibres known as fascicles. The length of the fascicle also determines the number of sarcomeres that are in series, and since sarcomeres contain the

Table 3.2 Summary of skeletal muscle differences accounting for the disparity in strength, mobility and locomotion between humans and chimpanzees.

	Forelimbs	Hind limbs	Relative muscle fascicle length	Effect	Relative PCSA (cm²)
Human	9%	38%	Short	Larger joint moments	Large
Chimpanzee	16%	24%	Long	Greater joint mobility	Small

Note: Percentage represents distribution of total body mass located in that region. PCSA is the relative physiological cross-sectional area when corrected for total body mass.

Source: Data taken from Zihlman (1992) and Thorpe et al. (1999).

contractile elements of skeletal muscle, the number of sarcomeres plays an important role in muscle shortening. Although human hind limbs have a larger muscle mass and, therefore, a greater physiological cross-sectional area (PCSA), we have comparably shorter fascicle lengths compared with chimpanzees. In fact, when comparing humans to other extant apes, including chimpanzees, bonobos, gorillas and orangutans, the fascicle length/body mass ratio for the majority of lower limb muscles is decidedly small (Payne et al. 2006). Interestingly, when the PCSA/body mass ratio is compared for the same species and muscles, this characteristic is much larger in humans (Payne et al. 2006). However, because of the greater PCSA we generally possess a larger number of sarcomeres in parallel.

When comparing the upper and lower limbs of chimpanzees and humans, it is evident that each is adapted for different kinds of locomotion since chimpanzees have a greater forelimb muscle mass with appreciably longer fascicle lengths. Although the shorter fascicle length in humans allows for large moments around a joint with limited mobility, the relative differences in fascicle length provide chimpanzees with the adaptation necessary for arboreal living. Thus, chimpanzees are adapted for power and strength in the upper limbs compared to humans. These discrete differences in muscle structure and function indicate that chimpanzees are uniquely adapted for fast, mobile climbing, whereas human skeletal muscle architecture is adapted primarily for bipedal walking. However, there is a caveat to this reasoning. Humans actually possess the ability to throw projectiles at high speed and with some accuracy. Other primates also throw objects but not in the same manner as humans. The major reason for this difference is that the structure of the human upper limb girdle provides for the storage and use of elastic energy, which has been shown to be the major contributor to the ability of human throwing (Roach et al. 2013). Interestingly, these skeletal features apparently appeared about 2 million years ago in *Homo erectus*, which also coincides with changes to the diet to include meat. No doubt the ability to throw would have benefited early hominins in their quest to source high-energy nourishment.

An apparent and interesting relationship also exists within the elite human population with respect to fascicle length. When comparing elite human sprinters and long distance runners with controls, lower limb skeletal muscle fascicle length was shown to be different among this group (Abe et al. 2000). Figure 3.6 shows the differences in fascicle length in this population, confirming that even within a select group, skeletal muscle architecture could play a significant advantage in human performance. In addition, this confirms that the longer fascicle lengths are more likely to be associated with individuals who can produce power and speed of contraction rather than endurance. A further question that arises from Figure 3.6 is whether training will produce the required effects on fascicle length such that adaptation would favour either power or endurance. For instance, it is noteworthy that the fascicle length in the controls is placed between the sprinters and distance runners, and it would be useful to know whether training could induce adaptations which could shift these controls into either the sprint or endurance group. In a recent study, resistance-trained subjects were compared with controls who had never participated in any resistance training (Fukutani & Kurihara 2015).

These authors found that while the training increased both muscle thickness and pennation angles, the fascicle length was not different between the trained and control groups. This is an important finding as it suggests that fascicle length

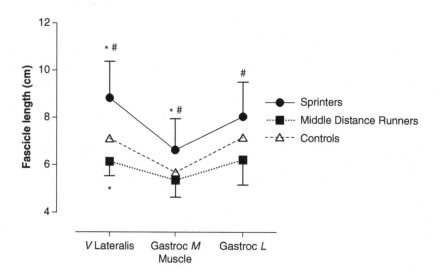

Figure 3.6 The fascicle length measured *in vivo* by ultrasound in 23 elite 100m sprinters (closed circles), 24 elite middle distance runners (closed squares) and 24 untrained (open triangles) males. *P < 0.01 sprinters vs middle distance runners vs controls, #P < 0.01 sprinters vs middle distance runners.

Source: Data redrawn from table 3.2 from Abe et al. (2000).

is predetermined, whereas adding more contractile material through training is a more likely result. However, this is somewhat controversial since there are studies in both animal models and in humans which show that specific training adds sarcomeres in series to muscle architecture (Franchi et al. 2016). Whether training provides the required stimulus for the development of fascicle length remains to be definitively proven, but the key aspect here is that the length of the fascicles is a critical element in determining the power and/or endurance capability of skeletal muscle.

Although comparison of skeletal muscle architecture provides some basis with which to understand human adaptation to bipedalism, further analysis of human neuromuscular adaptations shows distinct preferential characteristics for muscular endurance over power. The relationship between motor nerves and the variability of motor units is indicative of the preferential adaptation for the way in which muscular force is initiated, developed and maintained. The accepted Henneman size principle (Binder & Ruenzel 1983; Somjen & Carpenter 1965) posits that muscle contraction is always initiated by small motor units, followed in an orderly fashion by larger ones as greater force is produced. A key component of this principle establishes that the most fatigue-resistant muscle fibres (Type I) are recruited first, allowing for fine motor control, followed by the larger, less fatigue-resistant fibres (Type II) (Sale 1987). A fundamental aspect of the fibre type principle is the relationship that proportion and distribution of fibre types have with the needs of the species. For instance, in comparing the fibre type distribution of triceps surae between orangutan and the chimpanzee, the orangutan had a higher proportion of Type I fibres, which corresponds to the orangutan's adapted slow and controlled movements in their tree-dwelling habitat. In contrast, the higher proportion of Type II fibres in the chimpanzee reflects their compromise between controlled movements and the need for speed and power when terrestrial (Myatt et al. 2011). In humans, the estimate is that soleus and gastrocnemius muscles are about 70% and 50% Type I, respectively (Edgerton et al. 1975) which indicates a fibre type distribution in these muscles corresponding to fatigue resistance, especially in the soleus muscle.

However, the arrangement of the neuronal input from the CNS to the skeletal muscles between apes and humans provides an enticing hypothesis about the greater strength and power of apes versus the endurance and fatigue resistance of humans. In the classic studies by MacLarnon (1995, 1996) a difference in neuronal content was evident when comparing the relative quantity of white and grey matter in the brains and spinal cords of chimpanzees and humans. Recall that grey matter contains numerous cell bodies and relatively few myelinated axons, whereas white matter contains relatively very few cell bodies and is mainly composed of long-range tracts of myelinated axons. Add to this that the main function of the myelin layer is to increase the speed of conduction of an impulse along the myelinated fibre, and these studies established that chimpanzees have substantially less grey matter in their spinal cords when corrected for cross-sectional area and scaled according to muscle mass. In other words, chimpanzees have a greater preponderance of myelinated axons within the spinal cord in comparison to humans. Specifically, when segments of the spinal cord were scaled and compared, it was also evident that in both humans and chimpanzees there was increased white matter at the cervical and lumbosacral enlargements of the spinal cord (Percival 2013). This characteristic most likely corresponds to the increased nervous tissue supplying the upper and lower limbs. Since the large Type II motor units are innervated by myelinated neurons, chimpanzees have comparatively low numbers of small motor units (Type I) given that a preponderance of neuronal white matter is needed for faster conduction velocity. Thus, it is very likely, based on the evidence of relative distributions of grey and white matter, that apes will have a higher number of larger motor units which would serve their need for greater strength and power. Conversely, humans have a wide distribution of motor units which predictably allows us to have more control and exert less force during complex movements (Sale 1987). In fact, it has been shown that in human quadriceps, 52% of the muscle fibres are Type I, with the majority located in deeper regions compared with Type II fibre, located predominantly on the surface of the muscle.

An aspect of the relationship between muscle fibre types is the effect that ageing has on their ratio. In Chapter 2, the changes in skeletal muscle with age were discussed in relation to safety factor. It was noted that one of the changes with ageing was the loss of the larger, faster motor units with the re-innervation of the surviving Type II fibres by slow axons. In general terms this gives way to percentage increases in Type I fibres and a reduction in Type II fibres (Lexell et al. 1983). The critical aspect which strongly suggests that humans are adapted for fatigue resistance is the observation that with advancing age there is an increase in the size of the remaining low-threshold motor units (Stålberg & Fawcett 1982) but the total number of motor units decreases (Tomlinson & Irving 1977). This altered relationship supposedly reflects the necessity to be able to activate skeletal muscle with minimal, rather than increased, efferent drive since slow motor units have a lower threshold for activation where more rapid declines in muscle force would be expected. Finally, the question as to why animals are endowed with different skeletal muscle fibre types as opposed to any single muscle being of a singular type rests with the apparent need for animals to use different fibres to accommodate shortening velocities that are optimal for power production and efficiency (Funke et al. 1988). That is, during locomotion maximal movements are not possible without fast-twitch fibres as the slow-twitch fibres cannot shorten rapidly when needed. This suggests that different species have adapted different skeletal muscles with varying ratios of Type I and Type II fibres to maximise their distinctive locomotor behaviour.

The brain

In the preceding section, the relationship between skeletal muscle type and neuronal connection was discussed in relation to power and strength of chimpanzees versus the endurance of humans. However, of all the differences and similarities between humans and our closest living relatives, the brain remains the most studied anatomical feature for comparison. The main reason for this is the supposed relationship between brain size and intelligence, which has been debated for well over a century. Since it is generally accepted that the size of our brain distinguishes us from almost all of our ancestors and extant apes, the assumption is that this feature provides us with cognitive and intelligence advantage. It is now apparent that a bigger brain volume in modern humans correlates well with intelligence for all ages and genders (McDaniel 2005). However, this association should not be taken as a simple, perfect linear correlation. In fact, the overall correlation co-efficient when corrected for measurement error is moderate at 0.33, ranging from 0.4 for females to 0.34 for males (McDaniel 2005). Although this correlation is statistically significant, in reality it accounts for only about 10% of the variance, meaning that 90% of our intelligence is explained by other factors. Thus, in modern humans the association between intelligence and brain volume is a difficult one to make. Rather, the consensus is that brain expansion was a major factor in modern humans' cognitive capabilities. It is this difference in brain expansion which occurred during our evolutionary journey to becoming *Homo* that is important in understanding why we outperformed our hominin cousins. In Chapter 1 it was noted that the split from our last common ancestor between *Homo sapiens* and chimpanzees occurred around 5.3 MYA, and that around the same time there was a dramatic expansion in brain size. Thus, the key consideration here is what advantage the brain expansion provided us under the prevailing conditions. To answer this question, there are two aspects to consider. First, why is a bigger brain better? Second, in what way did we use the expanding brain size to differentiate us from other hominins? To begin to answer these seemingly basic questions, some fundamental aspects of brain size estimation need to be considered.

There are two fundamental methods to estimate brain size, one of which is direct and is not particularly practical since it requires dissection. The second is an indirect method by estimating the volume of the endocranial cavity (ECV), where regression equations relate the volume to mass corrected for other tissues and fluids within the cranial vault. This equation is given as:

$$\text{Brain mass} = 1.147 \times \text{ECV}^{0.976}$$

Details of the methods used to derive this equation are given in the work by Martin (1990). However, an important aspect for the comparison of brain size is how it scales to the body size since larger animals will have larger brains. For example, an elephant's brain mass will be about 5 kg, with a body mass up to 6,000 kg for fully grown males, compared to a dolphin's brain, which is about 1.6 kg, and a body mass of about 150 kg. The relationship between brain mass and body mass is known as the encephalisation quotient (EQ), and although there are a number of equations to estimate this relationship, the most commonly used regression has been proposed by Martin (1981), where mass is measured in grams:

$$EQ = \text{brain mass} / \left(0.059 \times \text{body mass}^{0.76}\right)$$

A selection of brain sizes is provided in Figure 3.7, which compares adult apes and hominins. As a way of illustration, there are at least two features which provide an interesting comparison between extant apes, early hominins and humans. First, the ECV of chimps, gorillas and *Au. afarensis* is very similar, ranging from approximately 390 to 450 cm³. This volume increased dramatically for *H. erectus* by almost doubling to approximately 970 cm³. A second feature suggests that Neanderthals had increased the ECV by almost another third to be approximately 1490 cm³, with the volume for *H. sapiens* being somewhat less at 1410 cm³.

However, Figure 3.7 also shows that the EQ changes dramatically when the ECV is scaled according to body mass. Notably, the EQ appears to have increased with early hominins, and even though Neanderthals may have had a larger brain volume, *H. sapiens* has a relatively higher EQ compared with all other hominins. This is an important distinction as it suggests that bigger brains alone are not

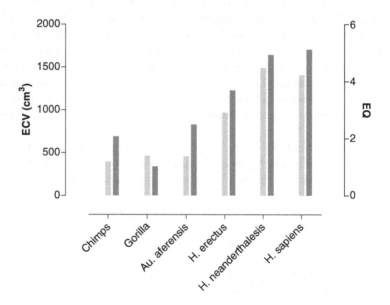

Figure 3.7 The endocranial volume (ECV, solid bars) estimated from brain mass = 1.147 × ECV^0.976 and the encephalisation quotient (EQ, unfilled bars) estimated from EQ = brain mass/(0.059 × body mass^0.76) for apes (chimps and gorilla), early hominins (*Australopithecus afarensis*, *Homo erectus*, *Homo neanderthalensis*) and *Homo sapiens*.

Source: Data are redrawn from Martin (1990), Robson (2008) and Lieberman (2011).

a prerequisite for survival, for if this was the only criteria for an evolutionary advantage, it cannot explain why we outperformed Neanderthals in particular, given their larger EVC.

Returning to the first key question: why is bigger better? Taking the ECV at face value as given in Figure 3.7, it is tempting to assume that the expansion was gradual over a long period of time. However, it is now apparent that brain expansion was not so much gradual as it was rapid with respect to the evolutionary timeframe. In fact, it is estimated that from the time of the split from the LCA around 5.3 MYA, the brain expansion continued for the next 3 million years at almost six times the rate of the previous 4 million years (Lieberman 2014; Hublin et al. 2015; Trinkaus & Holliday 1997). Understanding this acceleration in brain expansion as merely a purposeful trajectory towards greater cognitive capacity does not provide an adequate answer as to why bigger brains are better, since cognitive capabilities are an outcome and not a cause of the larger brain (Lynch & Granger 2008). Thus, brain expansion must have provided a reproductive advantage during the prevailing conditions.

As briefly discussed in Chapter 1, during the late Miocene, Africa was entering into a cooler and drier climate. The consequence of this climate change was an altered habitat, where the forest patches reduced in size, leading to more open woodlands. These open habitats were likely quite stressful for the hominids who relied mainly on fruit for their nourishment. The change in habitat must have also resulted in the selection of those individuals that were able to source alternative foods. This change to the climate and eventually to the habitat coincided with the expansion in brain size, as shown in Figure 3.8. Note that the expansion of the endocranial volume from the time *Homo* and chimpanzees split from the last common ancestor accelerated from approximately 2.5 MYA to the present, with major expansion occurring within the last 0.6 MYA. It is not definitively understood why this rapid brain expansion occurred (this will be discussed further in Chapter 8), but it is thought that the challenge for these hominins in a new habitat that had reduced their normal food supply forced them to acquire a different food – namely, meat (Pobiner 2016). The acquisition of meat most likely also required scavenging, graduating to tracking, capturing, killing and ultimately butchering. This seems to have occurred at least 2.5 MYA if not earlier (Pobiner 2016). Thus, as shown in Figure 3.8, if high-energy protein became available about 2.5 MYA just when the genus *Homo* appeared, the acceleration in brain size was very likely assisted greatly by the procurement of protein and other animal products, including fat. We are able to make this retrospective conclusion based on the *expensive tissue hypothesis* (Aiello & Wheeler 1995), which is based on the fact that the brain's mass is only about 2% of body mass but utilises 20% of the total body oxygen and 25% of the available energy as glucose (Zauner & Muizelaar 1997).

However, as per the discussion in Chapter 2 on trade-offs, the increase in animal products in the diet not only fuelled the expansion of the brain but also likely reduced the need to have a large gastro-intestinal tract, which is primarily

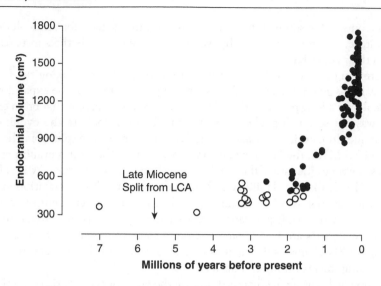

Figure 3.8 Millions of years before present time and the expansion of the endocranial volume. Note the split from the last common ancestor (LCA) by chimpanzees and *Homo* towards the end of the late Miocene (approx. 5.33 MYA). Early hominins (open circles) and genus *Homo* (filled circles, approx. 2.5 MYA).

Source: Data are redrawn from Lieberman (2014) and Hublin et al. (2015).

associated with omnivorous and vegetarian diets (Aiello & Wheeler 1995). This relationship holds that a large brain requires a small gut and vice versa in order to manage the energy requirement of these tissues. This relationship becomes apparent when considering that the human gut has a metabolic rate of at least 22% of the basal metabolic rate; a larger gut would most certainly require more energy with a likely trade-off for the brain and other tissues. However, this is but one hypothesis that has been advocated for explaining the trade-off between a large brain and a smaller gut. There are alternative views and data which explain this trade-off differently and which are discussed in more detail in Chapter 8.

A further consequence for a larger brain is the need to grow it during the post-natal period. Since the brain is highly metabolically active, it follows that there needs to be a sufficient energy supply and storage for this to occur. Whereas chimpanzees are born with almost no body fat, human babies are born with body fat accounting for up to 14% of body mass, which allows for the large storage of triglycerides and for the by-product of ketones, which are used for brain and lipid synthesis (Cunnane & Crawford 2003; Cunnane et al. 1993). This confirms that the metabolic basis for brain growth, development and maintenance is one that favours aerobic energy turnover. In fact, recent analysis comparing metabolic rates indicates that total energy expenditure of humans is well above those of extant apes by 1600–3400 kJ/day, and that this energy expenditure is sufficient to accommodate the larger brain of humans (Pontzer et al. 2016). However, there are two further interesting findings in this study: first, the extra total energy expenditure in humans is related to the basal metabolic rate due to the energy needed for organ maintenance, and second, humans apparently have greater body fat ranging from approximately 22% to 36% more than chimpanzees. These data indicate that humans are typically equipped to store fuel.

The preceding section establishes that there are some advantages to having bigger brains. However, recall that the second question to consider was in what way did we use the expanding brain size to differentiate us from other hominins? This question is the most difficult to answer since much of what we could consider is based on assumptions about what the larger brain could ultimately provide as an advantage. One of those assumptions is that the different areas of the brain can accomplish more because of their relative size. For example, the most anterior portion of the prefrontal cortex is associated with higher cognitive functions, such as undertaking initiatives, strategic processes in memory recall and a number of executive functions (Scott & Schoenberg 2011). It has been suggested that this area of the brain is able to provide humans with an advantage because of its relative size. In a comparative study of the prefrontal cortex (area 10) using histological sections, it was shown that in chimps, bonobos and gorillas the volume of this area was approximately only 15%–25% of that in humans (Semendeferi et al. 2001). However, in a follow-up study, it was also shown that the apparent size of this area of the brain is perhaps not the only important factor to consider. When comparing the cortices of this area in living extant apes by magnetic resonance imaging, it was found that the human frontal cortices were not disproportionately larger than those of great apes (Semendeferi et al. 2002). These authors suggested that the cognitive abilities of humans are more likely related to the preponderance of richer interconnectivity rather than the overall relative size of the frontal lobe.

Taking the evidence that interconnectivity could possibly play a key role in distinguishing humans from extant apes and possibly other hominins, some current evidence suggests that this greater sophisticated neural organisation might indeed play a role in determining how and why we stop exercising at a given point. Although the evidence is still developing, it has been shown that brain wave activity as measured by the electroencephalography (EEG) signal declines in the prefrontal cortex in response to exhausting exercise (Robertson & Marino 2015). Further to this observation, it has been suggested that the prefrontal cortex plays a key role in the decision to terminate exercise (Robertson & Marino 2016). This proposition is far from definitive, but it does provide an avenue to further elucidate the mechanisms responsible for the interpretation of the sensations related to fatigue during both performance and disease states (de Vries et al. 2010).

References

Abe, T., Kumagai, K. & Brechue, W.F., 2000. Fascicle length of leg muscles is greater in sprinters than distance runners. *Medicine and Science in Sports & Exercise*, 32(6), pp. 1125–1129.

Aiello, L.C. & Wheeler, P., 1995. The expensive-tissue hypothesis: the brain and the digestive system in human and primate evolution. *Current Anthropology*, 36(2), pp. 199–221.

Aiello, L.C. & Dean, C., 2002. *An introduction to human evolutionary anatomy*, New York: Elsevier Academic Press.

Bauman, J.E., 1923. The strength of the chimpanzee and orang. *The Scientific Monthly*, 16, pp. 432–439.

Bauman, J.E., 1926. Observations on the strength of the chimpanzee and its implications. *Journal of Mammalogy*, 7(1), pp. 1–9.

Binder, M.C. & Ruenzel, P., 1983. Does orderly recruitment of motoneurons depend on the existence of different types of motor units? *Neuroscience Letters*, 36(1), pp. 55–58.

Bradshaw, J.L., 1997. *Human evolution: a neuropsychological perspective*. Hove, UK: Psychology Press.

Bramble, D.M. & Lieberman, D.E., 2004. Endurance running and the evolution of *Homo*. *Nature*, 432, pp. 345–352.

Carrier, D.R. et al., 1984. The energetic paradox of human running and hominid evolution [and comments and reply]. *Current Anthropology*, pp. 483–495.

Cavagna, G.A., Saibene, F.P. & Margaria, R., 1964. Mechanical work in running. *Journal of Applied Physiology*, 19(2), pp. 249–256.

Cunnane, S.C. & Crawford, M.A., 2003. Survival of the fattest: fat babies were the key to evolution of the large human brain. *Comparative Biochemistry and Physiology – Part A: Molecular & Integrative Physiology*, 136(1), pp. 17–26.

Cunnane, S.C., Harbige, L.S. & Crawford, M.A., 1993. The importance of energy and nutrient supply in human brain evolution. *Nutrition and Health*, 9(3), pp. 219–235.

Dart, R.A., 1925. Australopithecus africanus: the man-ape of South Africa. *Nature*, 115(2884), pp. 195–199.

Dart, R.A. & Craig, D., 1959. *Adventures with the missing link*, London: Hamish Hamilton.

de Vries, J.M. et al., 2010. Fatigue in neuromuscular disorders: focus on Guillain-Barré syndrome and Pompe disease. *Cellular and Molecular Life Sciences: CMLS*, 67(5), pp. 701–713.

Edgerton, V.R., Smith, J.L. & Simpson, D.R., 1975. Muscle fibre type populations of human leg muscles. *The Histochemical Journal*, 7(3), pp. 259–266.

Fleagle, J.G., 2015. Major transformations in the evolution of primate locomotion. In K.P. Dial, N. Shubin & E.L. Brainerd, eds. *Great transformations in vertebrate evolution*. Chicago: University of Chicago Press, pp. 257–278.

Franchi, M.V. et al., 2016. Fascicle length does increase in response to longitudinal resistance training and in a contraction-mode specific manner. *SpringerPlus*, 5(94), pp. 1–3.

Fukutani, A. & Kurihara, T., 2015. Comparison of the muscle fascicle length between resistance-trained and untrained individuals: cross-sectional observation. *SpringerPlus*, 4(31), pp. 1–6.

Funke, R.P. et al., 1988. Why animals have different muscle fibre types. *Nature*, 335, pp. 824–827.

Higham, T. et al., 2014. The timing and spatiotemporal patterning of Neanderthal disappearance. *Nature*, 512(7514), pp. 306–309.

Hogervorst, T., Bouma, H.W. & de Vos, J., 2009. Evolution of the hip and pelvis. *Acta Orthopaedica Supplementum*, 80(336), pp. 1–39.

Hublin, J-J., Neubauer, S. & Gunz, P., 2015. Brain ontogeny and life history in Pleistocene hominins. *Philosophical Transactions of the Royal Society of London (Biological Sciences)*, 370(1663), pp. 20140062–20140062.

Indriati, E. et al., 2011. The age of the 20 meter Solo River Terrace, Java, Indonesia and the survival of *Homo erectus* in Asia. *PLoS ONE*, 6(6), pp. e21562–10. doi:10.1371/journal.pone.0021562

Kumar, S. et al., 2005. Placing confidence limits on the molecular age of the human-chimpanzee divergence. *Proceedings of the National Academy of Sciences of the United States of America*, 102(52), pp. 18842–18847.

Lexell, J., Henriksson-Larsen, K. & Sjostrom, M., 1983. Distribution of different fibre types in human skeletal muscles 2: a study of cross-sections of whole m. vastus lateralis. *Acta Physiologica*, 117(1), pp. 115–122.

Liebenberg, L., 2013. *The origin of science*, Cape Town: CyberTracker.

Lieberman, D., 2011. *The evolution of the human head*, Cambridge, MA: Harvard University Press.

Lieberman, D.E., 2012. Human evolution: those feet in ancient times. *Nature*, 483(7391), pp. 550–551.

Lieberman, D.E., 2014. *The story of the human body: evolution, health, and disease*, New York: Vintage Books.

Lieberman, D.E., 2015. Human locomotion and heat loss: an evolutionary perspective. *Comprehensive Physiolology*, 5(1), pp. 99–117.

Lynch, G. & Granger, R., 2008. *Big brain: the origins and future of human intelligence*, New York: Palgrave Macmillan.

MacLarnon, A., 1995. The distribution of spinal cord tissues and locomotor adaptation in primates. *Journal of Human Evolution*, 29(5), pp. 463–482.

MacLarnon, A., 1996. The scaling of gross dimensions of the spinal cord in primates and other species. *Journal of Human Evolution*, 30(1), pp. 71–87.

Marean, C., 2015. The most invasive species of all. *Scientific American*, 313(2), pp. 23–29.

Martin, R.D., 1981. Relative brain size and basal metabolic rate in terrestrial vertebrates. *Nature*, 293(5827), pp. 57–60.

Martin, R.D., 1990. *Primate origins and evolution: a phylogenetic reconstruction*, London: Chapman and Hall.

McDaniel, M., 2005. Big-brained people are smarter: a meta-analysis of the relationship between in vivo brain volume and intelligence. *Intelligence*, 33(4), pp. 337–346.

Myatt, J.P., Schilling, N. & Thorpe, S.K., 2011. Distribution patterns of fibre types in the triceps surae muscle group of chimpanzees and orangutans. *Journal of Anatomy*, 218(4), pp. 402–412.

Payne, R.C. et al., 2006. Morphological analysis of the hindlimb in apes and humans. I: muscle architecture. *Journal of Anatomy*, 208(6), pp. 709–724.

Percival, C.J., 2013. *The influence of angiogenesis on craniofacial development and evolution*. Pennsylvania State University, PhD Dissertation: Proquest LLC.

Pobiner, B., 2016. Meat-eating among the earliest humans. *American Scientist*, 104(2), pp. 110–117.

Pontzer, H. et al., 2016. Metabolic acceleration and the evolution of human brain size and life history. *Nature*, 533(7603), pp. 390–392.

Raichlen, D.A., Armstrong, H. & Lieberman, D.E., 2011. Calcaneus length determines running economy: implications for endurance running performance in modern humans and Neandertals. *Journal of Human Evolution*, 60(3), pp. 299–308.

Rightmire, G.P., 1995. Geography, time and speciation in Pleistocene Homo. *South African Journal of Science*, 91(9), pp. 450–454.

Roach, N.T., Venkadesan, M. & Rainbow, M.J., 2013. Elastic energy storage in the shoulder and the evolution of high-speed throwing in Homo. *Nature*, 498(7455), pp. 483–486.

Robertson, C.V. & Marino, F.E., 2015. Prefrontal and motor cortex EEG responses and their relationship to ventilatory thresholds during exhaustive incremental exercise. *European Journal of Applied Physiology*, pp. 1–10.

Robertson, C.V. & Marino, F.E., 2016. A role for the prefrontal cortex in exercise tolerance and termination. *Journal of Applied Physiology*, 120(4), pp. 464–466.

Robson, S.L., 2008. Hominin life history: reconstruction and evolution. *Journal of Anatomy*, 212(4), pp. 394–425.

Sale, D.G., 1987. Influence of exercise and training on motor unit activation. *Exercise and Sport Sciences Reviews*, 15(1), pp. 95–152.

Scholz, M.N. et al., 2006. Vertical jumping performance of bonobo (Pan paniscus) suggests superior muscle properties. *Proceedings of the Royal Society B: Biological Sciences*, 273(1598), pp. 2177–2184.

Scott, J.G. & Schoenberg, M.R., 2011. Frontal lobe/executive functioning. In M. Schoenberg & J. Scott (Eds.), *The little black book of neuropsychology: a syndrome-based approach*. Boston, MA: Springer, pp. 219–248.

Semaw, S. et al., 2003. 2.6-Million-year-old stone tools and associated bones from OGS-6 and OGS-7, Gona, Afar, Ethiopia. *Journal of Human Evolution*, 45(2), pp. 169–177.

Semendeferi, K., Armstrong, E. & Van Hoesen, G.W., 2001. Prefrontal cortex in humans and apes: a comparative study of area 10. *American Journal of Physical Anthropology*, 114(3), pp. 224–241.

Semendeferi, K. et al., 2002. Humans and great apes share a large frontal cortex. *Nature Neuroscience*, 5(3), pp. 272–276.

Shefelbine, S.J., Tardieu, C. & Carter, D.R., 2002. Development of the femoral bicondylar angle in hominid bipedalism. *Bone*, 30(5), pp. 765–770.

Somjen, G.G. & Carpenter, D.O., 1965. Functional significance of cell size in spinal motoneurons. *Journal of Neurophysiology*, 28, pp. 560–580.

Stålberg, E. & Fawcett, P.R., 1982. Macro EMG in healthy subjects of different ages. *Journal of Neurology Neurosurgery & Psychiatry*, 45(10), pp. 870–878.

Stern, J.T., 1972. Anatomical and functional specializations of the human gluteus maximus. *American Journal of Physical Anthropology*, 36(3), pp. 315–339.

Thorpe, S.K., Crompton, R.H., Guenther, M.M., Ker, R.F. & McNeill Alexander, R., 1999. Dimensions and moment arms of the hind-and forelimb muscles of common chimpanzees (Pan troglodytes). *American Journal of Physical Anthropology*, 110(2), pp. 179–199.

Tomlinson, B.E. & Irving, D., 1977. The numbers of limb motor neurons in the human lumbosacral cord throughout life. *Journal of the Neurological Sciences*, 34(2), pp. 213–219.

Trinkaus, E. & Holliday, T.W., 1997. Body mass and encephalization in Pleistocene Homo. *Nature*, 387(6629), pp. 173–176.

Walter, C., 2013. *Last ape standing: the seven-million-year story of how and why we survived*. New York: Walker and Company.

White, T.D. et al., 2009. Ardipithecus ramidus and the paleobiology of early hominids. *Science*, 326(5949), pp. 64–75–86.

Wood, B.A. & Pilbeam, D.R., 1996. Homoplasy and early *Homo*: an analysis of the evolutionary relationships of H. habilis sensu stricto and H. rudolfensis. 30(2), pp. 97–120.

Zauner, A. & Muizelaar, J.P., 1997. Brain metabolism and cerebral blood flow. In P. Reilly & R. Bullock, eds. *Head Injury*. London: Chapman Hall, pp. 89–99.

Zihlman, A.L., 1992. Locomotion as a life history character: the contribution of anatomy. *Journal of Human Evolution*, 22(4), pp. 315–325.

Chapter 4

Defining and measuring fatigue

The first virtue in a soldier is endurance of fatigue; courage is only the second virtue.

– Napoleon Bonaparte

Introduction

In the preceding chapters it was argued that the basis of human fatigue is the evolutionary adaptation that *Homo* 'opted' for endurance rather than power relative to other mammals, in particular other primates. If this proposition has merit, then the measurement of fatigue should confirm this view. This chapter will focus on two main concepts: the definition of fatigue and its measurement.

Normally, before anything is measured it is deemed essential to know what the actual measurement will convey, and in doing so provide us with an avenue to draw conclusions, predict future outcomes and even allow us to find a cause. Fatigue is still a concept used in physiology and in particular exercise physiology as it provides a basis on which to make a determination or describe performance in a certain way. As a concept, fatigue holds a central place in the exercise sciences and as such the need to define and measure this phenomenon is of utmost importance. To truly begin to understand the concept of fatigue and its measurement, it is critical to appreciate its historical development and the attempts scientists have made to quantify it.

The root of the term *fatigue* is from the Latin *fatigare*, which means to "tire out" (Stevenson 2010). If this was the strict usage of the term, there would likely be little confusion about its nature and consequence. However, alongside this strict definition are at least three others that are given:

1   Extreme tiredness resulting from mental or physical exertion or illness;
2   A reduction in the efficiency of a muscle or organ after prolonged activity;
3   A lessening in one's response to or enthusiasm for something, caused by overexposure.

These definitions of fatigue span the breadth of human capabilities, from mental to physical and even in disease states. Fatigue it seems can also be used to convey some perturbation in the skeletal muscle or any organ which we might believe to be functioning less than optimally. Interestingly, fatigue is also thought to be related to a lack of motivation since a lack of enthusiasm might affect one's optimal response to a given situation. These wandering definitions give rise to a particular problem in physiology, whereby agreement about the cause of reduced performance under either health or disease conditions may not be agreed upon. The outcome of this less than strict definition of fatigue is the development of select paradigms that are used to interpret observations of declining performance (Marino et al. 2011). Further to this is the inherent need to measure fatigue in a particular way, which then might not be useful in all circumstances. For example, measuring the maximal capacity of an athlete by having him or her run on a treadmill is unlikely to yield meaningful data if the same standard was applied to an individual who was suffering from a debilitating disease. In this instance, we would apply not only a different method of measuring fatigue but also a different standard. A further consideration is that fatigue is used in innumerable instances not just confined to humans. In addition to denoting the decline in physical effort, it is used in a different domain to describe weakness in physical materials and even the specific clothing worn by military personnel. This chapter will trace the history of the concept of fatigue in human performance and describe some of the methods available to observe and measure fatigue across the ways in which it is used.

Origins and fatigue concepts

Although it is difficult to trace the origins of the conceptual basis of fatigue, it is thought that Neapolitan physician Alfonso Borelli was the first to describe his observations relating to movement deterioration. Borelli's classic text from 1710, *De Motu Animalium* (Figure 4.1A), is regarded as the foundation for the understanding of human and animal motion and biomechanics (Figure 4.1B). Borelli's pivotal insight was that "The performances of animals are due to mechanical causes, instruments, and reasons" (Mosso 1904a, p. 32). In essence Borelli deduced that

> in the production of muscular contraction two causes concur, which one resides in the muscles themselves, and the other comes from without. The excitation of movement can be transmitted from the brain by no other route than by the nerves. All experiments agree in proclaiming this fact in a very evident manner. One rejects, however, the hypothesis that there is any question here of the action of any immaterial power or spirit; one must admit that some material substance is transmitted from the nerves to the muscles, or that the shock is communicated which is able, in the twinkling of an eye, to produce the swelling of the muscles.
>
> (Mosso 1904a, p. 33)

What is particularly prescient about Borelli's insight is that electricity as a method of transmission was not demonstrated until about half a century later by

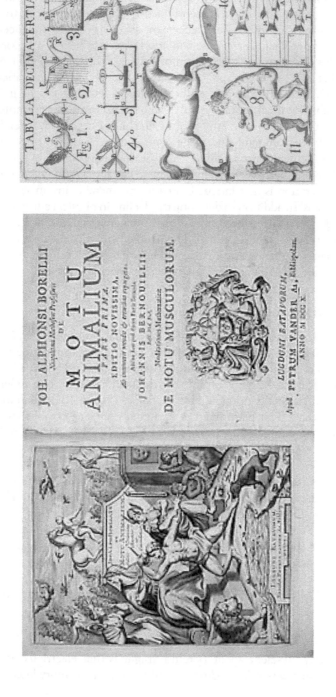

A

B

Figure 4.1 (A) The original foundation text of human motion and biomechanics by Alfonso Borelli, *De Motu Animalium*. (B) Borelli's analytical and geometrical methods in mechanics relating to the biology of motion illustrating his 'Propositions,' with sketches of the mechanics of man and animals during physical activities.

Luigi Galvani (McComas 2011). Thus, what is evident from Borelli and his contemporaries is that understanding the degradation of movement has its roots in the experiments and writings of the 1600s–1700s. This is perhaps the most salient point in the understanding of fatigue as its conceptual basis became synonymous with the observation that the reaction of skeletal muscle was what would need to be measured to infer a degree of reduced performance.

A cornerstone in the study of fatigue is the publication of Angelo Mosso's text *La Fatica* (Mosso 1891). This seminal text describes a detailed set of observations in both men and animals. In particular, Mosso was initially intrigued by his observations of migratory quails, which would seemingly kill themselves by hitting telegraph poles, trees and houses after their long journey. Mosso wrote,

> Taking them in my hand and blowing up the feathers, I perceived that they were not wasted. There was still fat under the skin in several parts of the body, and the pectoral muscles were in good condition. The poor creatures are so exhausted by the journey that their strength is just sufficient for flight.
> (Mosso 1904b, p. 2)

This observation underscores much of Mosso's later work on fatigue as he intuitively assumed that these migratory birds had sufficient energy reserves, which they were unable to access to avoid flying into structures. The conclusion that can be drawn from this observation was that energy availability was not likely to be the cause of the fatigue. Figure 4.2A shows the ingenious ergograph designed and used by Mosso. By fixing the forearm to the table and having the middle digit hold a 500g weight while stimulating the muscles of the forearm, Mosso was able to measure force output every 2 seconds.

The traces in Figure 4.2B show the level of force that was able to be produced on three different occasions in the same subject. Notably, when the subject was fresh (trace 1) the force produced was substantially higher and remained so for longer compared with when the subject had undertaken mental work (trace 2) and then rested for 2 hours (trace 3). Mosso also recognised that fatigue was unlikely to be attributed solely to what was observed from the skeletal muscle response. He wrote, "It is then not only the will, but also the nerves and the muscles which are fatigued in consequence of intense brain work. Let us remember this proof that fatigue due to intellectual labour affects the periphery of the body" (Mosso 1904b, p. 273).

A further pivotal insight by Mosso was that fatigue was not likely to be a function of just one physiological entity, such as skeletal muscle. He described his observation from his experiments as follows:

> On an examination of what takes place in fatigue, two series of phenomena demand their attention. The first is the diminution of muscular force. The second is fatigue as a sensation. That is to say, we had a physical fact

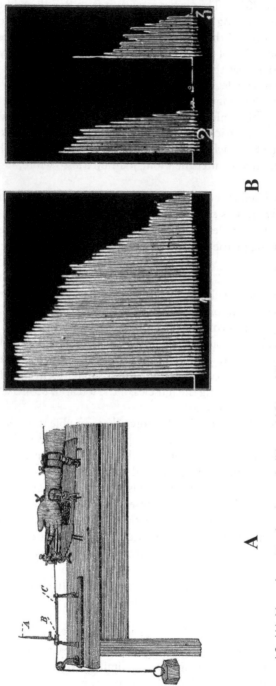

A

B

Figure 4.2 (A) Mosso's original ergograph (Moss 1891 p. 88) where skeletal muscle force output was measured by hanging a weight (W; 500g) from the middle digit and fixed forearm. (B) Involuntary contractions of the elbow flexors, which were directly stimulated every 2 s while the middle digit held a weight at three different times over the day (p. 272). Trace 1 at 9 a.m. when the subject was fresh. Trace 2 at 5:30 p.m. following 3.5 hrs of lecturing. Trace 3 and after a 2 hr rest from lecturing. The traces show the reduced skeletal muscle force produced as vertical spikes in the latter time periods when the subject was fatigued when compared to trace 1.

which can be measured and compared, and a psychic fact which eludes measurement.

(Mosso 1904b, p. 154)

Although not explicitly stated, this could be the first instance where fatigue was described as being a phenomenon that was either central or peripheral in origin. We shall return to the issue of dichotomising fatigue as either central or peripheral, but for the moment it suffices to say that there is a myriad of definitions of fatigue beyond what Mosso and his contemporaries suggested. Table 4.1 provides a few examples of the definitions used by authors since Mosso's initial suggestion.

The authors listed in Table 4.1 (Mosso 1904a; Fitts & Holloszy 1978; Bigland-Ritchie et al. 1986; Allen & Westerblad 2001; Vøllestad 1997) have used the individual definitions to suit a particular experimental context. Nevertheless, the overriding theme in each of these definitions is the reduction in performance of the skeletal muscle expressed as force or power. Importantly, the basis for these definitions is the less than obvious caveat that the reduction in performance must be *reversible* at some point. Thus, recovery from fatigue must also be a central component of its definition, since if recovery was not possible, then that would constitute a very different physiological phenomenon. Fatigue as a concept requires a relationship between at least two key components: first, that there is a reduction in performance which can be measured in some way, normally by altered skeletal muscle performance; and second, that there is recovery of that reduction in performance. These two components can lead only to the basic premise that what is actually imbedded in the working concept of fatigue is the capacity to *resist* fatigue rather than the decrement in performance *per se*. That is, the decrement

Table 4.1 Example definitions of fatigue

Author/s	Definition
Mosso (1904b)	The first is the diminution of the muscular force. The second is fatigue as a sensation. That is to say, we have a physical fact which can be measured and compared, and a psychic fact which eludes measurement.
Fitts and Holloszy (1978)	A reversible state of force depression, including a lower rate of rise of force and a slower relaxation.
Bigland-Ritchie et al. (1986)	A loss of maximal force-generating capacity.
Vøllestad (1997)	Any exercise-induced reduction in the maximal capacity to generate force or power output.
Allen and Westerblad (2001)	Intensive activity of muscles causes a decline in performance, known as fatigue.

Source: Fitts and Holloszy (1978), Bigland-Ritchie et al. (1986), Vøllestad (1997) and Allen and Westerblad (2001).

in performance alone is not a particularly useful measure on its own. Rather the attenuation in that performance decrement would signal a somewhat different meaning of fatigue. To make this point clearer, the seldom cited but likely most comprehensive definition of fatigue expresses this notion (Bartlett 1953, p. 1):

> Fatigue is a term used to cover all those determinable changes in the expression of an activity which can be traced to the continuing exercise of that activity under its normal operational conditions, and which can be shown to lead, either immediately or after delay, to deterioration in the expression of that activity, or, more simply, to results within the activity that *are not wanted*.

(Author's emphasis)

The current view and understanding of fatigue are that it is a multifactorial response which develops during or within a specific context. The interpretation of the resulting fatigue is dependent on the status of the individual: healthy or diseased. This has led researchers to continue studying the possible mechanisms and causes of fatigue by attempting to identify the actual site of physiological failure, since in disease states a physiological or mechanical disruption to tissues might be more easily identified at a particular site or point in time – for example, one of many glycogen storage diseases (GSD) which can lead to exercise-induced muscle weakness or intolerance and cramps. This returns us to the original dichotomy alluded to by Mosso – either *central* or *peripheral* in nature.

Regulation versus limitation

The fatigue response can also be thought of as a regulated process along a "chain" of overlapping biological structures. Figure 4.3 is a schematic of the biological structures involved in the chain of events that produce eventual skeletal muscle tension. In this schematic, the brain and spinal cord constitute the central nervous system (CNS), where the upper motoneurons are cortico-spinal interneurons that arise from the motor cortex and descend to the spinal cord. Here they activate the lower motoneurons through synapses. The term 'motor nerve' usually denotes those fibres that actually innervate muscles (lower motoneurons) at the neuromuscular junction (NMJ).

The relevance of this schematic is that skeletal muscle tension development is a regulated process reliant upon interconnected subsystems, which either singularly or collectively develop incapacity to produce a targeted effort. As shown in Figure 4.3, fatigue can develop at any one point in the system. Incapacity, or a change in the ability to generate the output along the chain, would also suggest that maintaining function or overriding the changes, either further up or down the chain of events, could modify the output. Therefore, the ability to resist any specific change at one or more of the structures in the chain could be possible. However, the caveat with this reasoning is that at either end of the chain the

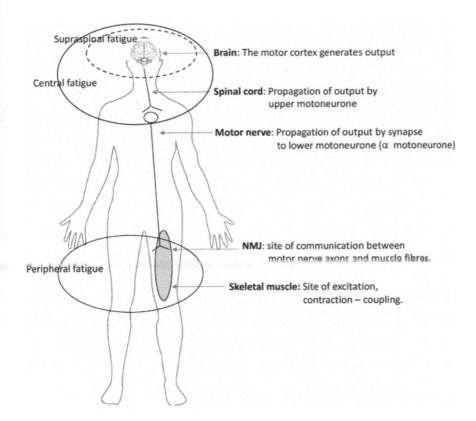

Figure 4.3 Basic schematic of the neuromuscular system. Supraspinal fatigue is the result of failure to generate output from the motor cortex (dashed oval), whereas central fatigue is related to progressive failure to activate skeletal muscle within the central nervous system down to the neuromuscular junction (NMJ). Peripheral fatigue is due to changes at or below the NMJ.

muscle cells and the supraspinal motoneurons represent the biological limits. Essentially, this means that changes between these two limiting structures can alter the output. We will return to this issue in Chapter 10 when discussing the potential effects of specific pathology on fatigue.

However, to illustrate the potential changes which can seemingly occur along the chain, Ikai and Steinhaus (1961) established that with diminishing muscular effort it was still possible to elicit increases in muscle contraction provided that sufficient motivation was given (Figure 4.4). These authors reasoned that muscular effort is always short of maximum due to the prevailing physiological state of the working muscles but subject to override by Pavlovian response – in

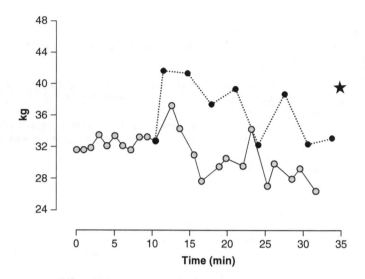

Figure 4.4 The effect of override on diminishing muscular tension over time. Participants were required to exert maximal forearm flexion once every minute for 30 min (open circles). The same protocol was used with unwarned gunshot from a starter's pistol when attempting maximal forearm flexion (filled circles) and when the participant shouted (star). Note original ordinate scale in *lb*, converted here into SI (kg) units.

Source: Data are redrawn from Ikai and Steinhaus (1961).

this example, the sound of a gunshot or a shout. These data suggest that fatigue was a central manifestation since the decreasing muscular force was restored by stimulation of some kind, for if peripheral changes at or below the neuromuscular junction were in operation, the muscle could not respond. Thus, this indicates that the biological "limits," at least at the muscle cell, were not achieved.

It has also been shown that if motivation for 'maximal' effort is provided from the beginning of the effort by visual and verbal cues, then extra stimulation seldom results in additional muscular force, although momentary interruption of maximal effort with percutaneous stimulation can briefly elicit increased muscular effort (Bigland-Ritchie 1981). Collectively, these findings (Ikai & Steinhaus 1961; Bigland-Ritchie 1981) show that human fatigue is a complex response dependent on the interaction of subsystems and a chain of physiological events that are seldom ever at their individual limits. Therefore, fatigue could be thought of as a product of interactions between subsystems working in unison, but when appropriate in "opposition," so that the net effect is either resistance to a reduction in muscular performance or uninterrupted muscular performance.

The dichotomy of central and peripheral fatigue is experimentally convenient as it allows researchers to identify to some extent where in the elaborate chain of events muscular fatigue might initiate, continue and come to cessation. However, humans or, for that matter, most other animals typically do not divide themselves into discrete functional components for the purpose of physical performance. Thus, it can be much more useful to consider fatigue from a whole-body performance perspective and as a *regulatory* process which is initiated the moment physical exertion commences and seldom ends with irreversible cellular death (Kay & Marino 2000). As Figure 4.5 shows, during an attempt to maintain a sustained maximal contraction, the force output begins to diminish almost immediately. The decline in force is observed to be gradual over the initial 50% of the time, but the decline becomes much more rapid thereafter. In this scenario fatigue is a regulated process and not one that ends in complete cellular breakdown or death, for if an appropriate rest period was provided at the end of this bout, recovery at least to some extent would be possible.

The popular school of thought is that fatigue is inferred from the observable reduction in skeletal muscle force. This is based on the fundamental physiological premise that biological systems have inherent limitations. However, as already discussed at length in Chapter 2, all biological structures also have

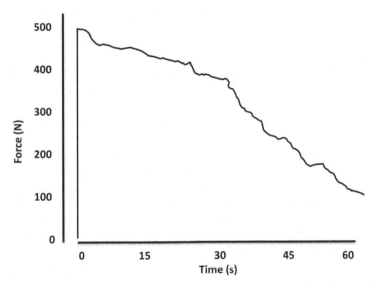

Figure 4.5 The typical reduction in force during a sustained muscle contraction over a 60s period when visual feedback of force progression was available, and the individual was afforded strong verbal encouragement to maintain the contraction. Note that at 50% of the contraction duration, force decline is 26% of the initial value, compared to 80% at the end of the contraction duration (60 min).

inherent safety factors which do not limit processes *per se* as much as they regulate to prevent catastrophic failure by seldom exceeding those safety factors. For instance, skeletal muscle has several safety factors which almost guarantee the cascade of events needed for contraction to occur. These include the number of acetylcholine receptors, post-synaptic folds and the abundance of neurotransmitter substance (see Chapter 2). On this basis, placing the process of fatigue in the traditional paradigm of physiological *limitation* negates the fact that cellular limitations are seldom attained. In other words, the traditional view holds that cellular processes will cause a cascade of cellular events and only termination of the fatigue-producing activity will prevent a catastrophic outcome (Noakes & St Clair Gibson 2004).

The concept of cellular catastrophe

The concept of cellular catastrophe as related to fatigue is based on the premise that muscle contraction terminates due to the combined loss of energy, excitation/activation and force. This eventually leads to cellular events where the biological system has reached its precipice and fatigue ensues, but crucially avoiding skeletal muscle rigor (stiffness). As indicated earlier (Table 4.1), a fundamental component of fatigue is the capacity for recovery. This component is known as *hysteresis*, which is the point when there is the possibility of recovery of excitation with little or no increase in force generation, until excitation-contraction coupling is restored (Edwards 1983). Essentially, the processes which culminate in the reduced capacity to generate muscle force have progressed to principally be thought of as cellular limitations or *catastrophe* as the final outcome. Although this is generally described as exhaustion, a state of extreme physical or mental tiredness, this conveys a substantially different meaning to the often-used term 'fatigue.'

The key component for the concept of cellular catastrophe is that the use of adenosine triphosphate (ATP) by contracting skeletal muscle exceeds its availability by the oxidative production for those same muscles (Bang 1936; Asmussen 1950). The classical teaching is that any deficit in oxidative production of ATP requires that anaerobic glycolysis provide the energy for continued muscular contraction, which in turn leads to premature reductions in intensity of muscular effort and fatigue. Importantly, the ATP concentrations of skeletal muscle are only very small at 20–27 mmol/kg of dry mass (DM). The level of ATP is well protected, as shown in Figure 4.6. When intense exercise is performed, the decrease in ATP is quite modest, from about 24 to 21 mmol/kg (13%) within 6 seconds (Gaitanos et al. 1993).

However, even after ten consecutive maximal sprints, interspersed by 30 s of recovery between each, the level of ATP failed to drop below 16 mmol/kg (dry mass; dm). By the end of sprint 10, ATP declined by about 33% from the initial values. Interestingly, this was matched by the decline in peak power output, which was also 33.4% of the initial value. These data show that the level of ATP

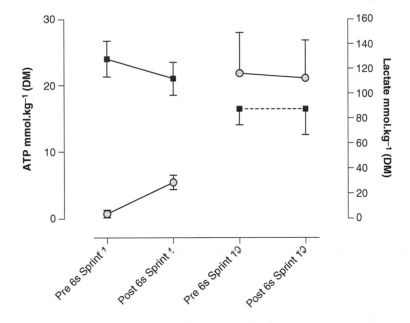

Figure 4.6 The level of ATP (*closed squares*, left ordinate) and muscle lactate (*open circles*, right ordinate) in mmol.kg⁻¹ dry mass (DM), before and after a 6s maximal sprint. Subjects performed ten maximal sprints with a 30s recovery between each sprint. The level of ATP dropped after sprint I by about 13%. After sprint 10 the level of ATP had fallen by 33% of the initial value but failed to drop any further, reaching a plateau when subjects became fatigued (post–sprint 10). The muscle lactate values increased after sprint I and then failed to increase after sprint 10.

Source: Data redrawn from table 4.1 in Gaitanos et al. (1993).

required to sustain intense exercise is well protected and that even after consecutive efforts, ATP level fails to fall to any level that would be considered dangerously low. Thus, the use and re-synthesis of ATP are, for all intents and purposes, exquisitely matched, since rates of maximal ATP production were about 15 mmol.kg dm⁻¹.s⁻¹ after the first sprint compared to 5.3 mmol.kg dm⁻¹.s⁻¹ after the last sprint (Gaitanos et al. 1993). However, a further finding in this study was that muscle lactate increased from ~3.8 mmol.kg⁻¹ pre-sprint 1 to ~28.6 mmol.kg⁻¹ post–sprint 1 (Figure 4.6). This indicates the ATP re-synthesis was predominantly from phosphocreatine (PCr) and anaerobic glycogenolysis. Conversely, after sprint 10, muscle lactate did not accumulate any further beyond the pre-sprint value (Figure 4.6), indicating that re-synthesis of ATP was predominantly from PCr and aerobic oxidation as power output was still 73% of that recorded at the start of the trials.

Although merely confirming the basic understanding of cellular energy use and supply, whereby initial re-synthesis of ATP is mainly supported from alactic and anaerobic metabolism with further re-synthesis requiring aerobic oxidation, confirms the preference for fatigue resistance. Since ATP is protected from precipitously falling to threatening levels by the exclusive use of anaerobic sources, there is a preferential switching to aerobic oxidation even when undertaking intense physical exercise. The trade-off for this energy supply preference is a reduction in power output in order to maintain a reasonable level of effort – in the example earlier, 73% of initial peak power (Gaitanos et al. 1993).

Even more compelling is the maintenance of ATP levels in individuals with GSD, such as McArdle's disease. In this type of disease, there is an enzyme deficiency which blocks the breakdown of glycogen in the muscle. As already discussed, the breakdown of glycogen by the process of glycogenolysis is essential during the initial moments of exercise (Gaitanos et al. 1993). As such, McArdle's patients have only about half the exercise capacity as normal people as sudden exercise results in the development of premature fatigue in addition to potential development of cramps and muscle injury. However, exercise tolerance in these patients is enhanced with additional energy availability. When McArdle's patients consumed a beverage with the addition of sucrose 30–40 min before exercising for 15 min at a constant workload, both heart rate and perceived exertion were lower compared with the placebo for the same workload (Vissing 2003). In fact, with the addition of sucrose, McArdle's patients had significantly elevated plasma lactate and pyruvate. Since McArdle's disease blocks glycogenolysis and limits the availability of glycolytic metabolites such as pyruvate, oxidative metabolism is limited because pyruvate is a metabolic intermediate needed in the tricarboxylic acid cycle for aerobic oxidation. Thus, when McArdle's patients are provided additional sucrose there is a spike in pyruvate, which results in an increase in the oxidative capacity of the skeletal muscle due to the extracellular energy supply, manifesting as a reduced heart rate and rating of perceived exertion (Haller & Vissing 2002; Vissing 2003).

Finally, when comparing the development of muscular fatigue between normal healthy individuals and those with GSD, the level of intramuscular ATP achieved during intense maximal voluntary contractions (MVC) is seemingly strictly defended (Cady et al. 1989). Figure 4.7 shows the change in muscular force during consecutive MVCs of the first dorsal interosseous muscle in both healthy normal subjects and those with GSD. It is clear that the level of ATP utilisation does not change between the normal and diseased subjects as force drops. Notably, the force decrement in each instance is accompanied by the utilisation of PCr. An interesting finding in the study described in Figure 4.7 is that the pH of the muscle over the course of the individual contractions not only remained stable but also remained elevated in the diseased muscle. At the very least this finding indicates that force generation is not particularly sensitive to increases in acidic (H^+, pH) levels, suggesting that this local environment might not be the only cause of muscular fatigue during repetitive high-force exercise (Cady et al. 1989).

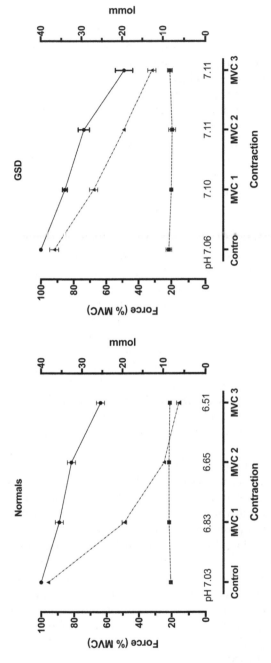

Figure 4.7 Data from normal healthy subjects (left) and in glycogen storage disease (GSD; right) for a control and three times maximal isometric contractions (MVC) of 15 s each for normals and 7 s each for GSD. Each contraction was separated with a 3-min rest period. The left ordinate is %MVC (*filled circles*) and right ordinate is metabolites phosphocreatine (*filled triangles*) and ATP (*filled squares*). The pH achieved for each MVC is shown above the x-axis.

Source: Data are redrawn from table 4.1 in Cady et al. (1989).

As mentioned previously, a key component of fatigue is the capacity for reversal and recovery (*hysteresis*). The findings as presented in Figure 4.7 also suggest that the metabolic changes experienced during this type of exercise do not involve processes that induce long-lasting damage or death – cellular catastrophe. In fact, as shown, the H^+ accumulation in GSD was less than that observed in the normal healthy muscle, and the degree of fatigue experienced for both was of a similar magnitude. Thus, the conclusion that can be drawn here is that force loss was independent of H^+ accumulation, and that there must be at least one other mechanism that accounts for this development of muscular fatigue beyond the observed metabolic perturbation.

One further possibility for the fatigue experienced in GSD, such as in McArdle's disease, is the impaired function of the enzymes known as the ATPases. These enzymes normally allow the coupling of ATP hydrolysis to other crucial cellular work, including the activation and processes associated with the operation of the skeletal muscle sodium-potassium pump (Na^+-K^+ pump). It has been established that Na^+-K^+ pump levels in McArdle's disease are significantly lower than in normal healthy muscles (Clausen & Vissing 1998). In addition, it was found that during 20 min of constant load exercise, the peak exercise increase in plasma $[K^+]$ over the resting levels in McArdle's patients was approximately two-fold higher than for controls (Clausen & Vissing 1998). Decreases in *intra*cellular $[K^+]$ when there are rises in both *extra*cellular $[K^+]$ and *intra*cellular $[N^+]$ influence sarcolemma excitability and muscle contractility. Thus, any decrease in the ratio of Na^+-K^+ pump to available sodium channels is associated with more rapid muscle fatigue during exercise (Harrison et al. 1997). A less than adequate coupling of the glycogen-dependent ATP supply for the Na^+-K^+ pumps in skeletal muscle might reduce their availability, which could potentially result in increased plasma K^+ levels (hyperkalemia) during exercise and an accelerated loss of membrane excitability (Lucia et al. 2008). Thus, one further potential factor in fatigue development in GSD is the premature loss of skeletal muscle membrane excitability.

Although development of muscular fatigue in GSD can be hastened by the metabolic milieu described earlier, its relationship to the potential alterations in membrane excitability should not be overlooked. This potential mechanism could explain the reduced ability to generate muscle force, but it can also explain why cellular catastrophe is unlikely to occur in these patients.

The purpose of the preceding discussion on cellular catastrophe was to highlight that even under the most strenuous efforts of skeletal muscle force output, including conditions where energy supply is limited, the biological system seldom fails. This clearly indicates that biological limits are very rarely achieved, and that the physiology associated with physical exertion is well regulated even in diseases which seemingly accelerate the development of fatigue. Finally, it is worth reiterating that ATP never achieves values which would cause muscle rigor. Therefore, there must exist another mechanism yet to be identified that controls the cessation of muscular effort before ATP levels are depleted and fall to the point when rigor would develop (Noakes et al. 2005). The only conclusion that can be drawn from this biological process is that cellular catastrophe cannot be the exclusive explanation for the development of fatigue.

Measuring fatigue

The measurement of fatigue can be complex and highly dependent on the criteria used to estimate the reduction in performance. Since the fundamental components of fatigue are two-fold – reduced performance and capacity to recover – it is useful to outline the basic techniques which are used to quantify these two components. In doing so there is also a need to differentiate between a reduction in power output during dynamic exercise and the assessment of maximal isometric muscle force before and after exercise. As discussed earlier, this is also complicated by the need to differentiate between central and peripheral components.

Reduction of power during exercise

The earliest attempt at quantifying the reduction in power during dynamic exercise is difficult to pinpoint. However, Margaria et al. (1966) proposed a test based on the individual's capacity to rapidly run up stairs. This type of test is able to show the decline in power over consecutive attempts, which indicates the development of fatigue. However, this type of test has been shown to be limited in its approach to quantifying fatigue based on a number of practical issues, such as run-up approach (Huskey et al. 1989).

In the field of exercise physiology, the most utilised method for observing fatigue in action is by measuring the response to exercise against a constant or fixed resistance. This model is essentially based on the understanding that the biological capacity is limited by the delivery and subsequent utilisation of energy, as discussed earlier with respect to the cellular catastrophe model of fatigue. Consequently, this is based on the premise that there is an apparent physiological limit which is normally measured to determine the individual maximum oxygen consumption (VO_{2max}) or peak power output (PO_{peak}). The resultant value of the VO_{2max} test is then used in a subsequent experimental trial to anchor the exercise load at a given percentage of the VO_{2max} (e.g. 70% VO_{2max}). This load is then maintained during exercise until there is a reduction in the prescribed intensity whereby exercise is terminated by the individual or by the experimenter, assuming the individual has attained the point of fatigue. Figure 4.8 shows the reduction in exercise intensity over time when expressed as a percentage of VO_{2max}. The data in Figure 4.8 are redrawn from the classic studies which evaluated the effects of carbohydrate feeding versus a placebo on strenuous exercise (Coyle et al. 1983). What is shown is that the addition of an exogenous energy source will delay the onset of fatigue. In this example, the carbohydrate feeding increased the time to fatigue from ~150 min in the placebo to ~180 min with carbohydrate feeding. However, fatigue in this example was defined as the time at which the exercise

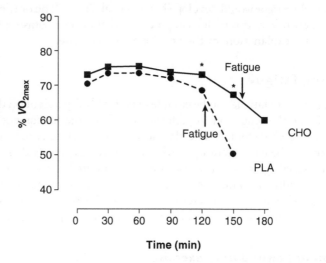

Figure 4.8 The exercise intensity (%VO$_{2max}$) that could be maintained with carbo-hydrate (CHO) feeding versus a placebo (PLA). The arrows denote the average time to fatigue as defined in the study (a reduction in intensity by 10% VO$_2$). *$P < 0.01$ versus PLA.

Source: Data redrawn from Coyle et al. (1983).

intensity could be maintained before subjects dropped below their initial work rate by 10% of VO$_2$. Exercise was terminated when intensity dropped below 50% of VO$_{2max}$ or after 180 min, whichever came first. In this example, the classic understanding of fatigue is defined as a reduction in exercise intensity rather than complete exhaustion. A further interpretation is that additional energy availability improved the capacity for fatigue resistance.

As per the findings depicted in Figure 4.8, there are numerous other studies which essentially describe the same phenomenon: a reduction in exercise intensity leading to premature termination of exercise or the improved capacity to resist fatigue as defined in the specific studies (Coggan & Coyle 1988; Parkin et al. 1999; Bergström et al. 1967; Montain et al. 1998; Nybo et al. 2001). Although this model of measuring fatigue during exercise has been very useful in clarifying what effects various interventions, such as carbohydrates and hydration, might have on the capacity for human performance, it is essentially based on the premise that there is a physiological limitation that when approached physical exertion must cease.

Regulation of power during exercise

A different approach to quantifying fatigue development during exercise has more recently been suggested based on the premise that the traditional model is less ecologically valid since very few pursuits require exercising at a constant or against a fixed resistance. Over the past two decades many studies have used self-paced exercise as a model to study fatigue (Marino 2012). Regardless of the actual putative mechanism limiting exercise performance, it is an unavoidable fact that sporting events require the individual to give an effort which will sustain him or her up to and well beyond the end of the event. On this basis alone, it is likely that during a sporting event requiring sustained effort, an individual will likely implement a strategy which will take into account the amount of energy required to complete the task. This understanding is not particularly new as many athletes recognise this as *pacing*. A prime example of pacing was the record-breaking mile run by Sir Roger Bannister in 1954. In his recording of that historic event, Bannister described the moments in the race where his friends and fellow runners Chris Brasher and Chris Chataway undertook a pacing strategy leading to success:

> We seemed to be going slowly! Impatiently I shouted "Faster!" But Brasher kept his head and did not change the pace. I went on worrying until I heard the first lap time, 57.5 seconds. In the excitement my knowledge of pace had deserted me. Brasher could have run the first quarter in 55 seconds without my realising it, because I felt so full of running, but I should have had to pay for it later. Instead, he had made success possible.
>
> (Bannister 2004, p. 165)

Although anecdotal, the events of 1954 provide some insight into the real possibility that there must be a strategy for resisting fatigue and eventual exhaustion.

Based on this concept, the self-paced model has provided novel insights into the regulation of exercise and more generally physical activity. For example, when subjects were required to sprint maximally for 1 min every 10 min while attempting to complete 60 min of cycling as fast as possible, the fatigue profile based on power output and muscle activity was not linear (Kay et al. 2001). Figure 4.9A shows the power output and muscle activity (integrated electromyography; IEMG) at each maximal sprint. What is evident is that power output was tracked by the muscle activity, indicating that muscle recruitment was commensurate with the changes in power output. What is particularly evident is the immediate reduction in muscle recruitment of about 30% from the initial sprint.

However, there are two additional findings from this study which merit further consideration. First, the peak heart rate response and rating of perceived exertion continued to increase and remained elevated for each sprint (Figure 4.9B), indicating that subjects gave a conscious maximal effort at each attempt. These findings coupled with the reduction in power output and EMG at the same time points indicate that power output was to some degree disconnected from the heart rate response and the perceived effort. Further to this is the observation that power and muscle recruitment were restored at almost initial values at the end of the trial, supposedly when subjects were most fatigued.

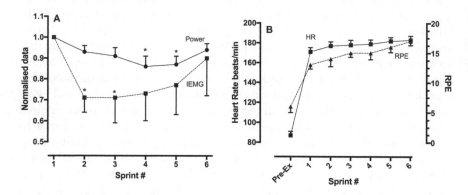

Figure 4.9 (A) Normalised power output and integrated electromyography (IEMG) at each maximal sprint. Sprint I was taken as the maximal effort. Note the return of power and muscle recruitment at sprint 6 to near initial values. (B) is the heart rate (left y-axis) and rating of perceived exertion (RPE; right y-axis). *$P < 0.05$ vs sprint I.

Source: Data are redrawn from Kay et al. (2001).

The salient point here is that the fatigue profile as measured by power output is not linear as predicted by the constant load model of exercise. That is, a reduction in exercise intensity as the indicator of fatigue was evident from only the initial stages, not the latter. Rather, the self-paced model describes a different fatigue phenomenon, a reduction in power output from the initial stages of the exercise, with a re-establishment of power output and muscle recruitment during the last moments of the exercise. This has typically been labelled the end-spurt. The question remains as to what the mechanism for this reduction and re-establishment of muscle activity might be.

Nevertheless, this response has also been shown under a number of varying conditions and modes of exercise (Amann et al. 2006; Marino et al. 2004; Amann et al. 2007; Billaut et al. 2010; Micklewright et al. 2010). In fact, when subjects performed a 5km cycle time trial with either 20% or 36% pre-existing locomotor muscle fatigue versus fresh non-fatigued locomotor muscle, power output and muscle recruitment (IEMG) reflected a dose-dependent inverse response (Amann & Dempsey 2008) (Figure 4.10). Most striking is the finding that power output was re-established at either the same or higher than the initial value by the end of the trial (Figure 4.10A). In addition, despite the difference in pre-existing fatigue the magnitude of the fatigue that was developed at the end of exercise was identical. These findings reflect a system that is regulated to avoid the development of locomotor muscle fatigue. Thus, these data also confirm that regardless of the existing level of fatigue, power and efferent drive are reduced in order to either prevent premature fatigue, thereby allowing the completion of

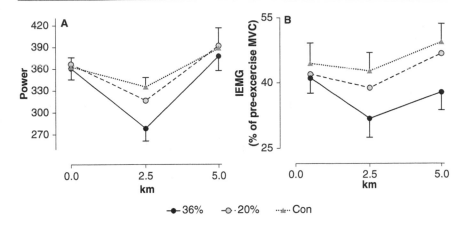

Figure 4.10 The power output (A) and the integrated electromyography (B; IEMG) as a percentage of the pre-exercise maximal voluntary contraction (MVC) for the *vastus lateralis* muscle over a 5km cycle time trial. Each trial was preceded by either no (Con) or 20% or 36% preexisting locomotor muscle fatigue.

Source: Data redrawn from Amann and Dempsey (2008).

the required task, or preserve a capacity to increase efferent drive when necessary. These findings as described in Figures 4.9 and 4.10 show a very different locomotor muscle fatigue response compared to the linear response that would be normally observed during the predetermined constant load model of exercise. Thus, locomotor fatigue is very dependent on the model used to quantify it. In the former constant load model, the ability to measure resistance to fatigue is removed, whereas in the self-paced model the resistance to the development of fatigue can be observed.

The findings from laboratory protocols are of greater value when similar phenomena are observed during competition, and as already mentioned humans, as do most other creatures, rarely perform physical activity at a near constant intensity. Thus, if the self-paced model of exercise is an ecologically valid method to measure the development of fatigue, similar observations should be evident in real-life performances. In an analysis of the world record times over a period of 83–85 years for the 5km and 10km distances, a similar profile emerges whereby the initial and last kilometre distances are the fastest, with the middle intervals being evenly paced (Tucker et al. 2006). However, when comparing these longer distances with the shorter 800 m, the initial 200 m was the fastest, with each consecutive 200 m either remaining similar or becoming slower, ending with the final 200 m as the slowest (Figure 4.11).

Recall from Chapter 1 that the capacity for endurance running, which was made possible by a myriad of other adaptations, also provided the possibility to hunt co-operatively by out-running or, more precisely, by running a large animal

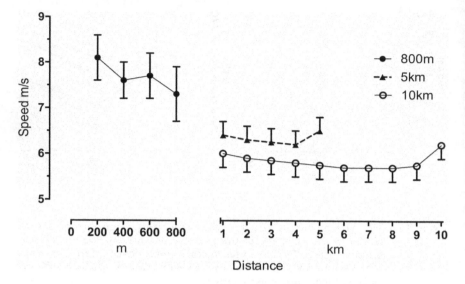

Figure 4.11 The mean running speed for individual intervals in world record running performances in the 800 m, 5k m and 10 km. Note the reduction in running speed from the start of each distance, with the re-establishment of running speed at the final interval for the 5 km and 10 km but not the 800 m.

Source: Data redrawn from Figures 4.2 and 4.5 from Tucker et al. (2006).

to exhaustion (Bramble & Lieberman 2004). Out-performing a competitor species because of a better endurance ability requires a strategy to also resist fatigue. Regardless of whether endurance running evolved because of the need to pursue prey or for other survival needs, just being able to run long distances without some implied strategy is not an appealing proposition. As previously suggested (Liebenberg 2006), tracking and then pursuing prey would be possible only if endurance running was a developed strategy. The data presented in Figures 4.9–4.11 provide evidence for a possible physiological strategy which fits the proposition not only that *Homo* is an exceptional endurance athlete but also that the physiology is such that it allows for appropriate pacing not necessarily observed in short distances. Thus, from an evolutionary perspective, the laboratory findings employing self-paced protocols coupled with the real-world findings from athletic events underscore the proposition that *Homo* favoured endurance over power and speed. Further to this is the observation that in the shorter 800 m there was no evidence of recovery from the intensity employed to facilitate the increase in speed for the last interval, as seen in the 5–10km distances. In contrast and most important is that in the longer distances not only is there a distinct increase in speed for the last interval but also this speed is faster than the starting speed, likely facilitated by a strategy which reduces intensity and locomotor muscle recruitment during the middle intervals (Figure 4.11).

In summary, measuring fatigue during dynamic exercise is highly dependent on the protocol. The use of a protocol that requires the individual to either run or cycle at a constant or fixed intensity will result in a linear response and the cessation of exercise when predetermined fatigue criteria are achieved. In contrast, a self-paced protocol will permit regulation of exercise intensity so that the task can be completed without the forced termination by predetermined fatigue criteria. Thus, the measurement of the fatigue profile is very different during dynamic exercise and based on the protocol that is employed.

Measurement of fatigue during static exercise

The measurement of skeletal muscle fatigue during static exercise requires a different methodology and approach compared with those for dynamic exercise. At the centre of the measurement of fatigue during static exercise is the evaluation of the maximal voluntary isometric contraction (MVIC) with superimposed electrical stimulation of the peripheral nerve supplying the skeletal muscle under investigation. As shown in Figure 4.3, the measurement of skeletal muscle fatigue is also highly dependent on the pathways under investigation. Although it is not in dispute that the processes related to excitation and contraction of the skeletal muscle contribute to the changes in maximal force production, the processes within the nervous system also contribute to the fatigue process, as outlined in the section earlier (regulation versus limitation). The neuromuscular changes which contribute to the fatigue process that can be measured are either central, which encompasses the processes above the level of the terminal branches of the motor axons, or peripheral, which includes the changes within the terminal branches, the neuromuscular junction and the actual muscle fibres. In practical terms, central fatigue is regarded as a reduction in the voluntary activation of the skeletal muscle during exercise (Gandevia et al. 1992). In relation to Figure 4.3, this means that the CNS has reduced its ability to continue to drive the muscle at a maximal capacity. However, it is important to note that the ability to drive the muscle from the motor cortex is regarded as supraspinal fatigue (Gandevia et al. 1992). The purpose of this section is to outline the basic methods used to measure neuromuscular performance, along with the interpretation of the changes that occur within the nervous system as a consequence of exercise.

Maximal voluntary contraction

The maximal voluntary contraction is usually measured while a subject is positioned so that a particular muscle group can be isolated and tested. Normally, this would be either the wrist flexors, elbow flexors or the quadriceps muscles, but can be done with almost any muscle group, including the small muscles of the hand. Once the limb is in a fixed position, the subject is asked to produce a maximal isometric contraction, usually for 3–5 seconds, which generates force output or torque that can be quantified as shown in Figure 4.12A. When the contraction has reached a plateau, an electrical current is delivered to the peripheral nerve supplying the muscle in question. The technique and equipment used to deliver the stimulus are beyond the scope of this discussion; however, the reader is referred to the methods and procedures outlined previously for a comprehensive description (Cannon et al. 2008). When the current is delivered during the plateau phase of the MVIC, a further increase in force output is observed, as shown in Figure 4.12A.

The muscle torques shown in Figure 4.12 indicate that despite a maximal effort by the individual to achieve a distinguishable plateau in torque, there was further torque developed with the superimposed electrical stimulus. This is typically referred to as voluntary activation and is calculated as:

$$\text{Voluntary activation} = (\text{voluntary torque/superimposed torque}) \times 100$$

Figure 4.12 also shows that the voluntary effort was submaximal since the torque was only about 90% of that achieved with the additional peripheral nerve stimulation. However, in Figure 4.12B already fatigued muscle was able to produce voluntary torque of only about 70% of that achieved with electrical stimulation. Regarding the data described in both Figure 4.12A and Figure 4.12B, three

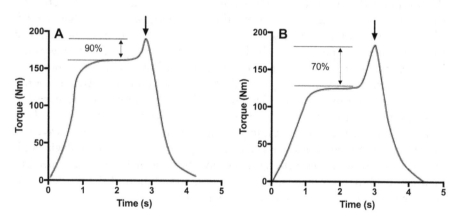

Figure 4.12 The development of muscle torque during a maximal voluntary isometric contraction (MVIC) with superimposed electrical stimulation (ES; downward arrow) and the resultant additional muscle twitch. Fresh unfatigued muscle (A) shows the difference between MVIC torque developed (plateau) versus that with ES, with the difference being 90% complete activation during the MVIC. Compare this to the fatigued muscle (B), where the voluntary activation was only 70% of maximum.

critical points need to be considered. First, extra peripheral stimulation when the muscle was either fresh or fatigued elicited further force, suggesting that the contractile apparatus was intact, and therefore a reduction in voluntary force was of central origin. Second, the development of skeletal muscle force is never truly maximal regardless of whether the muscle is fresh or fatigued. Third, the difference in force development before and immediately upon superimposed stimulation suggests that some motor units either are not recruited and are quiescent or are unable to fire at a rate required to form a fused contraction. Thus, these observations suggest that despite the availability of 100% of muscle fibres, the recruitment is always below that available.

In addition to the gross measurement model described in Figure 4.12, a further model can be used to infer whether locomotor muscle fatigue is of central origin. This is known as the potentiated twitch technique. This technique accounts for the possibility that ongoing contractions from a previous activity can potentiate the force evoked from a muscle. Thus, the superimposed twitch is potentiated by the preceding contraction and should be compared with a potentiated resting twitch elicited a short time following the MVIC. Using this method, the voluntary activation can be calculated by the following:

$$\text{Voluntary activation} = (1\text{-superimposed twitch/resting twitch}) \times 100$$

The potentiated twitch technique provides an added measurement of the effect of exercise on muscle contractile function. By evoking a potentiated muscle twitch, it is then possible to produce twitch torque-time curves, as shown in Figure 4.13.

These curves are able to provide information about specific aspects of the contractile function which can further elucidate what aspects of muscle performance impinge on the development of muscle fatigue. Since the twitch torque-time curve is produced with percutaneous stimulation of the peripheral nerve, it represents the potential contribution to muscle fatigue as a result of alterations to the excitation-contraction coupling apparatus, generally referred to as peripheral fatigue. The discrete components shown in Figure 4.13 provide the basis by which to draw conclusions about the level of peripheral fatigue. For example, a reduction in the peak twitch torque would indicate that the level of tension development is a result of changes in the contractile function rather than changes in neural drive. This was highlighted when comparing the evoked twitches before and after a set of 25 continuous isokinetic concentric and eccentric contractions (Martin et al. 2005). In this study, the authors found that regardless of the type of contraction (shortening or lengthening), the evoked twitches post-exercise were significantly reduced, indicating that the contractile function contributed to the fatigue profile. Similarly, when comparing young with older (25 vs 67 years) muscle function, researchers have found that the rate of twitch torque development, peak twitch torque and rate of twitch relaxation were all significantly less in the older group (Cannon et al. 2008). However, an interesting observation was that the ratio of peak twitch torque/maximal voluntary contraction and the time to

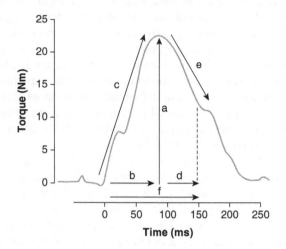

Figure 4.13 An example twitch torque-time curve produced during evoked testing labelled with the relevant time periods used to assess the twitch
contractile properties. (a) Peak twitch torque (PT), which is the highest isometric value achieved. (b) Time to PT as the time from torque
onset to PT. (c) Rate of torque development, which is defined as the
tangential slope of the curve between the onset and PT. (d) Half-
relaxation time (1/2 RT), which is the time required for PT to decline
by half. (e) Rate or relaxation is the mean tangential slope of the
curve between PT and 1/2 RT. (f) Contraction duration, which is the
time to peak torque plus 1/2 RT.

peak torque were comparable between the young and older group. These observations suggest that as ageing muscle loses its ability to develop peak torque due to
alterations at the contractile level, there is some compensation in the ratio and
the time taken to develop that tension. The reasons for this compensation are
speculative, but it is enticing to suggest that whatever tension can be developed,
nature has opted to at least maintain its ability to develop that tension as quickly
as possible.

There are several other methods and procedures used to derive the potential
site of neuromuscular fatigue. These include such methods as transcranial magnetic stimulation (TMS), which is able to assess the drive from the motor cortex
(Todd et al. 2007; Ross et al. 2007). There is also consideration of the effects of
other inputs to motoneurones which are likely to make these nerve fibres less
responsive during fatigue. These include afferents from muscle spindles (Groups
Ia and II), Golgi tendon organs (Ib) and small-diameter myelinated and unmyeli-
nated afferents (Groups III & IV) (Gandevia 2001). In addition, there is the relationship between the compound muscle action potential (M-wave) and the level
of fatigue developed. The integrity of the M-wave can apparently indicate the

integrity of neuromuscular transmission during sustained voluntary contractions (Merton 1954; Bigland-Ritchie et al. 1982). However, each of these methods and procedures, along with those discussed earlier, has limitations and interpretation difficulties when used to study fatigue. Nevertheless, the fundamental tenets of these methods that describe the outcomes of neuromuscular performance are still valid.

Evolutionary perspective

The overarching purpose of this book is to provide an avenue to understand fatigue from an evolutionary perspective. The preceding sections on the methods to measure fatigue during either dynamic or static exercise suggest that human physiology very seldom operates at maximal levels. In other words, there is always some reserve. From an evolutionary perspective this would make sense, since if the systems available to us do not generate a maximal effort from the start, then a "reserve" must exist. The question then is, why does a reserve exist? The obvious answer is that a reserve could be mobilised in extraordinary moments. Implicit in this is the survival value that a biological reserve could potentially provide. Thought of in another way, the question is, what would be the consequence of having no available reserve at the start of physical exertion? There are two possibilities according to the preceding section on the different methods to measure fatigue: voluntary activation continues maximally until peripheral fatigue ensues or central fatigue eventually develops. Intuitively, the problem with this scenario is that should one be faced with a dire circumstance in which extra force development would be required and not possible because of the initial maximal level of activation, the survival value would be compromised. On the other hand, since we have already established that voluntary activation is always submaximal to begin with, several more desirable possibilities exist. First, activation can increase by drawing on the reserve. Second, if activation is more than required there can be a decrease in the activation, thereby reducing the potential energy expended. Third, and most obvious, is the possibility of maintaining the voluntary activation at a submaximal level for longer than would otherwise be possible. These three possibilities are what evolutionary biology would predict since anything that would provide for an inherent survival value would be more desirable.

References

Allen, D. & Westerblad, H., 2001. Role of phosphate and calcium stores in muscle fatigue. *Journal of Physiology*, 536(3), pp. 657–665.

Amann, M. et al., 2006. Arterial oxygenation influences central motor output and exercise performance via effects on peripheral locomotor muscle fatigue in humans. *Journal of Physiology*, 575(Pt 3), pp. 937–952.

Amann M., Romer, L.M., Subudhi, A.W., Pegelow, D.F. & Dempsey, J.A., 2007. Severity of arterial hypoxaemia affects the relative contributions of peripheral muscle fatigue to exercise performance in healthy humans. *Journal of Physiology*, 581(1), pp. 389–403.

Amann, M. & Dempsey, J.A., 2008. Locomotor muscle fatigue modifies central motor drive in healthy humans and imposes a limitation to exercise performance. *Journal of Physiology*, 586(1), pp. 161–173.

Asmussen, E., 1950. Pyruvate and lactate content of the blood during and after muscular work. *Acta Physiologica*, 20(2–3), pp. 125–132.

Bang, O., 1936. The lactate content of the blood during and after muscular exercise in man. *Skandinavisches Archiv Für Physiologie*, 74(S10), pp. 51–82.

Bannister, R., 2004. *The first four minutes*, Phoenix Mill, UK: Sutton Publishing.

Bartlett, F., 1953. *Symposium on fatigue.* In W.F. Floyd & A.T. Welford, eds. *Psychological criteria of fatigue.* Oxford: H. K. Lewis & Co, pp. 1–5.

Bergström, J. et al., 1967. Diet, muscle glycogen and physical performance. *Acta Physiologica*, 71(2–3), pp. 140–150.

Bigland-Ritchie, B., 1981. EMG and fatigue of human voluntary and stimulated contractions. *CIBA Foundation Symposium*, 82, pp. 130–156.

Bigland-Ritchie, B., Furbush, F. & Woods, J., 1986. Fatigue of intermittent submaximal voluntary contractions: central and peripheral factors. *Journal of Applied Physiology*, 61(2), pp. 421–429.

Bigland-Ritchie, B. et al., 1982. The absence of neuromuscular transmission failure in sustained maximal voluntary contractions. *Journal of Physiology*, 330, pp. 265–278.

Billaut, F. et al., 2010. Cerebral oxygenation decreases but does not impair performance during self-paced, strenuous exercise. *Acta Physiologica*, 198(4), pp. 477–486.

Bramble, D.M. & Lieberman, D.E., 2004. Endurance running and the evolution of *Homo*. *Nature*, 432, pp. 345–352.

Cady, E.B., Jones, D.A. & Lynn, J., 1989. Changes in force and intracellular metabolites during fatigue of human skeletal muscle. *Journal of Physiology*, 418, pp. 311–325.

Cannon, J. et al., 2008. Reproducibility and changes in twitch properties associated with age and resistance training in young and elderly women. *Scandinavian Journal of Medicine & Science in Sports*, 18(5), pp. 627–635.

Clausen, T. & Vissing, J., 1998. Reduced levels of skeletal muscle Na+K+ -ATPase in McArdle disease. *Neurology*, 50(1), pp. 37–40.

Coggan, A.R. & Coyle, E.F., 1988. Effect of carbohydrate feedings during high-intensity exercise. *Journal of Applied Physiology*, 65(4), pp. 1703–1709.

Coyle, E.F. et al., 1983. Carbohydrate feeding during prolonged strenuous exercise can delay fatigue. *Journal of Applied Physiology*, 55(1 Pt 1), pp. 230–235.

Edwards, R., 1983. Biochemical bases for fatigue in exercise performance: catastrophe theory in muscular fatigue. In H.G. Knuttgen, J.A. Vogel & J. Poortmans, eds. *Biochemistry of exercise.* Champagne, IL: Human Kinetics, pp. 3–27.

Fitts, R.H. & Holloszy, J.O., 1978. Effects of fatigue and recovery on contractile properties of frog muscle. *Journal of Applied Physiology*, 45(6), pp. 899–902.

Gaitanos, G.C., Boobis, L.H. & Brooks, S., 1993. Human muscle metabolism during intermittent maximal exercise. *Journal of Applied Physiology*, 75(2), pp. 712–719.

Gandevia, S.C., 2001. Spinal and supraspinal factors in human muscle fatigue. *Physiological Reviews*, 81(4), pp. 1725–1789.

Gandevia, S.C. et al., 1992. Human motor output, muscle fatigue and muscle afferent feedback. In *Proceedings of the Australian physiological and pharmacological society.* Sydney: Ramsay Ware Stockland, pp. 59–67.

Haller, R.G. & Vissing, J., 2002. Spontaneous "second wind" and glucose-induced second "second wind" in McArdle disease: oxidative mechanisms. *Archives of Neurology*, 59(9), pp. 1395–1402.

Harrison, A.P., Nielsen, O.B. & Clausen, T., 1997. Role of Na (+)-K+ pump and Na+ channel concentrations in the contractility of rat soleus muscle. *American Journal of Physiology. Regulatory, Integrative and Comparative Physiology*, 272(5), pp. R1402–R1408.

Huskey, T. et al., 1989. Factors affecting anaerobic power output in the Margaria-Kalamen test. *Ergonomics*, 32(8), pp. 959–965.

Ikai, M. & Steinhaus, A.H., 1961. Some factors modifying the expression of human strength. *Journal of Applied Physiology*, 16(1), pp. 157–163.

Kay, D. & Marino, F.E., 2000. Fluid ingestion and exercise hyperthermia: implications for performance, thermoregulation, metabolism and the development of fatigue. *Journal of Sports Sciences*, 18(2), pp. 71–82.

Kay, D. et al., 2001. Evidence for neuromuscular fatigue during high-intensity cycling in warm, humid conditions. *European Journal of Applied Physiology*, 84(1–2), pp. 115–121.

Liebenberg, L., 2006. Persistence hunting by modern hunter-gatherers. *Current Anthropology*, 47(6), pp. 1017–1026.

Lucia, A., Nogales-Gadea, G. & Pérez, M., 2008. McArdle disease: what do neurologists need to know? *Nature Clinical Practice*, 4(10), pp. 568–577.

Margaria, R., Aghemo, P. & Rovelli, E., 1966. Measurement of muscular power (anaerobic) in man. *Journal of Applied Physiology*, 21(5), pp. 1662–1664.

Marino, F.E., 2012. The limitations of the constant load and self-paced exercise models of exercise physiology. *Comparative Exercise Physiology*, 7(04), pp. 173–178.

Marino, F.E., Gard, M. & Drinkwater, E.J., 2011. The limits to exercise performance and the future of fatigue research. *British Journal of Sports Medicine*, 45(1), pp. 65–67.

Marino, F.E., Lambert, M.I. & Noakes, T.D., 2004. Superior performance of African runners in warm humid but not in cool environmental conditions. *Journal of Applied Physiology*, 96, pp. 124–130.

Martin, P.G. et al., 2005. Reduced voluntary activation of human skeletal muscle during shortening and lengthening contractions in whole body hyperthermia. *Experimental Physiology*, 90(2), pp. 225–236.

McComas, A.J., 2011. *Galvani's spark: the story of the nerve impulse*, New York: Oxford University Press.

Merton, P.A., 1954. Voluntary strength and fatigue. *Journal of Physiology*, 123(3), pp. 553–564.

Micklewright, D. et al., 2010. Previous experience influences pacing during 20 km time trial cycling. *British Journal of Sports Medicine*, 44(13), pp. 952–960.

Montain, S.J. et al., 1998. Hypohydration effects on skeletal muscle performance and metabolism: a 31P-MRS study. *Journal of Applied Physiology*, 84(6), pp. 1889–1894.

Mosso, A., 1891. *La fatica*, Milano: F. lli Treves.

Mosso, A., 1904a. *Fatigue*, London: Swan Sonnenschein & Co. Ltd.

Mosso, A., 1904b. *Fatigue*, New York: G. P. Putnam's Sons.

Noakes, T.D. & St Clair Gibson, A., 2004. Logical limitations to the "catastrophe" models of fatigue during exercise in humans. *British Journal of Sports Medicine*, 38(5), pp. 648–649.

Noakes, T.D., St Clair Gibson, A. & Lambert, E.V., 2005. From catastrophe to complexity: a novel model of integrative central neural regulation of effort and fatigue during exercise in humans: summary and conclusions. *British Journal of Sports Medicine*, 39(2), pp. 120–124.

Nybo, L. et al., 2001. Effects of marked hyperthermia with and without dehydration on VO_2 kinetics during intense exercise. *Journal of Applied Physiology*, 90(3), pp. 1057–1064.

Parkin, J.M. et al., 1999. Effect of ambient temperature on human skeletal muscle metabolism during fatiguing submaximal exercise. *Journal of Applied Physiology*, 86(3), pp. 902–908.

Ross, E.Z. et al., 2007. Corticomotor excitability contributes to neuromuscular fatigue following marathon running in man. *Experimental Physiology*, 92(2), pp. 417–426.

Stevenson, A., 2010. *Oxford dictionary of English*, Oxford: Oxford University Press.

Todd, G. et al., 2007. Use of motor cortex stimulation to measure simultaneously the changes in dynamic muscle properties and voluntary activation in human muscles. *Journal of Applied Physiology*, 102(5), pp. 1756–1766.

Tucker, R., Lambert, M.I. & Noakes, T.D., 2006. An analysis of pacing strategies during men's world-record performances in track athletics. *International Journal of Sports Physiology and Performance*, 1(3), pp. 233–245.

Vissing, J., 2003. The effect of oral sucrose on exercise tolerance in patients with McArdle's disease. *New England Journal of Medicine*, 349(26), pp. 2503–2509.

Vøllestad, N.K., 1997. Measurement of human muscle fatigue. *Journal of Neuroscience Methods*, 74(2), pp. 219–227.

Chapter 5

Morphology and skeletal muscle

All organs of an animal form a single system, the parts of which hang together, and act and re-act upon one another; and no modifications can appear in one part without bringing about corresponding modifications in all the rest.

– Baron Georges Cuvier (1789)

Introduction

In Chapter 1 habitual bipedality was discussed as one distinguishing characteristic of *Homo*, and although this characteristic is distinct among mammals, there is another universal similarity among all mammals and indeed most other animals, regardless of their individual locomotor characteristics: the skeletal muscle. This is the organ of choice since other life forms, such as plants, do not require moving to another location to source their nourishment. Plants acquire what they need from the soil, air and sunlight. Animals must obtain their nourishment by moving to acquire it. In some circumstances movement is required over large distances, and in others less so. This movement is obviously accomplished with skeletal muscle, which also provides the movement required for breathing and other actions which tend to reflect our emotions and other needs. Simply put, skeletal muscle provides for the voluntary actions that sustain our existence through the development of the force exerted against a given resistance. However, there is one important aspect of skeletal muscle that also needs to be considered and which determines its capacity to exert tension: the length and shape of bones.

In previous chapters, specific elements of skeletal muscle were discussed in some detail, in particular the typical safety factor associated with force production and its relationship to muscle fibre types (Chapter 2). Further to this was the gross comparison of skeletal muscle attributes of primates and how this might account for the observation that humans selected endurance rather than power and strength when compared with other extant primates (Chapter 3). In Chapter 4 the basic methods used to measure fatigue during dynamic and static exercise were discussed and what elements we are able to utilise to infer whether fatigue is of central or peripheral origin.

In this relatively short chapter, two critical aspects of skeletal muscle will be discussed. First, the relationship between morphology and skeletal muscle adaptability will provide a background for why *Homo* compromised absolute power for endurance and fatigue resistance. In this case, a comparison with our extinct ancestors, such as Neanderthals, and early modern humans might provide the clues for the choices we made along our evolutionary journey. Second, there is a distinct relationship between skeletal muscle performance and local temperature. Evidence seems to suggest that warmer muscles are better muscles, and the way in which this is typically achieved is by increasing the muscle temperature through physical activity, generally known as "warming up." Although the reasons for considering this characteristic are not immediately obvious, the fact that "warming up" is a prerequisite for better-performing muscles means that sudden and immediate physical exertion cannot lead to optimal performance. How this might relate to morphology will be discussed.

Muscle morphology

Like many anatomical structures, form and function are intimately tied. In Chapter 3 a comparison of the muscle morphology between humans and chimpanzees was used to illustrate that we are adapted more for endurance than for power. The reasons for favouring this adaptation seem obvious when we make the stark, yet useful comparison with our closest living relatives. Specifically, the skeletal muscle fascicle length seems to be a significant feature, with humans opting for shorter rather than longer fascicles compared with chimps (see Table 3.1). Interestingly, this characteristic seems to also be significant in the human athletic population, with sprinters having comparatively longer fascicles than middle distance runners and controls (see Figure 3.6). However stark the musculoskeletal differences seem to be between humans and chimpanzees, this provides only a partial understanding of the adaptation favouring endurance over power. A better comparison could be ascertained between *Homo sapiens* and the distant extinct species which were either partially or fully adapted for bipedal locomotion. Table 5.1 (and repeated in Table 3.1) provides the timeline for the appearance of *Homo*, which emphasises the overlap between species and that hominids likely lived side by side for extended periods (Walter 2013). However, any direct comparison between extinct hominids and *Homo* is fraught with limitations since biological material has long gone. Nevertheless, by reconstructing skeletons from partial remains of these extinct species, it is possible to draw some useful conclusions about muscle morphology and whether this played a part in our own evolution and eventual choice of endurance over power.

The estimated average masses and heights of the extinct species and modern humans are shown in Table 5.1. What is clear from these data is that average and lean body mass is generally associated with stature. However, these gross approximations are difficult to interpret since the current trends for mass for modern-day humans are skewed by the great number of people now classified as obese. Nevertheless, as plotted in Figure 5.1 these data show that the increase in both mass

Table 5.1 The average estimated heights and masses of the closest extinct *Homo* species versus *Homo sapiens*. The last three columns show estimated lean body mass as an index of muscle mass.

Species	Million years ago	Average height (m)	Average mass (kg)	BF (kg)	JF (kg)	HM (kg)	SM (kg)
Ard. ramidus*	4.4	1.20	50	33.2	32.8	27.6	7.5
Aus. afarensis	3.9–2.9	1.51	42	38.2	36.3	35.5	6.3
Aus. africanus	3.3–2.1	1.38	41	34.3	33.8	30.7	6.1
H. habilis#	2.4–1.5	1.30	32	28.5	27.4	25.1	4.8
H. erectus#	1.9–0.7	1.65	54	46.8	45.7	44.2	8.1
H. Heidelbergensis	0.6–0.2	1.75	62	52.8	52.1	50.2	9.3
Neanderthals	0.4–0.3	1.64	65	51.0	51.4	47.4	9.7
H. sapiens	0.2 –	1.73	75	57.3	58.2	53.5	11.2

Note: The lean body mass was calculated using three separate equations, where BF is the Boer formula (Boer 1984), JF is the James formula (Engbers et al. 2010) and HM is the Hume formula (Hume 1966). SM is the estimated skeletal mass (15% of average mass). In all cases data are for males except for *female, #average for the available skeletal specimens.

Source: Average height and mass for extinct species taken from data provided by the Smithsonian Museum of Natural History: http://humanorigins.si.edu/evidence/human-fossils/species. Data for *H. sapiens* taken as an average for male from Walpole et al. (2012).

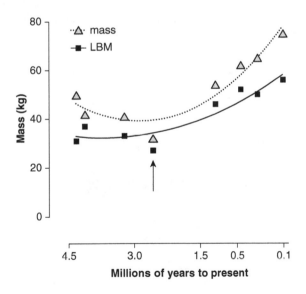

Figure 5.1 The estimated mass and lean body mass (LBM) over millions of years to present of the species listed in Table 5.1. The lines represent a second-order polynomial where mass (kg) = $54.23 - 8.55(x) + 1.44(x^2)$ where $R^2 = 0.83$ and LBM (kg) = $31.36 - 0.31(x) + 0.45(x^2)$ where $R^2 = 0.76$. The arrow indicates genus *Homo*.

and lean body mass is a non-linear phenomenon. The reasons for this relation-ship remain unclear.

However, when the plot in Figure 5.1 is compared with that plot in Figure 3.8, which estimates the increase in endocranial volume (ECV) over a similar time period, it is apparent that the increase in both ECV and body mass occurred approximately 2.5 million years ago. Most important to note with these plots is that the changes in the ECV and body mass do not imply causation; rather the plots simply confirm that morphology began to change around the same time as brain size began to change. Even more salient is the observation that the increase in lean body mass was not as dramatic as the increase in ECV. In fact, others have calculated and concluded that the most dramatic changes in these two parame-ters occur with the appearance of modern *H. sapiens* about 100,000 years ago with a relative decrease in body mass and an increase in relative brain size, seemingly driven by selection for a smaller body mass (Kappelman 1996). This conclusion suggests that a smaller body mass, which results in a relatively smaller skeletal muscle mass, provided some advantage for *H. sapiens* compared with our distant relatives. As an example of this difference, Figure 5.2 is a comparison of the *H. sapiens* and Neanderthal skeletons. What is notable about this comparison is not only the shorter stature and the larger cranium of Neanderthals (as discussed in Chapter 3; Figure 3.7) but also a distinctly more robust skeleton with larger joints, broader rib cage and hips, and shorter forearms and legs. These features must have altered the skeletal muscle morphology compared to what modern humans now possess. Thus, Neanderthals provide a robust model from which to make comparisons.

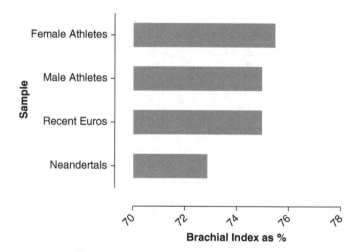

Figure 5.2 A comparison of the brachial index from Neanderthals, recent humans (Holliday 1999) and male and female athletes competing in a variety of sports (Norton & Olds 1996).

Considering the lengths and overall shapes of the limbs of Neanderthals provides interesting comparisons which allow us to speculate about the muscle morphology and their physical abilities. Whether Neanderthals had more robust bones is still debated (Pearson et al. 2006), but initial clues suggest that Neanderthals were perhaps not as dextrous as modern humans (Musgrave 1971). This question was largely based on the observation that metacarpals and phalangeal bones generally had wider heads and were distinctly more robust. Neanderthals apparently also possessed radius and ulna bones that were shorter compared to modern humans (Holliday 1999; Porter 1999). This proportion is commonly known as the brachial index (BI), which is calculated by the following:

$$BI = (\text{length of radius} / \text{length of humerus}) \times 100$$

The significance of the BI is that it is a measure of lever ratio between arm and forearm and that a smaller BI would provide a mechanical advantage (Stewart et al. 2011). That is, by reducing the length of the lever on which the biceps brachii exerts its tension, but maintaining muscular force, the required work is reduced. Figure 5.2 compares the BI of Neanderthals, recent Europeans and male and female athletes competing in a variety of sports. What can be seen is that the BI increased by approximately 2%–2.5% from that of Neanderthals. Since it is estimated that Neanderthal radii were approximately 22.7 cm (De Groote 2011b) with a BI index of 73% (Holliday 1999), a positive change to the BI to 75% would result in an approximate 1cm increase in forearm length. An increase in BI does not necessarily convey an advantage as far as skeletal muscle is concerned, since a lever that is 1 cm longer will require approximately 4% greater torque to be produced for a given resistance.

It is also important to note that within the modern athletic population, the BI has a range for males between 71.8% and 79.5%, and for females between 72.0% and 76.8%. What is particularly notable about these data is that individuals engaged in sports requiring power and forceful movements that need full extension of the forearm tend to have a lower BI compared with those individuals that engage in sports that are more endurance-dependent (Norton & Olds 1996; Stewart et al. 2011).

However, the BI alone cannot account for the seemingly muscular adaptation of the Neanderthals. In fact, along with a smaller BI, the Neanderthal radius also possessed a significant lateral shaft curvature and a more medially located radial tuberosity (De Groote 2011b). These features suggest a much better mechanical advantage for Neanderthals since the lateral curvature of the radius allows for a larger muscle belly, with the muscle insertion maintained close to the axis of rotation. In addition, the larger and more medially placed radial tuberosity makes the biceps a stronger supinator (De Groote 2011b; Trinkaus & Churchill 1988). Furthermore, Neanderthal ulnae have a more distal brachialis insertion and larger mid-shaft and proximal epiphyses, all indicating that the joint reaction forces were likely much larger compared with modern humans (De Groote 2011b). Figure 5.3 also shows that Neanderthals had broader shoulders coupled

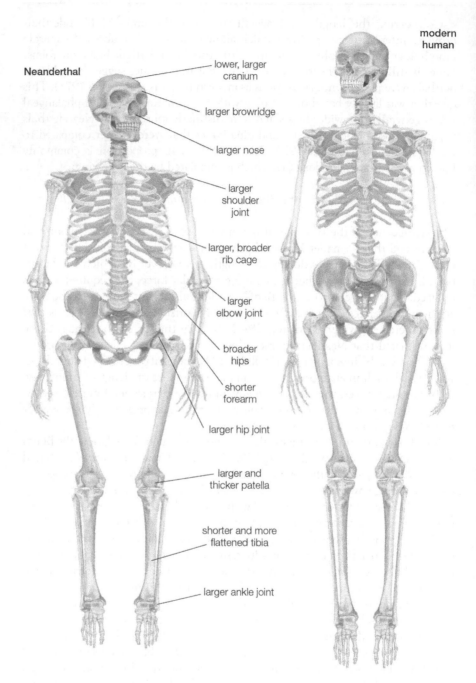

Figure 5.3 Neanderthal (left) and modern human (right) skeleton. With permission from Alamy Australia Pty Ltd.

with the larger shoulder joint. It has also been shown that the glenoid fossa in Neanderthals is elongated and shallow with less projecting articular rims compared to the deeper and broader glenoid fossa of modern humans (Macias & Churchill 2014). These distinct features necessitated larger muscle attachments and likely larger muscles generally. If this was the case, the one conclusion that can be drawn is that our closest extinct relatives certainly had a stronger, more powerful upper body.

The comparison of the upper limb morphology presents us with some useful points to speculate about our strength compared to that of the Neanderthals. Similarly and perhaps more salient is that the lower limb morphology of Neanderthals presents features suggesting quite different adaptations to our own: larger hip joint, larger and thicker patella and larger ankle joint (Figure 5.2). Not unlike the brachial index, the relative length of the lower leg to that of the thigh provides us with a measure known as crural index (CI):

$$CI = (\text{length of tibia} / \text{length of femur}) \times 100$$

Interestingly, the CI was also found to be smaller in Neanderthals compared with modern *H. sapiens* (Holliday 1999). Figure 5.4 compares the CI of Neanderthals, recent Europeans and male and female athletes competing in elite-level sports.

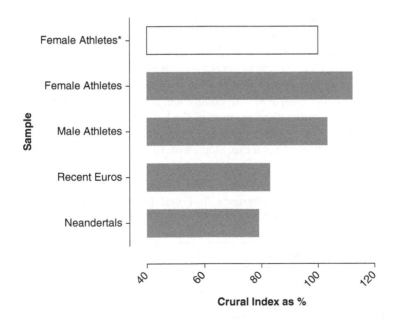

Figure 5.4 The crural index for male and female athletes from two different sports (basketball, *cricket) (Ackland et al. 1997; Stuelcken et al. 2007), recent Europeans and Neanderthals (Holliday 1999).

Unlike the BI, a wide array of data for the CI in various sports is somewhat scarce. Nevertheless, the CI for Neanderthals has been estimated to have been approximately 79%–80%, whereas this value increases to approximately 83% for recent Europeans (Holliday 1999). In Figure 5.4 the CI for male and female athletes is provided from two different sports (Ackland et al. 1997; Stuelcken et al. 2007). What is clear is that there is a seemingly remarkable increase in CI over time, commencing with Neanderthals, through to our elite athletic population. This increase illustrates the biomechanical differences and the probable morphology of skeletal muscle along with the potential advantages this might have provided these distinct groups. These data do not specifically permit any firm conclusions to be drawn as to whether the CI varies greatly from early to modern *Homo*, as far as the general population goes – only that our elite athletic population is likely to exhibit a very different CI.

For instance, Stewart et al. (2011) compared 1,146 athletes (829 males, 317 females) across endurance, speed, strength and combined sporting activities to 108 healthy controls. Their unique data shows that the CI varies overall by ~9% between the athletic group compared with controls. Generally, the athletic group has a larger CI, which also varies among sporting activity and by gender within each sport. Table 5.2 shows these per cent variations for each of the athletes within a sport and by gender.

Taking the data in Table 5.2 and extrapolating back to whether the CI in the modern human general population might vary compared to Neanderthals suggest that this is indeed the case, for if the largest variation from controls is ~9% as per the data provided by Stewart et al. (Stewart et al. 2011), this suggests that the CI for average modern humans is likely to be ~90% since the modern athletic population has a CI of ~100% as per the data in Figure 5.4. What is perhaps even more interesting, however, is that the CI associated with speed and strength is consistently smaller compared with endurance, at least for males. If we accept the general premise that the distal segment of the lower limb is comparatively shorter than the femur for activities that require speed and strength, then this characteristic must have a distinct advantage along with the accompanying skeletal muscle

Table 5.2 The percentage difference in crural index from the control group for each of the competitive athletic groups in different sports and by gender.

	Endurance	Speed	Strength	Combined
Male	6.8	1.2	0	7.0
Female	8.7	6.9	2.6	−0.23

Note: Combined is a group of athletes who participate in sports where endurance, speed and strength are requirements. The total N = 1146 (829 males, 317 females), Controls N = 108, Endurance N = 235, Speed N = 338, Strength N = 132, Combined N = 231.

Source: Data from Stewart et al. (2011).

morphology. Given that the evidence strongly suggests that Neanderthals possessed a smaller CI, it is then possible to speculate about their physical abilities and the kinds of activities that they likely engaged in.

A key element in the relationship between limb morphology and movement capability is the altered mechanics which accompany varying leg length. From a biomechanical perspective, changing the length of the tibia will effectively shift the centre of mass of the leg and its moment of inertia (square of the distance between the centre of mass and the axis of rotation) either proximally or distally to the knee joint. Since the knee joint provides the axis of rotation for extension and flexion of the leg, the inertial properties of the leg will be altered. Thus, if angular acceleration is increased by reducing the moment of inertia but with a concurrent maintenance of muscle torque by the quadriceps and hamstrings, the result will be greater speed and efficiency in locomotion.

A further consideration is not only the ratio of tibia to femur but also, not unlike the forearm, that the shape of the bones can play a significant part in the skeletal muscle morphology and the torque that can be developed. When comparing the femora of Neanderthals to those of early and recent modern humans, the Neanderthal femora exhibited the highest degree of anterior curvature followed by early modern humans, whereas the least curvature was observed in recent modern humans (De Groote 2011a). In addition to this characteristic, Neanderthals displayed a relatively larger femoral head, longer femoral neck, larger distal epiphyses and rounded femoral shaft and lacked a clear linea aspera (De Groote 2011a). These characteristic differences of the femur together with a shorter tibia suggest that Neanderthals had adapted a locomotor strategy for alternative needs. The resulting skeletal muscle morphology must have been adapted for carrying a relatively larger body mass with a better mechanical advantage because of a longer femoral neck. It is now also apparent that the terrain in which Neanderthals lived provides the clues as to their adapted skeletal and muscle morphology. A biomechanical analysis suggests that a shorter distal limb (tibia) length would be advantageous, since it provides for similar stride frequency to that of modern humans when moving over sloped and rugged terrain – a characteristic of bovines that inhabit such geography (Higgins & Ruff 2011). If one accepts that Neanderthals inhabited areas which were sloped and rugged, it follows that their lower limb skeletal muscle morphology was very likely adapted for strength and power rather than for endurance *per se*. This inference is partly supported by data which show that a reduced crural index is an advantageous feature, also possessed by athletic individuals that are agile and are capable of fast transition (Ackland et al. 1997). However, it is important to note that the lower limb morphology of the Neanderthals is not meant to imply that they did not possess the ability to develop endurance; rather, the need to develop such a capacity was perhaps not likely to be particularly useful.

From a biomechanical perspective, shorter limbs require the individual to either take more strides to cover a given distance or take strides more quickly to travel at the same speed as those individuals with longer limbs (Higgins & Ruff

2011). It is also apparent that the energy cost per kilogram per stride is almost the same for similar speeds over a range of animals (30g mouse – 200kg horse), and that the rate of energy consumption per kilogram of active muscle is directly proportional to stride frequency (Heglund & Taylor 1988). In considering this biomechanical principle, there are two fundamental processes that contribute to the energy cost of locomotion (Heglund & Taylor 1988). First, muscle activation itself amounts to approximately 30% of total energy cost, and second, force generation by cross-bridge recycling accounts for approximately 70% of the total energy cost. Thus, the cost of activation will be relative to how many times the muscles will need to be turned on and off, which will increase with stride frequency. In addition, a higher stride frequency will require faster rates of cross-bridge cycling for greater rates of force generation and decay (Heglund & Taylor 1988). Thus, the lower crural index of the Neanderthals at the very least meant that the energy cost of locomotion was higher than in modern humans, whose crural index is substantially larger (Steudel-Numbers & Tilkens 2004).

To elucidate the difference between early hominids and modern *Homo* with respect to energy cost of locomotion, an analysis of expired gases of human subjects with varying limb lengths while walking at various speeds (4.2, 4.5, 4.8 and 5.1 km/h) for 12 minutes, reveals an interesting relationship between limb length and mass (Steudel-Numbers & Tilkens 2004). When comparing these findings to published data on limb lengths, body mass and estimates of oxygen consumption for a number of species including *A. afarensis*, *H. habilis*, *H. erectus/ergaster*, Neanderthal, near modern and modern *Homo*, the total cost of oxygen per km was similar for Neanderthals only when accounting for the body mass with the additional lower limb length (Figure 5.5).

Conversely, in modern *Homo* the oxygen cost of locomotion increased substantially when the length of the lower limb was removed, and mass alone was used to estimate the efficiency. This study also showed that a smaller body mass

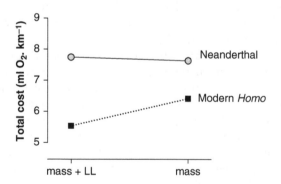

Figure 5.5 The total cost (ml O$_2$ m^{-1}) for locomotion when accounting for the body mass and lower limb length (LL) and body mass alone.

Source: Data taken from table 5.4 in Steudel-Numbers and Tilkens (2004).

with shorter limb lengths, such as in the *Australopiths*, would have reduced their overall locomotor efficiency; however, this reduced efficiency was likely mitigated by their need to retain some arboreal capabilities (Tilkens 2004).

To this point it seems that a lower CI would benefit locomotion on more rugged and sloping terrain as it allows for more enhanced agility through reduced angular inertia. In contrast, the low CI would be less advantageous for those individuals engaging in endurance running. Although lower limb length data and specifically CI data are scarce for modern-day long distance runners, the available evidence does indicate that a relative higher CI would be an advantage. The limited data on lower limb lengths indicate that for well-conditioned 18–40-year-old male runners, the CI was 85.6% (Kram 1989). This number is still relatively larger than the estimate for Neanderthals, which stands at around 80% (Figure 5.4). It is also interesting to note that there may be an optimal body morphology suited to endurance running, since it appears that heights and masses of males winning the Boston Marathon have remained relatively constant for over a century (Norton & Olds 1996). That is, the mean height has remained stable at 171.3 ± 5.4 cm and mass at 61.6 ± 5.1 kg, which is in contrast to the secular trend for the general population, where the increase in height seems to be ~1 cm per decade (Norton & Olds 1996). Although studies have shown that body morphology is a determining factor for successful endurance running, the reasons for this are not fully understood. It appears that beyond the biomechanical advantage that comes with different limb lengths, morphology could also play a role in the regulation of temperature during endurance running (Havenith 2001; Marino et al. 2004; Marino et al. 2000).

Although the comparison between modern humans and Neanderthals provides some basis on which to extrapolate why muscle morphology could have played a decisive role in the choice between power and endurance, there is a further comparison to be made between the Neanderthal and Cro-Magnon (originally named after its location of discovery, *Abri de Cro-Magnon*), now regarded as European Early Modern Humans (EEMH) living around 45,000–43,000 years ago. This is an important comparison as it provides clues as to not only the different morphology but also differences in culture. Figure 5.6 provides a summary of the known cultural and physical similarities and differences between the Neanderthal and EEMH. The cultural similarities give some insight into the lifestyles of these two distinct groups, but it is perhaps the physical differences that provide further evidence for their preferences in acquiring nourishment. Note that both were meat eaters and by definition likely to be hunters. Since EEMH existence spans some 45,000–40,000 years ago, a key difference was that projectile weaponry was available to them since this artefact is dated at most 100,000–71,000 years ago (Marean 2015). The differences in hunting methods between EEMH and Neanderthals are an important distinction. The available evidence from the fossil remains of Neanderthals indicates significant trauma to the head and neck but less so to the upper limb (Trinkaus & Zimmerman 1982). It is also postulated that this kind of trauma was related to their normal means

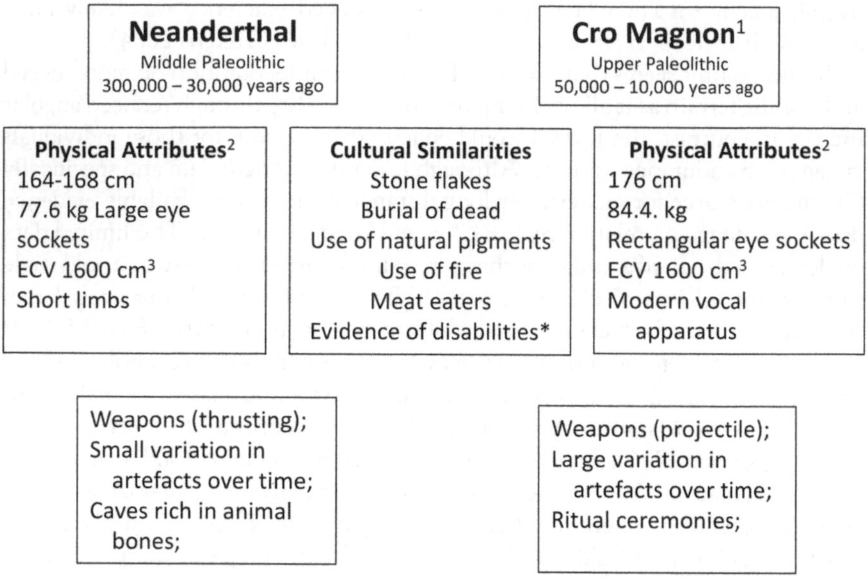

Neanderthal Middle Paleolithic 300,000 – 30,000 years ago		Cro Magnon[1] Upper Paleolithic 50,000 – 10,000 years ago

Physical Attributes[2] 164-168 cm 77.6 kg Large eye sockets ECV 1600 cm³ Short limbs	Cultural Similarities Stone flakes Burial of dead Use of natural pigments Use of fire Meat eaters Evidence of disabilities*	Physical Attributes[2] 176 cm 84.4. kg Rectangular eye sockets ECV 1600 cm³ Modern vocal apparatus

Weapons (thrusting); Small variation in artefacts over time; Caves rich in animal bones;		Weapons (projectile); Large variation in artefacts over time; Ritual ceremonies;

Figure 5.6 A comparison of the culture and physical attributes of Neanderthal and Cro-Magnon. [1]Current terminology uses the term 'European Early Modern Humans' (EEMH) instead of Cro-Magnon. [2]For males only for the purpose of comparison. *There is evidence for debilitating disease suggesting care for elderly and sick members. ECV is endo cranial volume.

Source: From Klein (2003).

of predation, whereby Neanderthals mainly hunted medium-sized ungulates and large-sized bovines at close quarters because of the weaponry available to them (Berger & Trinkaus 1995). That is, the fact that Neanderthals very likely did not have projectile weaponry available or used it sparingly, coupled with short powerful limbs, suggests that thrusting and close-quarter hunting were their method of procuring food (Churchill 1993). As such, these physical attributes – lower brachial and crural indices, being agile over rugged and sloped terrain but likely inefficient with endurance – together with the apparent inability to utilise projectile weaponry other than at close encounters with large animals, would have made the Neanderthal existence more difficult compared with the EEMH.

Thus far we have discussed the advantages and disadvantages of limb size and shape and the accompanying muscle morphology with respect to the strength, power and endurance capabilities of our distant relatives compared with modern *Homo*. It is apparent that our ancestors, particularly Neanderthals, had shorter limbs mainly due to the length of the distal segment of both the upper and lower limbs. The resulting biomechanics suggest that shorter limbs were likely a disadvantage if the goal was to achieve a useful endurance capacity, but advantageous if strength and power were the preferred adaptation. It also seems that Neanderthals had a distinct advantage if the ecology was sloped and rugged since this would require better agility rather than endurance *per se*. However, shorter limbs must have provided further distinct advantages beyond the biomechanics since Neanderthals lived for a relatively long period – some 400,000 years ago before their sudden disappearance about 40,000 years ago (Pinhasi et al. 2011).

It has been thought for some time that there is a direct relationship between limb morphology and the ambient temperature conditions in which animals live. This was first suggested by Joel Allen in 1877 and is commonly referred to as Allen's rule (Allen 1877). This hypothesis in its simple form suggests that animals adapted for cold climates have relatively shorter limbs, or more precisely that in cold climates limbs tend to exhibit high volume-to-surface and low surface-to-volume ratios. This observation is particularly important as it can potentially explain, in part, the adaptations that were required by different species of *Homo* at different times for different environments. For example, in a detailed analysis of the available fossil data at the time, it was shown that brachial and crural indices were higher in populations living in the tropics (Trinkaus 1981). Thus, individuals with longer limbs will have a greater relative surface area compared with individuals with shorter limbs, and since the avenues of heat loss and/or gain are highly dependent on surface area, the capacity to offload or retain heat can be a distinct advantage in a given climate (Havenith et al. 1995). In essence, the ability to either offload heat or retain heat is a critical component for survival in warmer and colder climates, respectively.

However, the hypothesis that limb length adaptation is due to climatic selection has been challenged. It is apparent that Upper Paleolithic populations (see Figure 5.6, European Early Modern Humans) do not particularly show evidence of shorter distal limb adaptation. Thus, if this population was indeed descended from a population that was from Africa and heat-adapted, one would expect that they exhibit an adjustment towards shorter limb lengths if this feature was indeed a thermal advantage and driven by climate (Frayer et al. 1993). In an effort to clarify this apparent discrepancy others have measured the average oxygen consumption (VO_2) during rest in both males and females with a gradient of ~15°C between the ambient temperature and body core, thus allowing for body heat loss to occur (Tilkens et al. 2007). Figure 5.7 shows three different regression lines for thigh length, shank length and total limb length against the resting metabolic rate (Tilkens et al. 2007).

Crucially, the analysis of the three lengths shows that the thigh length and not the shank length was the predictive characteristic, indicating that the total limb length is the most critical factor with respect to driving the metabolic rate. In other words, changing the length of the shank (tibia) did not seem to provide a thermal advantage, whereas maintaining the length of the thigh and hence the total length of the lower limb provided the thermal advantage, with the correlation being $r = 0.79$. This result was further confirmed when accounting for lean

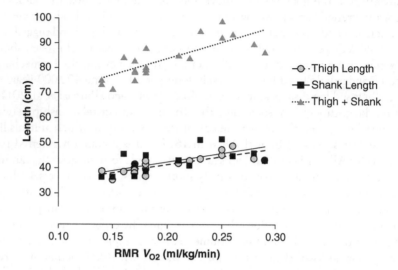

Figure 5.7 Regressions for the prediction of resting metabolic rate (RMR) with respect to thigh length, shank length and total length (thigh + shank). The data represent 20 (11 males 75.39 ± 10.95 kg and 9 females 70.53 ± 11.6) volunteers while sitting exposed to 21.9°C ambient temperature. The regression for thigh length is $y = 62.56 \times RMR + 28.85$ ($R^2 = 0.66, P < 0.0001$), shank length is $y = 68.10 \times RMR + 28.73$ ($R^2 = 0.47, P < 0.0008$) and total length (thigh + shank) is $y = 130.7 \times RMR + 57.57$ ($R^2 = 0.63, P < 0.0001$). Note that lengths were collected with the use of callipers.

Source: Data redrawn and reanalysed from table 5.1 in Tilkens et al. (2007).

mass and percent body fat, whereby no significant correlation was found for the shank and resting metabolic rate. Therefore, shorter overall limbs may not be as useful as longer limbs with respect to locomotion over long distances, but the fact that the resting metabolic rate was lower with shorter limbs suggests that Neanderthals when compared with modern *Homo* may have had a distinct thermoregulatory advantage in colder climates (Tilkens et al. 2007).

Finally, although the morphology of limbs and their accompanying skeletal muscle structure play a key role in the biomechanics and metabolic and thermoregulatory capacities of individuals, it is the total cost of having shorter limbs, such as the Neanderthals, or longer limbs, as seen in modern *Homo*, that is critical to understanding the choice between power and endurance, and therefore fatigue resistance. By using the estimated mass, stature and body surface area of fossil remains of Neanderthals (5 females, 16 males) from separate studies, it was estimated that the absolute surface area of Neanderthals was greater than modern humans (Churchill 2006). Specifically, these data show Neanderthals as having

5%–6% more skin and being 11%–13% more massive for a given stature, resulting in a lower surface area to mass ratio. If this was the case and applying the known estimations of basal metabolic rate (BMR) as previously proposed (Sorensen & Leonard 2001), then Neanderthals needed somewhere between 3,500 and 5,500 kcal per adult.d^{-1}. In putting this energy estimate into context, it has been suggested that the energetic needs of Neanderthals likely required at least 2 kg of meat per day, which would be equivalent to a hunting return of 3.8–7.6 kg hunter^{-1}.d^{-1}, depending on whether both males and females were engaged in the practice (Churchill 2006). On this basis alone, it indicates that Neanderthal existence was more energy costly and would likely be more so in colder environments. However, the critical point here is that given the robustness of Neanderthals, as suggested by their skeleton and their musculature, their body density would have been relatively higher compared to modern humans. Ultimately, this would have required higher energy yields for the higher energy needs. Whether Neanderthals could meet this demand has been the subject of intense investigation and indeed posited as one potential contribution for their extinction (Bar Yosef 2004; Hockett & Haws 2005). However, the potential reasons for Neanderthal extinction are beyond the scope of this discussion.

What is most important is whether the energy usage and yield potential can in some way account for the preference between endurance and power as a method of subsistence. Since Neanderthal populations lived for many thousands of years, their ability to acquire nourishment was likely enough for their high metabolic turnover. Nevertheless, when comparing modern-day foragers and hunter populations to Neanderthals, the difference in total energy expenditure per day is striking. Modern-day foragers and hunters require 2,000–3,670 kcal/d compared with the 4,422–6,633 kcal/d for Neanderthals (Sorensen & Leonard 2001). Thus, as already mentioned, the total energy requirement to sustain Neanderthal subsistence was markedly higher, and when coupled with the likelihood that Neanderthals had higher thermoregulatory costs and acquired their energy from hunting at close range, suggests that conservation of energy would have been imperative. Since it has already been established that Neanderthal limb and body morphology was adapted for power, strength and agility rather than for endurance, their higher energy requirements along with the need to obtain higher energy yields from the environment meant that apportioning any energy to other survival needs, such as reproduction and growth, was critical. This is an important mechanism to consider since with very few exceptions there is an apparent negative correlation between the energy invested in reproduction and the subsequent survival and/or reproductive performance of the parent (Calow 1979; Walker et al. 2008). The central tenet of this hypothesis is that energy required for reproduction will trade off with the nutrient allocation for metabolism, immune function and most other cellular processes. In fact, experimental evidence corroborates that when an animal has its capability for reproduction removed, such as with ovariectomy, the result is increased survival and growth and enhanced energy storage and immune function (Cox et al. 2010).

There are two further pieces of evidence to consider with respect to the nutrient trade-off mechanism. As discussed in Chapter 1, an increase in brain size escalated the energy needs, since larger brains consume up to 25% of the metabolic demand in humans (Zauner & Muizelaar 1997). In addition, the ECV of Neanderthals has been estimated to be 1,490 cm^3 compared to the 1,410 cm^3 for *H. sapiens* (Chapter 3, Figure 3.7). Whether this extra ECV alone significantly increased the energy demands of Neanderthal brain tissue is unknown. However, when this characteristic is added to other adaptations, such as more massive bodies, shorter limbs, more robust skeletal muscle structure and higher thermoregulatory costs, the higher energy requirements for Neanderthals resulted in a constant choice that modern *Homo* may have been better equipped to make. Modern *Homo* morphology (longer limbs, heat dissipation, smaller gut) is adapted for endurance, and since modern foragers and hunters seemingly use less energy, there is greater potential for energy to be apportioned for growth and reproduction. The fact that modern *Homo* was adapted for endurance and fatigue resistance may represent a better option for conservation and the acquiring of energy needs.

Morphology, skeletal muscle and temperature

The relationship between morphology, skeletal muscle and temperature is not an obvious one with respect to adaptation and performance. Yet, we intuitively understand that warmer skeletal muscles are likely to perform better compared to cooler muscles. Although this understanding is supported by long-standing empirical evidence, it is the trade-off between limb morphology and temperature that is perhaps most important to consider. We have already discussed the advantages that shorter limbs provide in terms of biomechanics, skeletal muscle force production and thermoregulation, in particular how shorter distal segments are adapted for power rather than for endurance. Thus, using the Neanderthal limb morphology as a comparative model presents an enticing relationship to explore with respect to the choice between endurance and power. In order to explore this potential relationship a key assumption is required – that Neanderthals primarily lived in an ecology that was habitually cold, so that shorter limbs and wider bodies were necessary adaptations for this climate (Ruff 1991). Although advantageous for the conservation of heat, this limb morphology comes at a cost in relation to performance.

An accepted physiological phenomenon is that muscle temperature alters the force-generating capacity of skeletal muscle. In basic terms, skeletal muscle produces greater forces when closer to a core temperature of 37°C. There are a variety of ways in which to achieve higher skeletal muscle temperatures, although the main method involves physically warming up, which in turn increases the metabolic heat production and muscle blood flow. The outcome of warming up is based on the findings from many studies that show reduced force production as muscle temperature decreases, as shown in Figure 5.8. The data in this figure indicate that between muscle temperatures of 35°C and 25°C, the reduction in

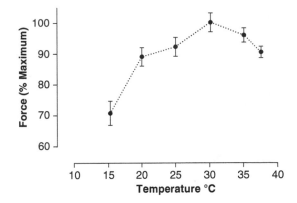

Figure 5.8 The percentage of maximum force produced by the first dorsal interosseous muscle of humans at different skin temperatures. Note that
muscle temperature was estimated from skin temperature as is usually
the case with good agreement normally reported, especially for the
hand.

Source: Data redrawn from Ranatunga et al. (1987).

isometric force production changes little, but as temperature approaches 20°C
and below, there are significant reductions in force production, as has also been
observed in other animals (Lännergren & Westerblad 1987; Johnston & Gleeson
1984). This observation also suggests that there is a high degree of tolerance in
maximal force production as muscle temperature drops from normal physiological
values. This tolerance appears to be as much as 15°C (James 2013). However, the
limitation to consider here is that the majority of studies that report this tolerance in muscle temperature reduction before force is significantly reduced do so
while measuring muscular force by isometric contractions. Although useful, isometric muscular contractions limit our understanding, since movement requires
dynamic contractions.

It appears that when examining the effect of temperature on skeletal muscle
performance during concentric contractions, force output and angular velocity
are reduced as muscle temperature decreases from 37°C to 22°C (de Ruiter 2000)
(Figure 5.9). The reasons for the decrease in both force and velocity with reductions in muscle temperature are varied.

One potential reason could be that slow-twitch muscle fibres are more sensi-
tive to temperature changes than fast-twitch muscle fibres (Bottinelli et al. 1996).
Thus, as the adductor pollicus muscle is mainly composed of slow-twitch fibres
(Round et al. 1984) it may be that changes in force are related to the specific
muscle characteristic and temperature interaction than just temperature alone.
However, this may not be the case with all skeletal muscles, particularly those

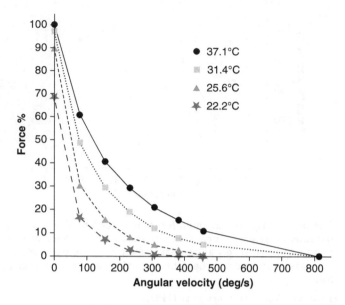

Figure 5.9 The force/velocity relationship of the adductor pollicus muscle at temperatures from 37.1°C to 22.2°C.

Source: Data redrawn from de Ruiter (2000).

muscles with larger bellies and composed of mixed fibre types, such as the triceps surae (Davies & Mecrow 1982). Nevertheless, the effects of temperature on the hand muscles are pertinent to this discussion since this area is more likely to be influenced by large fluctuations in ambient temperature. However, when other gross movements, such as jumping and sprinting, were evaluated when muscle temperatures ranged between 30°C and 39°C, jump heights and sprinting speeds were significantly reduced at the lower temperatures (Asmussen et al. 1976; Bergh & Ekblom 1979). A curious observation reported by others (Sargeant 1987) is that when muscle temperature was reduced to around 26°C, the rate of fatigue was approximately half that observed when muscle temperature was increased to 40°C (12 W.s^{-1} vs 33 W.s^{-1}). In other words, even though a lower muscle temperature produced lower maximal power output, the rate of fatigue was also lower with lower muscle temperatures. The reasons for this remain unclear, although it has been suggested that there is a greater energy turnover when muscle temperature is higher. However, this does not mean that depletion of adenosine triphosphate is faster under these higher muscle temperature conditions; rather it is likely to be due to the reduced rate of replenishment of energy stores (Edwards et al. 1972).

In considering the relationship between skeletal muscle temperature and survival, recall that shorter limbs are more able to conserve heat, thereby allowing the underlying skeletal muscles to maintain an adequate temperature. Maintaining adequate muscle temperature is essential in force development, and although studies evaluating the effect of muscle temperature on force output generally suggest that there is a 15°C tolerance before tension development is reduced, it also seems that during dynamic contractions the tolerance for temperature reductions is likely to be of less magnitude (see Figure 5.9). The capacity for shorter limbs to develop greater tension and to reduce heat loss is an advantage. Conversely, longer limbs provide for better heat dissipation and are advantageous in developing endurance. The choice for longer limbs by modern *Homo* seems to have favoured endurance capacity.

References

Ackland, T.R., Schreiner, A.B. & Kerr, D.A., 1997. Absolute size and proportionality characteristics of World Championship female basketball players. *Journal of Sports Science and Medicine*, 15(5), pp. 485–490.

Allen, J.A., 1877. The influence of physical conditions in the genesis of species. *Radical Review*, 1, pp. 108–140.

Asmussen, E., Bonde-Petersen, F. & Jørgensen, K., 1976. Mechano-elastic properties of human muscles at different temperatures. *Acta Physiologica Scandinavica*, 96(1), pp. 83–93.

Bar Yosef, O., 2004. Eat what is there: hunting and gathering in the world of Neanderthals and their neighbours. *International Journal of Osteoarchaeology*, 14(3–4), pp. 333–342.

Berger, T.D. & Trinkaus, E., 1995. Patterns of trauma among the Neandertals. *Journal of Archaeological Science*, 22(6), pp. 841–852.

Bergh, U. & Ekblom, B., 1979. Influence of muscle temperature on maximal muscle strength and power output in human skeletal muscles. *Acta Physiologica*, 107(1), pp. 33–37.

Boer, P., 1984. Estimated lean body mass as an index for normalization of body fluid volumes in humans. *American Journal of Physiology-Renal Physiology*, 247(4), pp. F632–F636.

Bottinelli, R. et al., 1996. Force-velocity properties of human skeletal muscle fibres: myosin heavy chain isoform and temperature dependence. *Journal of Physiology*, 495(2), pp. 573–586.

Calow, P., 1979. The cost of reproduction – a physiological approach. *Biological Reviews*, 54(1), pp. 23–40.

Churchill, S.E., 1993. Weapon technology, prey size selection, and hunting methods in modern hunter-gatherers: implications for hunting in the Palaeolithic and Mesolithic. *Archeological Papers of the American Anthropological Association*, 4(1), pp. 11–24.

Churchill, S.E., 2006. Bioenergetic perspectives on Neanderthal thermoregulatory and activity budgets. In K. Harvati & T. Harrison, eds. *Neanderthals revisited: new approaches and perspectives*. Dordrecht, The Netherlands: Springer, pp. 113–133.

Cox, R.M. et al., 2010. Experimental evidence for physiological costs underlying the trade-off between reproduction and survival. *Functional Ecology*, 24, pp. 1262–1269.

Davies, C. & Mecrow, I.K., 1982. Contractile properties of the human triceps surae with some observations on the effects of temperature and exercise. *European Journal of Applied Physiology*, 49(2), pp. 255–269.

De Groote, I., 2011a. Femoral curvature in Neanderthals and modern humans: a 3D geometric morphometric analysis. *Journal of Human Evolution*, 60(5), pp. 540–548.

De Groote, I., 2011b. The Neanderthal lower arm. *Journal of Human Evolution*, 61(4), pp. 396–410.

de Ruiter, C.J., 2000. Temperature effect on the force/velocity relationship of the fresh and fatigued human adductor pollicis muscle. *Pflügers Archives*, 440(1), pp. 163–170.

Edwards, R.H.T., Hultman, E. & Koh, D., 1972. Effect of temperature on muscle energy metabolism and endurance during successive isometric contractions, sustained to fatigue, of the quadriceps muscle in man. *Journal of Physiology*, 220(2), pp. 335–352.

Engbers, F.H. et al., 2010. Pharmacokinetic models for propofol: defining and illuminating the devil in the detail. *British Journal of Anaesthesia*, 104(2), pp. 261–264.

Frayer, D.W. et al., 1993. Theories of modern human origins: the paleontological test. *American Anthropologist*, 95(1), pp. 14–50.

Havenith, G., 2001. Human surface to mass ratio and body core temperature in exercise heat stress – a concept revisited. *Journal of Thermal Biology*, 26(4–5), pp. 387–393.

Havenith, G., Luttikholt, V.G. & Vrijkotte, T., 1995. The relative influence of body characteristics on humid heat stress response. *European Journal of Applied Physiology*, 70(3), pp. 270–279.

Heglund, N.C. & Taylor, C.R., 1988. Speed, stride frequency and energy cost per stride: how do they change with body size and gait? *Journal of Experimental Biology*, 138(1), pp. 301–318.

Higgins, R.W. & Ruff, C.B., 2011. The effects of distal limb segment shortening on locomotor efficiency in sloped terrain: implications for Neandertal locomotor behavior. *American Journal of Physical Anthropology*, 146(3), pp. 336–345.

Hockett, B. & Haws, J.A., 2005. Nutritional ecology and the human demography of Neandertal extinction. *Quaternary International*, 137(1), pp. 21–34.

Holliday, T.W., 1999. Brachial and crural indices of European late Upper Paleolithic and Mesolithic humans. *Journal of Human Evolution*, 36(5), pp. 549–566.

Hume, R., 1966. Prediction of lean body mass from height and weight. *Journal of Clinical Pathology*, 19(4), pp. 389–391.

James, R.S., 2013. A review of the thermal sensitivity of the mechanics of vertebrate skeletal muscle. *Journal of Comparative Physiology B*, 183(6), pp. 723–733.

Johnston, I.A. & Gleeson, T.T., 1984. Thermal dependence of contractile properties of red and white fibres isolated from the iliofibularis muscle of the desert Iguana (Dipsosaurus dorsalis). *Journal of Experimental Biology*, 113(1), pp. 123–132.

Kappelman, J., 1996. The evolution of body mass and relative brain size in fossil hominids. *Journal of Human Evolution*, 30(3), pp. 243–276.

Klein, R.G., 2003. Whither the Neanderthals? *Scientific American*, 299(5612), pp. 1525–1527.

Kram, R., 1989. Stride length in distance running: velocity, body dimensions, and added mass effects. *Medicine and Science in Sports & Exercise*, 21(4), pp. 467–479.

Lännergren, J. & Westerblad, H., 1987. The temperature dependence of isometric contractions of single, intact fibres dissected from a mouse foot muscle. *Journal of Physiology*, 390(1), pp. 285–293.

Macias, M.E. & Churchill, S.E., 2014. Functional morphology of the Neandertal scapular glenoid fossa C. Terhune, S.B. Cooke & J.T. Laitman, eds. *The Anatomical Record*, 298(1), pp. 168–179.

Marean, C., 2015. The most invasive species of all. *Scientific American*, 313(2), pp. 23–29.

Marino, F.E., Lambert, M.I. & Noakes, T.D., 2004. Superior performance of African runners in warm humid but not in cool environmental conditions. *Journal of Applied Physiology*, 96, pp. 124–130.

Marino, F.E. et al., 2000. Advantages of smaller body mass during distance running in warm, humid environments. *Pflügers Archives*, 441(2–3), pp. 359–367.

Musgrave, J.H., 1971. How dextrous was Neanderthal man? *Nature*, 233(5321), pp. 538–541.

Norton, K. & Olds, T., 1996. *Anthropometrica: a textbook of body measurement for sports and health courses*, Sydney: UNSW Press.

Pearson, O.M., Cordero, R.M. & Busby, A.M., 2006. How different were Neanderthals' habitual activities? A comparative analysis with diverse groups of recent humans. In J.-J. Hublin, K. Harvati & T. Harrison, eds. *Neanderthals revisited: new approaches and perspectives*. Vertebrate Paleobiology and Paleoanthropology. Dordrecht, The Netherlands: Springer, pp. 135–156.

Pinhasi, R. et al., 2011. Revised age of late Neanderthal occupation and the end of the Middle Paleolithic in the northern Caucasus. *Proceedings of the National Academy of Sciences*, 108(21), pp. 8611–8616.

Porter, A.M.W., 1999. Modern human, early modern human and Neanderthal limb proportions. *International Journal of Osteoarchaeology*, 9(1), pp. 54–67.

Round, J.M. et al., 1984. The anatomy and fibre type composition of the human adductor pollicis in relation to its contractile properties. *Journal of the Neurological Sciences*, 66(2), pp. 263–272.

Ranatunga, K.W., Sharpe, B. & Turnbull, B., 1987. Contractions of a human skeletal muscle at different temperatures. *Journal of Physiology*, 390(1), pp. 383–395.

Ruff, C.B., 1991. Climate and body shape in hominid evolution. *Journal of Human Evolution*, 21(2), pp. 81–105.

Sargeant, A.J., 1987. Effect of muscle temperature on leg extension force and short-term power output in humans. *European Journal of Applied Physiology*, 56(6), pp. 693–698.

Sorensen, M.V. & Leonard, W.R., 2001. Neandertal energetics and foraging efficiency. *Journal of Human Evolution*, 40(6), pp. 483–495.

Steudel-Numbers, K.L. & Tilkens, M.J., 2004. The effect of lower limb length on the energetic cost of locomotion: implications for fossil hominins. *Journal of Human Evolution*, 47(1–2), pp. 95–109.

Stewart, A.D., Benson, P.J. & Olds, T., 2011. Self selection of athletes into sports via skeletal ratios. *Journal of Contemporary Athletics*, 5(2), pp. 153–167.

Stuelcken, M., Pyne, D. & Sinclair, P., 2007. Anthropometric characteristics of elite cricket fast bowlers. *Journal of Sports Science and Medicine*, 25(14), pp. 1587–1597.

Steudel-Numbers, K.L. & Tilkens, M.J., 2004. The effect of lower limb length on the energetic cost of locomotion: implications for fossil hominins. *Journal of Human Evolution*, 47(1), pp. 95–109.

Tilkens, M.J. et al., 2007. The effects of body proportions on thermoregulation: an experimental assessment of Allen's rule. *Journal of Human Evolution*, 53(3), pp. 286–291.

Trinkaus, E., 1981. Neanderthal limb proportions and cold adaptation. In C.B. Stringer, ed. *Aspects of human evolution*. London: Taylor & Francis, pp. 187–224.

Trinkaus, E. & Churchill, S.E., 1988. Neandertal radial tuberosity orientation. *American Journal of Physical Anthropology*, 75(1), pp. 15–21.

Trinkaus, E. & Zimmerman, M.R., 1982. Trauma among the Shanidar Neandertals. *American Journal of Physical Anthropology*, 57(1), pp. 61–76.

Walker, R.S. et al., 2008. The trade-off between number and size of offspring in humans and other primates. *Proceedings of the Royal Society B: Biological Sciences*, 275(1636), pp. 827–833.

Walpole, S.C., Prieto-Merino, D., Edwards, P., Cleland, J., Stevens, G. & Roberts, I., 2012. The weight of nations: an estimation of adult human biomass. BMC *Public Health*, 12(1), p. 439.

Walter, C., 2013. *Last ape standing: the seven-million-year story of how and why we survived,* New York: Bloomsbury Publishing.

Zauner, A. & Muizelaar, J.P., 1997. Brain metabolism and cerebral blood flow. *Head Injury*, pp. 89–99.

Chapter 6

The brain

The emotional aspect of fatigue

There is no instinct like that of the heart.

– Lord Byron (1788–1824)

Introduction

In the preceding chapters, fatigue was discussed in relation to biological structures and processes identified as either limiting human performance or precipitating the process of fatigue, and how evolutionary theory can help explain the
fatigue phenomenon. The cornerstone of this understanding is the measurement
of the decline in skeletal muscle performance (see Chapter 4). In reality, the
measurement and evaluation of that performance are only a manifestation of processes originating elsewhere in the body. In an attempt to further understand the
fatigue phenomenon, scientists now believe there is enough evidence to suggest
that fatigue could also be related to emotion – a relationship with the feelings of
tiredness, malaise and depression which in turn are able to heighten the sensations of fatigue. This makes evolutionary sense since the expression of emotion
contributes in any number ways to fulfilling needs and ultimately survival. It is
not inconsequential that the expression of emotions will provide cues to onlookers about what is needed at critical times by the individual expressing that emotion; pain, for example, can be expressed in a number of ways which will signal
a need to be removed from that stimulus causing the pain or for others to render
assistance. In fact, emotions expressing pain are thought to enhance social interactions (Craig 2009) and potentially heighten cortical activity of the observer
(Reicherts et al. 2012).

Understanding fatigue as an emotion has its roots in the concept outlined by
Mosso's classic text (Mosso 1891), which is likely to be the first such attempt to
describe a central nervous system component to fatigue. When translated from
the original Italian, the text suggests that

> in raising a weight we must take account of two factors, both susceptible to
> fatigue. The first is of central origin and purely nervous in character – namely,

the will; the second is peripheral, and is the chemical force which is transformed into mechanical work.

(Mosso 1904, pp. 152–153)

Mosso also recognised that his experiments indirectly showed that the reduction of muscular force was one observation, but critically fatigue can also be a sensation since there can be a reduction in force output even when there is no apparent or organic reason for its decline. Perhaps the most prescient observation by Mosso was that fatigue, which

> at first sight might appear an imperfection of our body, is on the contrary one of its most marvelous perfections. The fatigue increasing more rapidly than the amount of work done saves us from the injury which lesser sensibility would involve for the organism.
>
> (p. 156)

Thus, fatigue was thought of as a protective mechanism rather than one of catastrophe. In fact, the influential exercise physiology text by Bainbridge (1931) also recognised at the time that fatigue arising from the nervous system is "superadded" by the fatigue arising from the skeletal muscles (p. 228). This at least suggested that fatigue was likely to be multifaceted and involved the brain. Since the extent and the type of involvement from the nervous system were yet to be defined, a generation of exercise physiologists seemingly concentrated on the fatigue originating from the periphery – namely, the skeletal muscle. Thinking of fatigue as a sensation was lost until relatively recently, when studies began to show that muscular fatigue was also influenced by other less well-defined factors, such as perceived effort. It is now apparent that fatigue could also have an emotional aspect, adding to the complexity of this human response.

What are emotions?

To understand whether fatigue could in fact be an emotion, the first question to answer is, what is an emotion? This is perhaps the most difficult question to answer in all of physiology and psychology. We constantly use the term to convey a particular meaning ascribed to behaviour and to some of the decisions we make. The often used phrases "don't let your emotions get the better of you" and "I've been on an emotional rollercoaster" convey a deep connection between the mind, decisions and our eventual actions. It is also no wonder that society establishes rules and regulations which, in spirit, attempt to detach decisions from emotions since we recognise that decisions made under duress or euphoria can ultimately be biased rather than reasoned. Even the legal profession requires that a lawyer represent his or her client zealously within the bounds of the law. On the other hand, we might ask whether it is even remotely possible to make any decision without an emotional element.

Emotions have long been recognised as an intimate expression of who we are individually and collectively. In fact, Darwin's text titled "The Expression of the Emotions in Man and Animals" (Darwin 1993[1872]) stands as a comprehensive description outlining in great detail how behaviour reflects emotions in any given context. Darwin's text comes complete with line drawings of animal expressions which we recognise as pleasure, disappointment, fear or defence, among others. These are emotions which we predict and assess from observing expressions. For instance, when footballers clash in a tackle, we can immediately recognise from either their expression or body language whether there is pain, and whether the pain is excruciating or moderate. Similarly, when a runner crosses the finish line we can immediately recognise whether he or she is experiencing relief, exhaustion or ecstasy. These examples provide us mainly with intuitive and anecdotal evidence that there is at least an emotional component which we can interpret as being related to some level of fatigue. But this would be a simplistic understanding of the emotional relatedness of fatigue, since it does not explain whether an emotion can be triggered with or without some change in the physiological state. This is a conundrum which has plagued psycho-physiology for at least two centuries. Even though modern investigative techniques, such as functional neuroimaging, have provided us with a window into the various regions of the brain that might be involved with emotion, we are still grappling with what defines those feelings that we identify as emotions. Before considering the potential brain structures that might be involved in generating emotions, we need first to acknowledge the two most influential theories of emotion which have been used to study this complex phenomenon. Regardless of which regions of the brain are involved, we still require a construct to apply our understanding.

In 1884, William James, independently of Carl Lange in 1885, developed a theory of emotion based on the premise that we experience emotion in response to physiological changes occurring in the body (Dalgleish 2004). This became known as the James-Lange theory of emotion. Essentially, this theory proposed that the physiological changes are indeed the emotion and when these are extinguished or dampened the emotion is also removed. In simple terms, we might feel sad because we cry, not the other way around. The James-Lange theory was debated for many years as it seemed to be the complete opposite to the common experience, where a given situation would evoke the emotional response, giving rise to the physiological changes associated with that emotion. An example which would argue against the James-Lange theory is that the emotions we identify as love or even sympathy can still be experienced even when the physiological changes usually associated with these, such as a fast heart rate, sweaty palms and crying, are no longer exhibited. In other words, we do not stop loving a person because our heart rate is no longer racing in their presence. This rather intuitive observation led others to challenge the James-Lang theory, and by 1927 Walter Cannon published a critique proposing a new theory of emotion, which was subsequently modified by Philip Bard (Dalgleish 2004). This theory became known as the Cannon-Bard theory of emotion. The cornerstone of this theory was that emotions can be experienced even if physiological changes cannot be sensed. As proof, Cannon offered animal studies where the transection of the spinal cord eliminated sensory input, but the emotion was not abolished. That is, if emotional experience is due to the brain sensing a change in physiological status, then removing that sensation should also remove the capacity to experience the emotion, as predicted by the James-Lange theory. However, Cannon's and Bard's observations only seemed to confirm the opposite.

A further observation by Cannon was the consistent paradox between emotion and any given physiological response. For instance, anger is accompanied by increased heart rate and sweating but so are fear and other illnesses. How can these physiological responses be associated with a multitude of other emotions as well as anger? The answer to this may be found partly in the classic study by Ax (1953), who found a difference in the response pattern between fear and anger with respect to respiratory rate and the number of skeletal muscle action potentials. Fear showed an increase in breathing rate and more muscle action potentials, whereas anger was dominated by increases in blood pressure and a decrease in heart rate. The author concluded that fear was likely influenced by the effects of the hormone epinephrine, whereas anger was influenced by the combined effects of both epinephrine and norepinephrine. Subsequently, it was shown in pilots that epinephrine was elevated before, during and after being subjected to a stressful experience, but norepinephrine seemed to be elevated only during and after the experience (Goodall 1962). The inference that can be drawn here is that specifically norepinephrine secretion is more likely to be associated with active physical effort, whereas epinephrine under these conditions is more likely to be related to anxiety. The relationship between hormonal regulation, emotions and the physiological responses that are seemingly an outcome of this relationship is highly complex. Making sense of how emotions, performance and fatigue are related is extremely difficult since separating measurable physiological responses and attaching those to a particular emotion are challenging, as recognised by the early researchers.

Nevertheless, others have shown that the expression of emotion is intimately connected with and can also be independent of a particular stimulus generating the sensation. For example, pain and emotion are thought to be intimately connected, as was shown when individuals were simultaneously subjected to painful thermal stimuli and typical facial expressions categorised as either joy, neutral, fear or pain (Reicherts et al. 2013) (Figure 6.1). First, the data in Figure 6.1 shows the pain intensity rating did not change when pain stimuli were not matched to any facial expressions. Second, in the pain exposure trial when simultaneously exposed to painful stimuli with specific facial expressions, the pain intensity rating increased significantly. Third, when individuals were required to attend to the pain stimulus in the control fixation trial rather than facial expression, the pain intensity rating was further increased.

These results also indicate that there is an emotion-specific modulation of pain perception by faces that express pain, whereby perceived arousal of negative

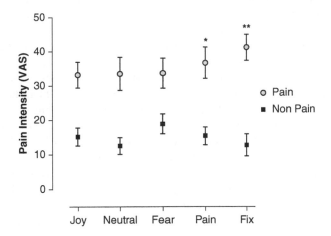

Figure 6.1 The mean pain intensity rating for each of the facial expressions and
the control condition (fix; fixation on a cross) when subjects were subjected to painful thermal stimulation. The pain ratings were increased
during control trials compared to all visual stimuli. During presenta-
tion of pain faces, pain ratings were higher compared to all other facial
expressions revealing emotion-specific modulation of pain; *P < 0.05,
compared with other facial expressions; **P < 0.01, compared with all
facial expressions.

Source: Redrawn from data from figure 6.3 in Reicherts et al. (2013).

facial expressions can be augmented with painful stimulation. These findings
demonstrate mutual effects of pain and the processing of that emotion. However, a critical observation is that pain rating is reduced when presented with
emotional expressions compared to no expression. This strongly indicates that
the expression of emotion may be associated with attentional diversion, which
might reduce or alter the perception of the intensity of the stimulus or at least be
manipulated by affective (attention) allocation to other stimuli. As a practical
application, perhaps the more elite or seasoned performer is able to reduce the
perception of the symptoms of fatigue, such as tiredness, malaise and even pain
and discomfort, by reducing the amount of attention allocated to these related
emotions (Pennebaker & Lightner 1980). However, this has yet to be studied in
any great detail in elite athletes. Nevertheless, in diseases that are known to produce or heighten the feelings associated with fatigue, any strategy distracting the
individual by allocating attention elsewhere could potentially be of therapeutic
use, although even this approach has apparent limitations (McCaul et al. 1992).

From an evolutionary perspective the function of expressing emotion would
be advantageous in a number of ways. Overtly expressing an emotion could
provide observers with cues and instructions about actions to follow and assist

in protection from danger, aiding in obtaining basic needs, recovery and many aspects of survival (Williams 2002). Expressing fatigue as an emotion could incorporate, for example, malaise or tiredness, signalling the need for assistance, particularly for those that are not apparently healthy. However, in the healthy individual who might otherwise express fatigue as an emotion might be quite a complex process and not be particularly obvious. The photos shown in Figure 6.2 are likely to be some of the most recognisable moments in marathon running history. Beyond their historical significance of the moment, there are distinct features of these individuals which provide some insight into the emotional aspect of fatigue. From Figure 6.2A through to 6.2E, what is discernable is the evolving expression of fatigue as a facial expression but more obvious in terms of a strong, stable posture (Figure 6.2A) to less stable, requiring assistance (Figure 6.2B & 6.2C and 6.2E) and leading to eventual collapse (Figure 6.2D). These photos also show that emotion through either facial expression or body posture and position signals a level of fatigue which is interpreted by the onlookers as requiring assistance.

Consciousness and fatigue

As already discussed in Chapter 1 and in more detail in Chapter 4, fatigue is defined in many ways depending on its relevance to the performance or health status of an individual or group. A curious aspect of human fatigue is that we know little about the way the "sensation" we describe as fatigue is generated regardless of health status. One of the lurking problems in this field of study is what we believe "consciousness" to be. This particular idea has been debated and written about for millennia by both philosophers and scientists. To expand on the meandering history of this debate would take several volumes and its own textbook to do it justice. However, the purpose here is not the debate between philosophy and science; rather it is to arrive at a workable definition of consciousness so that we can begin to understand how the sensation of fatigue is either generated or at least interpreted by the brain. From a practical perspective, "'consciousness' refers to those states of sentience or awareness that typically begin when we wake from a dreamless sleep and continue through the day until we fall asleep again, die, go into a coma or otherwise become 'unconscious'" (Searle 1998, p. 1936). There are many levels to this definition, but the crucial aspect that should be considered is that consciousness and attention are not necessarily the same thing since any one of us can be conscious of a host of things around us but paying very little attention to them (Searle 1998).

Since this book is primarily concerned with the evolutionary basis of fatigue, it is appropriate to ask what significance or purpose consciousness has from an evolutionary perspective. In more "simplistic" terms, was consciousness useful in our distant past? Before exploring this question, recall that our working definition of consciousness refers to states of sentience or awareness. Therefore, as Searle (1998) suggests, consciousness is not necessarily a phenomenon separate from all

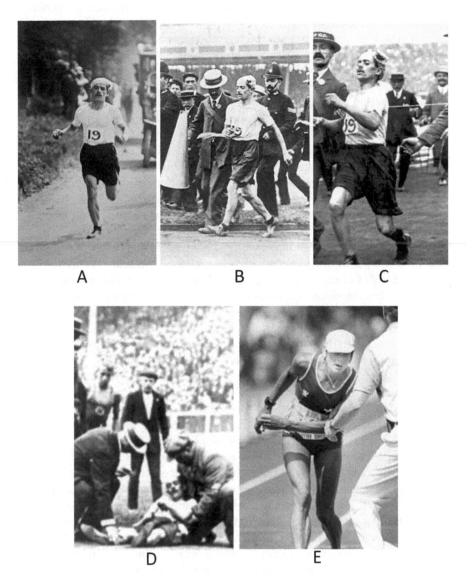

Figure 6.2 Photographs of Dorando Pietri during (A) and at the end (B–D) of the 1908 London Olympic Marathon. Gabrielle Andersen-Schiess (E) moments before finishing the 1984 Los Angeles Women's Marathon. In both instances complete recovery was achieved within hours.

Source: Images freely available from Google Images.

other aspects of life, but it includes all of the activities that humans undertake, including those which have survival value: walking, running, eating, thinking, speaking, avoiding danger and almost anything we consider to be a human activity. If we think of consciousness in this way, then its evolutionary significance and its relationship to fatigue reveal themselves. Each of these activities generates a range of sensations, and when an individual becomes aware of those sensations, a change in perception ensues. The perception is unique for that individual and the interpretation is also unique. This makes the study and quantification of sensation difficult since an observer cannot exactly feel what another individual might feel when undertaking a range of activities generating a myriad of sensations. Nevertheless, recent advancements in the study of neural networks have allowed us to correlate a range of activities with consciousness (Rees et al. 2002). Since physical activity generates a conscious sensation, there will be changes in the activity of the neural networks of the brain. As such, fatigue can potentially be studied by examining changes in the neural networks within brain structures which we now believe to be associated with awareness and sensation.

However, the study of neural networks in isolation from a theory of consciousness does not get us any closer to what consciousness is and how the feelings associated with fatigue are either generated or interpreted. For instance, since physical activity produces conscious sensations, we still require a way to understand how a sensation experienced by one person is interpreted and whether this would be the same for another person. For example, why does a sprint to the finish line feel so different to the start of the same race? Are these sensations similar or different for the individuals in the same race? If the sensations generated are different either between the two points of the race or even between individuals, what function do these sensations have? To begin answering these complex questions two contemporary and popular theories of consciousness have emerged: the global neuronal workspace (GNW) theory, proposed by Baars (1988), and the integrated information theory (IIT), proposed by Tononi (2004).

The GNW theory proposes that when we are conscious of something there are many different parts of the brain that have access to that specific information. This suggests that once there is sensory content it is then distributed to the neural networks, which then allow the brain to integrate, access and coordinate the functioning of specialised networks which would otherwise operate autonomously (Baars 2005). However, for this to work the assumption is that some information has already been written onto a 'workstation' or 'blackboard' from some previous experience. The GNW essentially proposes that consciousness emerges when the sensory information comes in and is then broadcast from this 'workspace' to other cognitive areas of the brain. Once this happens, execution such as speaking, motor action or the like will take place. This theory potentially solves the issue of space on the 'workspace' whereby storage of every conceivable action or execution would seem impossible. Therefore, once the information is sent from the workspace to the vast neural network to be dealt with, we become conscious of the sensory input, or rather we are aware of it.

In contrast to the GNW theory, the IIT proposes that we accept consciousness as the starting point and that individual experiences are integrated. That is, each experience has some essential elements or properties which exist only for the individual (Koch 2018). The IIT suggests that any particular experience cannot be deconstructed into individual parts, that an experience has all of the elements which make it conscious. For example,

> when you sit on a park bench on a warm, sunny day, watching children play, a different part of the experience – the breeze playing in your hair or the joy of hearing your toddler laugh – cannot be separated into parts without the experience ceasing to be what it is.
>
> (Koch 2018, p. 60)

The originator of the IIT suggests that if this is indeed how consciousness is derived, it would be theoretically possible to measure consciousness since it would correspond to the capacity to integrate information (Tononi 2004). In basic terms, it is suggested that if there is no consciousness then it is possible to assign a non-negative number (Φ; fy) which can quantify consciousness. On this basis, the larger Φ becomes, the more conscious the system or we become. Thus, as the amount of information increases that can be integrated by the neural network, the more conscious we become of the vast array of sensory information. Clearly, the human brain has a high level of Φ, which indicates a high level of consciousness.

Although the GNW theory and IIT require their own interrogation in terms of validity and application to the study of consciousness, they both have elements that can shed light on the evolution of fatigue as a human condition. The fundamental proposition of the GNW theory is that consciousness emerges when the incoming information is broadcast to the rest of the brain to make sense of and eventually execute an action. Thus, those inputs which are sent from the 'workspace' which then generate sensations such as tiredness and malaise perhaps manifest as fatigue. This could explain why individuals with varying pathologies report fatigue as a common symptom since the 'workstation' already has some experience to utilise. On the other hand, the IIT proposes that the level of consciousness is relative to the capacity to integrate information. In this scenario, a myriad of sensations originating from changes in respiration, heart rate, local metabolic milieu and skeletal muscle tension would heighten the consciousness of the situation, leading to the manifestation of fatigue. How these two theories might explain fatigue as a phenomenon during exercise or physical exertion has not been described. Nevertheless, the GNW theory and IIT provide fertile ground to further understand the relationship between fatigue and consciousness.

Sensations and effort

There is a large body of literature dedicated to the relationship between an array of sensations as cues for effort or exertion. Since we have already established that many human activities generate sensations, then it is not unreasonable to posit that these sensations are or indeed form the basis for the sensation we interpret as fatigue. The cornerstone of this body of work is the proposition that there are 'local' and 'central' cues for sensing exertion (Golobarg 1971). Figure 6.3 lists the various cues from local and central physiological responses that are thought to be inputs to sensing the level of exertion. However, it is important to not ascribe any one of these responses as a putative cause for the sensation of exertion or even fatigue, since it is thought that combined physiological responses account for about 66% of the variance in the perception of exertion, whereas the remaining variance is likely to be accounted for by psychological variables (Morgan 1973).

An intriguing aspect of the dichotomy of effort sense arising from the cues listed in Figure 6.3 is not so much their apparent total contribution but the level at which either central or peripheral cues might be at play for a given exercise bout. For example, it has been suggested that local factors play a significant part in the perception of effort in the early stages of exercise, whereas central factors are thought to amplify the sensation as intensity or the exercise time continues beyond the initial 30–180 s (Robertson 1982). However, this view is not based on overwhelming experimental evidence and is still very much based, it seems, on an historical consensus view about how the physiological responses to exercise are thought to be used as feedback. This issue will be discussed in more detail in the subsequent section dealing with perceived exertion.

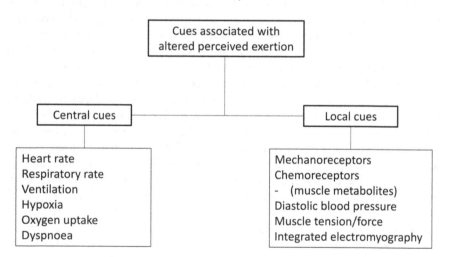

Figure 6.3 The sensory cues that have been reported and thought to be inputs for the perception of exertion and fatigue. These cues have been shown to be dichotomised based on central versus local (peripheral) inputs generated at various levels of responses to physical exertion.

Source: Based on work reported by Golobarg (1971), Morgan (1973), Robertson (1982), Pandolf (1983), Pandolf (1982), Pandolf (1978), Mihevic (1981) and Cafarelli (1982).

Since we are mainly concerned with movement as an outcome of skeletal muscle coordination, the way in which sensations are generated during movement is critical in establishing whether fatigue is indeed a sensation that can be studied and quantified. Exactly how the brain interprets the input from skeletal muscle is still not completely understood, having been a question for researchers for well over a century (Bell 1826). Nevertheless, there is consensus that information from such inputs as joint angle, velocity of shortening and level of force generation is relayed to the central nervous system in the form of feedforward, feedback and a combination of these two processes (Figure 6.4) (Cafarelli 1982).

There is little opposition to the notion that movement generates feedback via sensory input, which is then used by the central nervous system to make certain the movement is carried out in the intended manner, but more importantly

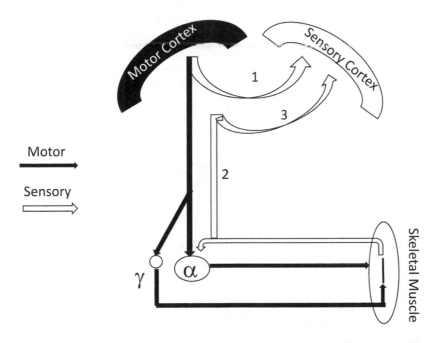

Figure 6.4 A classic schematic of the potential mechanisms which are thought to generate sensations from skeletal muscle. (1) Relates the feedforward component of motor outflow from the cortex which has a corollary discharge to the sensory cortex. (2) Relates the feedback component from the peripheral receptors which provide information about the muscle contraction to the sensory cortex. (3) Relates the combined feedforward and feedback component where the afferent inflow is compared to the copy of the efferent outflow. As such, when there is misalignment between these signals there will be adjustments made to the movement.

Source: Redrawn from original figure in Cafarelli (1982).

feedback allows for the correction of errors if the movement is not as intended. On the other hand, the basis for a feedforward mechanism has been contentious for some time since it is unknown how feedforward command to the sensory cortex (Figure 6.4) actually works or if indeed it actually occurs. However, there is strong evidence to suggest that adjustments to the skeletal muscle responsible for the maintenance of posture are indeed likely to be of feedforward origin. In fact, it has been shown that anticipatory postural movements are detectable in the lower limbs and the pelvis well before the upper limbs are engaged, suggesting that they are specific to the forthcoming movement and are preprogramed (Bouisset & Zattara 1981).

Brain structures involved in the fatigue sensation

Physiologists will quickly identify the basic senses as touch, taste, smell, hearing and sight where each of these can be evaluated, respectively by varying degrees, by subjecting the specific sense organs to pressure, food, odour, sound and light. However, beyond these basic senses are others which physiologists study in order to further understand human behaviour and perception. For example, other sensations are derived from temperature, pain, balance and proprioception. In the exercise sciences, there is considerable interest in the movement sense commonly referred to as kinesthesis. Although there is broad agreement that kinesthesis is a derived sensation, it is not typically classified as one of the basic sensations. There are brain structures that have been identified which mediate kinesthesis. The problem with this is that we are not able to identify a unique receptor or structure within the nervous system from which we are able to determine a measure of exertion or muscular effort. We are only able to infer from various instruments what the effort sense might be. For example, the effort expended by a runner or cyclist in a competitive race is a complex phenomenon derived from physiological, psychological and social inputs and a variety of other cues.

The difficulty in isolating specific brain structures which could be involved in generating or interpreting the sensation of fatigue is likely related to the relative contribution of peripheral factors thought to contribute to afferent input to the brain. These factors can be but are not limited to the local metabolic milieu, energy substrate availability or limitations and cardiorespiratory alterations, such as heart rate and respiratory frequency (Fitts 1994; St Clair Gibson et al. 2005; Peltonen et al. 2001). In addition to these peripheral changes and responses, there are those intrinsic factors which alter motivation and perception. Thus, these peripheral and intrinsic factors form part of an integrated input which either generates a sensation of fatigue or allows brain structures to interpret the input as leading to fatigue.

In order to assemble a picture of the possible nervous system structures involved in the fatigue sensation, there are three assumptions that need to be made. First, since all sensations can be altered, the level of fatigue that is experienced must also be able to be altered. Second, expectations of the demands of a task or situation have potential to alter the interpretation of fatigue. Third, and most important, is that in clinical cases where the sensation of fatigue is described as a constant and debilitating condition, indicates that this feeling of fatigue is generated independently of physical activity so that fatigue must be generated by structures within the brain (St Clair Gibson et al. 2003). If these three assumptions are met, then it becomes possible to elucidate the structures involved in the generation or the perception of fatigue. There is at least one important caveat to these assumptions. Attempting to distinguish between those biological, psychological and cultural aspects of behaviour and the associated responses is not likely to be easy, since these aspects are totally intertwined (Sapolsky 2017) (pp. 4–5). In order to be able to describe the relationship between the brain and any behavioural outcome, it is critical to constrain this relationship to the time immediately before the observed behaviour or response in question. This will, on balance, place the emphasis on neurobiology rather than the psychological or cultural realm (Sapolsky 2017) (pp. 10–12). This not to assert that these latter inputs are not important, but rather the moment before the behaviour occurs means that we have a reference point in relation to the neurophysiology.

Based on our current understanding of what areas of the brain are involved with generating emotions, it is possible to identify the key brain structures central in the emotional side of fatigue (Figure 6.5).

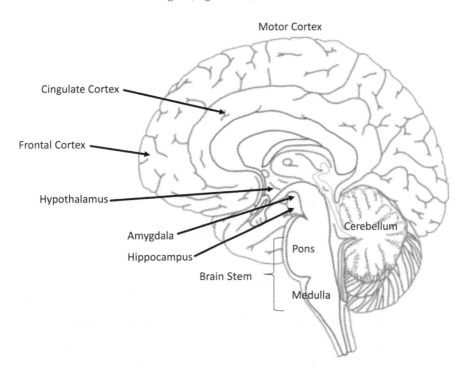

Figure 6.5 Brain regions thought to be involved in the sensation of fatigue.

Evidence for fatigue as a potential emotion comes from innovative studies in which subjects cycled at a constant load for 15 min after being hypnotised to respond to either uphill, downhill or level gradient (Williamson et al. 2001). In these studies, the mere suggestion of uphill gradient altered the heart rate response significantly, even though under all three conditions of resistance the gradient was actually identical. Interestingly, the perceived exertion was commensurate with the suggestion of the gradient rather than the heart rate response *per se*. These findings indicate that physiological responses might be related to an 'expectation' and not necessarily to only what needs to be accomplished physiologically. In terms of what regions of the brain were involved in response to expectations, measures of regional cerebral blood flow (rCBF) distribution during the three different hypnotic exercise tests changed according to whether there was a suggestion of downhill or uphill cycling. The suggestion of downhill cycling produced decreases in rCBF in a region of the anterior cingulate cortex, as shown in Figure 6.6 (see Figure 6.5 for anatomical location). In fact, the difference compared with the control condition was -6.6 ± 4.4 % for downhill and 4.6 ± 3.0% for uphill. Importantly, the suggestion of a different gradient also resulted in higher heart rates and perceived exertion for the uphill condition.

Curiously, the heart rate did not change between control and downhill suggestions, but the perceived exertion decreased only for the downhill suggestion.

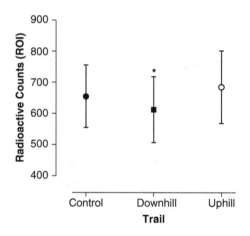

Figure 6.6 The change in radioactive counts for the region of interest (ROI), which in this case was the *Ant.* cingulate cortex (ACC; see Figure 6.5 for anatomical site) during cycling with the hypnotic suggestion of either downhill, uphill or control trials when the actual resistances were identical across all trials. The reductions in radioactive counts for the ACC were equivalent to -6.6 ± 4.4 % (downhill) and 4.6 ± 3.0% (uphill) compared with the control condition. *$P < 0.05$.

Source: Data redrawn from table 6.1 in Williamson et al. (2002).

This discrepancy is indicative of at least two possibilities with respect to fatigue as an emotion. One, there is likely to be a minimum sympathetic response for the maintenance of cardiorespiratory and metabolic demands for the exercise, given that heart rate did not decrease for the control and downhill condition. Two, perceived exertion decreased without any adjustment to heart rate, suggesting a powerful disconnect from what is perceived versus what is normally thought to be physiologically required for exercise to continue. These two key observations mean that whether we perceive a given effort to be higher or lower is clearly intertwined with both the response to that effort and the expectation of what that effort entails, even though the actual required effort is not necessarily different.

This observation and the fact that the anterior cingulate cortex, the region involved in the reaction to the "required" effort and thought to be involved in the modulation of emotion (Jackson et al. 2006; Decety & Jackson 2016), suggest that fatigue may indeed be interpreted as an emotion. In addition, it has been shown that activation of the anterior cingulate cortex is closely related to perceived change in unpleasantness of painful stimuli (Rainville et al. 1997). Therefore, the diminution in perceived exertion with the suggestion of downhill cycling might indicate that specific brain regions are related to the interpretation of unpleasantness and are activated by not solely the actual physical effort but also the perceived effort. Conversely, with the suggestion of uphill cycling there were increases in rCBF to the right thalamic region and the insular cortex, which we now understand to be linked to emotion, consciousness and the regulation of homeostasis.

Central command

The previous section outlined the problem of fatigue as a sensation and the brain structures thought to be involved. Although we have been able to identify a number of brain regions which give rise to sensations which might be interpreted as fatigue, there is an additional phenomenon which needs to be considered – that of central command. In its original proposition this was termed cortical irradiation, which essentially described how the descending motor command influences the increase in cardiovascular and respiratory responses, such as blood pressure, heart rate and ventilation (Krogh & Lindhard 1913). Subsequently, this was termed central command, as it described the relationship between the central signals originating from the higher brain centres which were observed to influence cardiovascular responses during exercise (Goodwin et al. 1972). These authors observed that when submaximal (20% of maximum) isometric contractions of the biceps brachii were augmented with 100 Hz vibration to achieve the same level of tension as with voluntary activation, both systolic and diastolic blood pressures were attenuated along with the heart rate and ventilation. Since the vibration can be a powerful stimulus for muscle spindle primary endings, it will elicit reflex pathways, assist in maintaining the contraction and reduce the level of central command required for that contraction – termed 'command assisted' skeletal muscle effort (see Figure 6.7). This finding suggested that cardiovascular responses are indeed altered by muscle afferent activity during skeletal muscle contraction.

However, subsequent studies observed that perception of effort has a decidedly strong influence on the relative magnitude of central command rather than being a response that is solely dependent on the actual physical effort, as extensively described by Mitchell (1990). When a small dose of curare or similar is administered, a drug inducing neuromuscular junction blockade, there is a decrease in the force-generating capacity of the muscle (Iwamoto et al. 1987; Leonard et al. 1985). Figure 6.8 shows the heart rate response when human subjects attempted a maximal voluntary contraction with and without the partial blocking agent. What is typically observed is the increase in heart rate with blockade when subjects attempted to achieve maximal isometric force. In panel A of Figure 6.8, the heart rate increased as soon as voluntary contraction commenced for both control and neuromuscular blockade. The reduction in voluntary force with blockade was 39%

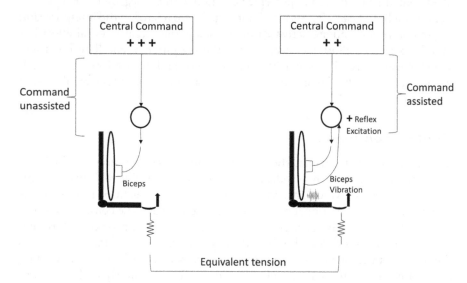

Figure 6.7 The theoretical design for the assisted central command using biceps vibration (right) which achieves the same tension as in the normal condition when the biceps is contracting voluntarily (left). Note that the level of central command on the left is given by + + + whereas the assisted central command is given by + +, which is supplemented by the biceps vibration of +. This vibration contributes to the overall contraction by exciting the primary afferents from muscle spindles of the contracting muscles, which achieves the same tension with less central command.

Source: Redrawn from Goodwin et al. (1972).

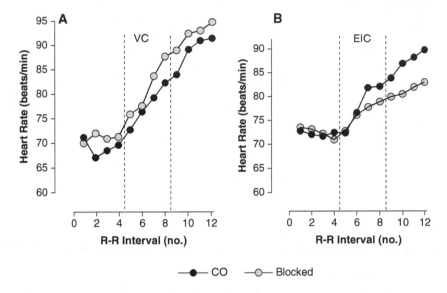

Figure 6.8 The heart rate response (expressed as the R-R intervals in the electrocardiogram) during voluntary contractions (VC) of the quadriceps muscle in A, and electrically induced contractions (EIC) in B when administered curare for partial neuromuscular block (blocked) or control (CON). Muscle contractions were evoked between the dashed lines. Note the same increase in heart rate response when there is partial neuromuscular block during voluntary contraction (A) when electrically elicited (B).

Source: Data redrawn from Figure 6.4 in Iwamoto et al. (1987).

of the control effort, which did not result in any significant change in heart rate response over the course of the voluntary contraction. This result indicates that the heart rate response was not driven by muscle afferent activity *per se*. As such, this observation is strong evidence that it was the perceived effort which augmented the heart rate via an increase in central command. Critically, when the muscular contraction was induced by electrical stimulation eliciting 75% of maximum (Figure 6.8 panel B), under the same control and drug conditions, and presumably with no effort required by the individual, the magnitude of the heart rate increase was delayed but similar as per the voluntary contractions, albeit attenuated with blockade. It is now widely accepted that perception of effort is a significant driver of central command with and without the accompanying physical exertion.

These observations and many like these have been interpreted as central command being a feedforward mechanism with the capability of activating motor and cardiovascular responses in parallel but possibly independently. As discussed earlier (see Figure 6.4 and associated text), it seems plausible that the level of central command required to elicit cardiovascular responses during exercise is able to be somewhat independent of the actual exercise itself, implying that there exists a feedforward mechanism where no continuous feedback is needed. In fact, when subjects attempted 7 min of dynamic cycling exercise at 20% of maximal oxygen uptake (VO_{2max}) and a static one-legged exercise at 20% maximal voluntary contraction with and without neuromuscular blockade, heart rate, mean arterial pressure, lactate and rating of perceived exertion (RPE) all increased significantly with the blockade (Gallagher et al. 2001) (Figure 6.9). These findings indicate that perceived effort is a strong stimulus for central command in the regulation of cardiovascular control during dynamic and static exercise, since the force produced in both modes of exercise was less than 50% of the control force.

It appears that central command has two parallel neural networks: one for cardiovascular activation and the other for motor control. How or why this parallel system evolved remains unclear, but arguably very important since it is known to also exist in lower animals (Jansen et al. 1995; Matsukawa 2011). Nevertheless, there are at least two possible advantages to having this parallel yet integrated neural circuitry. First, if there was a complete integrated system where cardiovascular control was dependent solely on muscle afference, then there would be no need for a sense of effort to play any role. However, as we have already seen, the

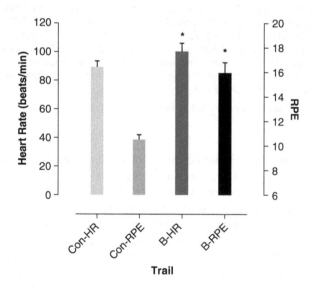

Figure 6.9 The mean (± S.E.) heart rate (HR; left ordinate) and mean rating of perceived exertion (RPE; right ordinate) during control (Con) and with neuromuscular blockade with curare (B) when undertaking 7 min of dynamic cycling exercise. * $P < 0.05$ compared with corresponding variable in control trial.

Source: Data derived from table 6.1 and figure 6.2 in Gallagher et al. (2001). Data from static exercise not shown.

possibility exists that central command generates corollary discharge to the sensory cortex (Figure 6.4), which could produce a sense of effort (Marcora 2009). Thus, when there is an increase in the central motor command in an attempt to meet the required force output, there is an increase in perceived exertion possibly due to the corollary discharge. Second, since sense of effort through the expression of perceived exertion seems to drive the cardiovascular response, it makes sense that the 'need' for metabolic turnover and delivery is available well before the effort is undertaken. These possibilities suggest that the two parallel neural circuits would be advantageous in times of escape (Jansen et al. 1995) and when a specific target force is required to be achieved based on the perceived effort rather than the actual force that is accomplished. Thus, the evolutionary forces that selected for this independent and parallel neural circuitry have included effort sense as fine-tuning for physiological control. Finally, this parallel circuitry could potentially explain why individuals suffering from chronic conditions such as multiple sclerosis or Parkinson's disease report a higher perceived effort and higher resting heart rates (Savci et al. 2009) even without muscular exertion. An increased perception of effort with attenuated motor drive in these pathologies would be similar to what is experienced with neuromuscular blockade and would be a counter-measure to augment the magnitude of central command.

The relevance of perceived exertion

Thus far we have explored the meanings and the possible ways in which the global terms 'emotion,' 'consciousness' and 'sensation' are defined and their relationships with fatigue. Table 6.1 is a summary of the terms and their respective definitions used in the preceding sections.

Table 6.1 Terms and definitions of concepts used to describe the understandings of and relationships to fatigue.

Term/concept	Description
Emotion	A feeling generated by a physical or psychological stimulus, potentially detected and interpreted by others as conveying a specific feeling or mood.
Consciousness	A state of sentience and awareness.
Sensation	Physiological changes derived from touch, taste, smell, hearing and sight in addition to other responses from temperature, pain, balance and proprioception, which are interpreted as sensations by the central nervous system.
Effort sense	A complex sensory experience which is not directly connected to a specific receptor or nervous system structure but integrated to generate a sensation of effort.
Perceived exertion	A complex, subjective experience based on physiological and psychological inputs which generate the perception of exertion or effort.

However, there are some overlapping and interchangeable terms when describing these concepts which require further elaboration with respect to their relationship with fatigue. Specifically, perceived exertion and effort sense are concepts that not only are used interchangeably but also carry some implied relationship with physical exertion since both require sensory and psychophysiological inputs to generate the perception.

In the exercise sciences, the measurement of perceived exertion was popularised by Borg (1962) as a construct which could indicate the degree of physical strain during exercise. This assertion was based primarily on the notion that "The overall perception of exertion rating integrates various information, including the many signals elicited from the peripheral working muscles and joints, from the central cardiovascular and respiratory functions, and from the central nervous system" (Borg 1982, p. 377). Crucially, Borg considered the integration of these signals to be a "Gestalt" of the perceived exertion. In this sense, Gestalt is used in its original meaning in which the whole is *something else* than the sum of its parts (Koffka 1935, p. 176). The original rating of perceived exertion (RPE) scale ranged from 6 to 20, which was a convenient way of assigning numbers to heart rates ranging from 60 to 200 beats.min^{-1} (Borg 1982). This was mainly based on the observation that heart rate was a linear function of the % VO_{2max} (Figure 6.10A). However, when blood lactate is plotted against the increasing oxygen consumption (VO_2) the relationship is no longer linear but curvilinear regardless of training status (Figure 6.10B).

Although the ratings on the original RPE scale were found to increase linearly with power output and heart rate and with almost any physiological variable

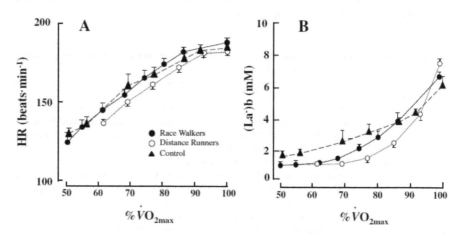

Figure 6.10 The typical heart rate (A) and blood lactate (B) response during incremental exercise as a percentage of maximal oxygen consumption (%VO_{2max}) in three different groups (Abe et al. 2015).

Source: With permission from BioMed Central Ltd under the terms of the Creative Commons Attribution License.

during exercise, RPE was found to be deficient in its linearity with blood lactate. This relationship is shown in Figure 6.11A, whereby the blood lactate when plotted against the RPE shows an exponential rise regardless of whether individuals are trained or untrained (Abe et al. 2015). Since blood lactate is related to exercise intensity, and if perceived exertion is a way to measure the sensations which are generated during exercise, the scale used to measure perceived exertion must be representative of those inputs which generate the sensations.

The curvilinear response of blood lactate during exercise presented a particular problem for the RPE, since the scale must be representative of how those physiological responses and their associated sensations grow during exercise. The observation that sensations grow during exercise indicate that perceptual scales used to measure sensations are likely tied to an exponent. To address this problem, the Category Ratio Scale (CR-10) was developed so that perceptual ratings would increase as a positively accelerating function. Thus, the CR-10 scale is anchored at "0" (nothing at all) at the low end, versus the symbol "•," which represents a maximal rating at the high end (Noble et al. 1983). Comparing this scale between untrained and trained individuals results in a linear response for blood lactate at ratings above moderate intensity (Figure 6.11B), and an almost linear response with heart rate (data not shown) (Abe et al. 2015).

The question as to how sensations grow during exercise and why perceptual scales must reflect this phenomenon needs careful consideration. Studies which examine these relationships reveal the effect that increasing sensations have on

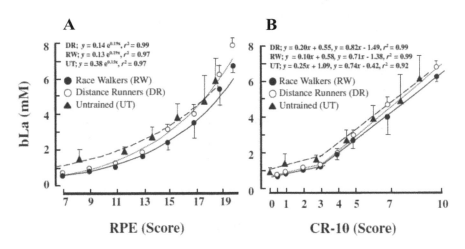

Figure 6.11 The blood lactate (bLa) response plotted against the rating of perceived exertion (RPE; A) and the category ratio scale (CR-10; B) for trained and untrained groups (Abe et al. 2015).

the brain. This was shown in individuals exercising for 15 min at 50% VO_{2max} with acidosis or alkalosis induced by ingestion of appropriate compounds, resulting in no difference in the sensory intensity to the placebo condition (Kostka & Cafarelli 1982). However, when exercise increased to 80% VO_{2max} for the subsequent 15 min, the sensory intensity also increased by about 20% with acidosis but not in either alkalosis or placebo (Kostka & Cafarelli 1982). In terms of magnitude, the change in exercise intensity from 50% to 80% VO_{2max} accelerated the subjective sensation of the load by six-fold in alkalosis and placebo but nine-fold in acidosis. This suggests that there needs to be careful consideration about how perceived exertion is generated and subsequently measured. The fact that a physiological response such as blood lactate rises in a non-linear fashion is an example of how and why a perceptual scale must account for the way in which the sensations are derived from such a response. If we take the blood lactate response as an example, it is now apparent that this metabolic "by-product" has the capacity to enhance sensitivity via neurons that express acid-sensing ion channels (ASICs), thereby potentiating sensitivity during high exercise intensities (Immke & McCleskey 2001).

In addition to ASICs, increases in blood lactate have been associated with increased motor excitability even when lactate is infused and not just produced during exercise alone (Coco et al. 2010; Ishii & Nishida 2013). Figure 6.12 shows the blood lactate response plotted against the oxyhaemoglobin response at three

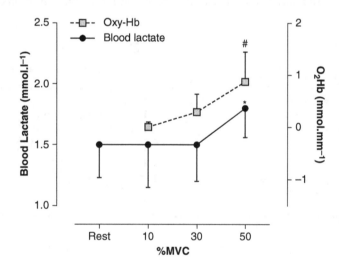

Figure 6.12 The blood lactate and oxyhaemoglobin response (O_2Hb) during each of the percentage maximal voluntary contractions (%MVC) of the wrist flexors. *$P < 0.05$ compared with resting value. #$P < 0.05$ compared with 10% and 30% values.

Source: Data redrawn from table 6.2 in Ishii and Nishida (2013).

different percentages of maximal voluntary muscle contractions performed during 120 s of handgrip exercise. What is remarkable about these data is the 68-fold increase in oxy-haemoglobin when contractions were raised from 10% to 30% and the 207-fold increase from 30% to 50% of maximum. Further to these data, it has been shown that blood lactate can be a significant contributor to brain blood flow explaining over half the variance (r^2 = 0.56) (Ishii & Nishida 2013). Finally, when subjects were administered lactate by intravenous infusion and compared with exercise-induced levels of lactate, both conditions resulted in enhanced motor cortex excitability as measured by transcranial stimulation (Coco et al. 2010).

The evolutionary significance of perceived exertion

It should now be clear that an increase in perceived exertion is dependent on the growth of the physiological response and presumably the growth of the associated sensations. The example given in the previous section was based upon the relationship between RPE, metabolic load as inferred by lactate and its potentiating effects at the periphery by ASICs, and centrally by its influence on motor cortex excitability. Importantly, similar relationships have been described, particularly with respect to temperature (Stevens & Stevens 1960). In fact, subjective warmth is an accelerating function so that it grows more rapidly as temperature increases. As a rule, the growth of a sensation can be described by the power function or exponent generally observed in almost all psychophysical relationships, including metabolic, temperature and skeletal muscle force (Stevens & Stevens 1960; Stevens & Mack 1959; Borg 1982).

However, regardless of what the exponent might be (noting that previous research has suggested exponents ranging from 0.3 to 3.0; Stevens 1957), it is worthwhile understanding (1) what purpose the exponent plays in psychophysical relations beyond its quantification, and (2) what advantage this relationship provided during our evolutionary past and how it relates to fatigue. The answers to these questions are not particularly apparent, but we are able to infer from previous work that has established an allometric law that pervades biological diversity (Porter & Brand 1993; West et al. 1997). Although allometry specifically describes relations of size of different organs or parts of an organism, it is now accepted that a 3/4 scaling law has been established by nature as a way of placing constraints on body size relative to the rates at which resources are used from the environment, transported and transformed within the body (West et al. 1997). Similarly, an exponent related to apparent and perceived exertion based on the accelerating growth of sensation would also constrain the organism within its biological limitations.

In considering the evolutionary significance of perceived exertion, two aspects are key. First, beyond the quantification of the exponent, the accelerating nature of the sensation relative to the physiological response would provide the organism with the opportunity to integrate the related sensory signals within appropriate time limits, well before any impending cellular disruption can occur. The prime example is the acceleration of apparent temperature. This makes intuitive sense as it would be of no use if higher temperatures were not sensed as an accelerating function since impending thermal limits are critical for survival. Similarly, blood lactate provides accelerating sensitivity with respect to metabolic load potentially signalling higher energy usage. Second, recall that in Chapters 2 and 3 it was postulated that our species opted for structure and function that are adapted more for endurance than for power. As such, an accelerating function with respect to subjective rating of sensory information would potentially explain why sensations typically grow at the higher rather than the lower exercise intensities (see Figures 6.8A, 6.9B, 6.10), for if the growth in the perceived sensation occurred at the lower exercise intensities then periods of prolonged exercise would be less likely to be achieved. Therefore, the relation of the sensory exponent to the apparent rating must have been advantageous in providing the gauge by which we were able to judge our effort under a range of conditions without exceeding biological limitations.

A further piece of evidence for the evolutionary significance of perceived exertion comes from studies which show a time lag in heart rate response during the initial stages of high-intensity exercise. When subjects commence exercise at an RPE of 14 to 20 (hard – very, very hard) the heart rate response does not reach a plateau until approximately 10 min after the commencement of exercise (Ulmer 1996). However, at any intensity between an RPE of 8 and 11 (very light – fairly light) the heart rate achieved a plateau within the first few minutes of exercise and was maintained until completion. These observations indicate that the heart rate response alone cannot be the sole input which achieves the RPE, as described in Figure 6.3. In addition, this observation provides further evidence that feedback from skeletal muscle, heart and lungs has a limited contribution to the perception of effort, at least during exercise (Marcora 2009). If this is indeed the case, then it makes sense from an evolutionary point of view that accelerated growth of sensation would be desirable since afferent feedback from particular organs would be lagging.

References

Abe, D. et al., 2015. Relationship between perceived exertion and blood lactate concentrations during incremental running test in young females. *BMC Sports Science, Medicine and Rehabilitation*, 7(1), pp. 2621–2629.

Ax, A.F., 1953. The physiological differentiation between fear and anger in humans. *Psychosomatic Medicine*, 15(5), pp. 433–442.

Baars, B.J., 1988. *A cognitive theory of consciousness*. Cambridge, UK: Cambridge University Press.

Baars, B.J., 2005. Global workspace theory of consciousness: toward a cognitive neuroscience of human experience. *Progress in Brain Research*, 150, pp. 45–53.

Bainbridge, F.A., 1931. *The physiology of muscular exercise*, 3rd ed., New York: Longmans, Green and Co.

Bell, C., 1826. On the nervous circle which connects the voluntary muscles with the brain. *Philosophical Transactions of the Royal Society of London (Biological Sciences)*, 116(1/3), pp. 163–173.

Borg, G.A., 1962. *Physical performance and perceived exertion*, Oxford: University of Lund.

Borg, G.A., 1982. Psychophysical bases of perceived exertion. *Medicine and Science in Sports & Exercise*, 14(5), pp. 377–381.

Bouisset, S. & Zattara, M. (null), 1981. A sequence of postural movements precedes voluntary movement. *Journal of Human Evolution*, 22(3), pp. 263–270.

Cafarelli, E., 1982. Peripheral contributions to the perception of effort. *Medicine and Science in Sports & Exercise*, 14(5), pp. 382–389.

Coco, M. et al., 2010. Elevated blood lactate is associated with increased motor cortex excitability. *Somatosensory & Motor Research*, 27(1), pp. 1–8.

Craig, K.D., 2009. The social communication model of pain. *Canadian Psychology*, 50, pp. 22–32.

Dalgleish, T., 2004. The emotional brain. *Nature Reviews Neuroscience*, 5(7), pp. 583–589.

Darwin, C., 1993[1872]. The expression of the emotions in man and animals. In D. Porter & P. Graham, eds. *The portable*. London: Penguin Random House.

Decety, J. & Jackson, P.L., 2016. The functional architecture of human empathy. *Behavioral and Cognitive Neuroscience Reviews*, 3(2), pp. 71–100.

Fitts, R.H., 1994. Cellular mechanisms of muscle fatigue. *Physiological Reviews*, 74(1), pp. 49–94.

Gallagher, K.M. et al., 2001. Effects of partial neuromuscular blockade on carotid baroreflex function during exercise in humans. *Journal of Physiology*, 533(Pt 3), pp. 861–870.

Golobarg, A.N., 1971. The influence of physical training and other factors on the subjective rating of perceived exertion. *Acta Physiologica*, 83(3), pp. 399–406.

Goodall, M., 1962. Sympathoadrenal response to gravitational stress. *Journal of Clinical Investigation*, 41(2), p. 197.

Goodwin, G.M., McCloskey, D.I. & Mitchell, J.H., 1972. Cardiovascular and respiratory responses to changes in central command during isometric exercise at constant muscle tension. *Journal of Physiology*, 226(1), pp. 173–190.

Immke, D.C. & McCleskey, E.W., 2001. Lactate enhances the acid-sensing Na+ channel on ischemia-sensing neurons. *Nature Neuroscience*, 4(9), pp. 869–870.

Ishii, H. & Nishida, Y., 2013. Effect of lactate accumulation during exercise-induced muscle fatigue on the sensorimotor cortex. *Journal of Physical Therapy Science*, 25(12), pp. 1637–1642.

Iwamoto, G.A. et al., 1987. Cardiovascular responses at the onset of exercise with partial neuromuscular blockade in cat and man. *Journal of Physiology*, 384(1), pp. 39–47.

Jackson, P.L. et al., 2006. Empathy examined through the neural mechanisms involved in imagining how I feel versus how you feel pain. *Neuropsychologia*, 44(5), pp. 752–761.

Jansen, A.S.P. et al., 1995. Central command neurons of the sympathetic nervous system: basis of the fight-or-flight response. *Science*, 270(5236), pp. 644–646.

Koch, C., 2018. What is consciousness? *Scientific American*, 318(6), pp. 57–60.

Koffka, K., 1935. *Principles of Gestalt psychology*, New York: Harcourt Brace.

Kostka, C.E. & Cafarelli, E., 1982. Effect of pH on sensation and vastus lateralis electromyogram during cycling exercise. *Journal of Applied Physiology*, 52(5), pp. 1181–1185.

Krogh, A. & Lindhard, J., 1913. The regulation of respiration and circulation during the initial stages of muscular work. *Journal of Physiology*, 47(1–2), pp. 112–136.

Leonard, B. et al., 1985. Partial neuromuscular blockade and cardiovascular responses to static exercise in man. *Journal of Physiology*, 359(1), pp. 365–379.

Marcora, S., 2009. Perception of effort during exercise is independent of afferent feedback from skeletal muscles, heart, and lungs. *Journal of Applied Physiology*, 106, pp. 2060–2062.

Matsukawa, K., 2011. Central command: control of cardiac sympathetic and vagal efferent nerve activity and the arterial baroreflex during spontaneous motor behaviour in animals. *Experimental Physiology*, 97(1), pp. 20–28.

McCaul, K.D., Monson, N. & Maki, R.H., 1992. Does distraction reduce pain-produced distress among college students? *Health Psychology*, 11(4), p. 210.

Mihevic, P.M., 1981. Sensory cues for perceived exertion: a review. *Medicine and Science in Sports Exercise*, 13(3), pp. 150–163.

Mitchell, J.H., 1990. Neural control of the circulation during exercise. *Medicine and Science in Sports & Exercise*, 22, pp. 141–154.

Morgan, W.P., 1973. Psychological factors influencing perceived exertion. *Medicine and Science in Sports*, 5(2), pp. 97–103.

Mosso, A., 1891. *La fatica*, Milano: F. lli Treves.

Mosso, A., 1904. *Fatigue*, London: Swan Sonnenschein & Co. Ltd.

Noble, B.J. et al., 1983. A category-ratio perceived exertion scale: relationship to blood and muscle lactates and heart rate. *Medicine and Science in Sports & Exercise*, 15(6), pp. 523–528.

Pandolf, K.B., 1978. Influence of local and central factors in dominating rated perceived exertion during physical work. *Perceptual and Motor Skills*, 46(3), pp. 683–698.

Pandolf K.B., 1982. Differentiated ratings of perceived exertion during physical exercise., *Medicine and Science in Sports & Exercise*, 14(5), pp. 397–405.

Pandolf K.B., 1983. Advances in the study and application of perceived exertion. *Exercise and Sports Science Reviews*, 11(1), pp. 118–158.

Peltonen, J.E., Tikkanen, H.O. & Rusko, H.K., 2001. Cardiorespiratory responses to exercise in acute hypoxia, hyperoxia and normoxia. *European Journal of Applied Physiology*, 85(1–2), pp. 82–88.

Pennebaker, J.W. & Lightner, J.M., 1980. Competition of internal and external information in an exercise setting. *Journal of Personality and Social Psychology*, 39(1), pp. 165–174.

Porter, R.K. & Brand, M.D., 1993. Body mass dependence of H+ leak in mitochondria and its relevance to metabolic rate. *Nature*, 362(6421), pp. 628–630.

Rainville, P. et al., 1997. Pain affect encoded in human anterior cingulate but not somatosensory cortex. *Science*, 277(5328), pp. 968–971.

Rees, G., Kreiman, G. & Koch, C., 2002. Neural correlates of consciousness in humans. *Nature Reviews Neuroscience*, 3(4), pp. 261–270.

Reicherts, P. et al., 2012. Electrocortical evidence for preferential processing of dynamic pain expressions compared to other emotional expressions. *Pain*, 153(9), pp. 1959–1964.

Reicherts, P. et al., 2013. On the mutual effects of pain and emotion: facial pain expressions enhance pain perception and vice versa are perceived as more arousing when feeling pain. *Pain*, 154(6), pp. 793–800.

Robertson, R.J., 1982. Central signals of perceived exertion during dynamic exercise. *Medicine and Science in Sports & Exercise*, 14(5), pp. 390–396.

Sapolsky, R.M., 2017. *Behave: the biology of humans at our best and worst.* New York: Penguin Books.

Savci, S. et al., 2009. Six-minute walk distance as a measure of functional exercise capacity in multiple sclerosis. *Disability and Rehabilitation*, 27(22), pp. 1365–1371.

Searle, J.R., 1998. How to study consciousness scientifically. *Philosophical Transactions of the Royal Society of London (Biological Sciences)*, 353(1377), pp. 1935–1942.

St Clair Gibson, A. et al., 2003. The conscious perception of the sensation of fatigue. *Sports Medicine*, 33(3), pp. 167–176.

St Clair Gibson, A. et al., 2005. Metabolic setpoint control mechanisms in different physiological systems at rest and during exercise. *Journal of Thermal Biology*, 236(1), pp. 60–72.

Stevens, J.C. & Mack, J.D., 1959. Scales of apparent force. *Journal of Experimental Psychology*, 58, pp. 405–413.

Stevens, J.C. & Stevens, S.S., 1960. Warmth and cold: dynamics of sensory intensity. *Journal of Experimental Psychology*, 60(3), pp. 183–192.

Stevens, S.S., 1957. On the psychophysical law. *Psychological Review*, 64(3), pp. 153–181.

Tononi, G., 2004. An information integration theory of consciousness. *BMC Neuroscience*, 5(1), pp. 42–23.

Ulmer, H.V., 1996. Concept of an extracellular regulation of muscular metabolic rate during heavy exercise in humans by psychophysiological feedback. *Experientia*, 52(5), pp. 416–420.

West, G.B., Brown, J.H. & Enquist, B.J., 1997. A general model for the origin of allometric scaling laws in biology. *Science*, 276(5309), pp. 122–126.

Williams, A.C. de C., 2002. Facial expression of pain: an evolutionary account. *Behavioral and Brain Sciences*, 25(4), pp. 439–55 – discussion 455–488.

Williamson, J.W. et al., 2001. Hypnotic manipulation of effort sense during dynamic exercise: cardiovascular responses and brain activation. *Journal of Applied Physiology*, 90(4), pp. 1392–1399.

Williamson, J.W., McColl, R., Mathews, D., Mitchell, J.H., Raven, P.B. & Morgan, W.P., 2002. Brain activation by central command during actual and imagined handgrip under hypnosis. *Journal of Applied Physiology*, 92(3), pp. 1317–1324.

Chapter 7

The environment

Temperature and the human
capacity to resist fatigue

Heat not a furnace for your foe so hot that it do singe yourself.

– Shakespeare

Introduction

In his classic paper which examined the myriad of potential heat disorders from sunburn to hyperpyrexia, Ladell (1957) concludes that

> heat stroke or hyperpyrexia, hitherto regarded almost as an act of God and the most fatal of heat disorders, is, I believe, a purely physiological phenomenon; whenever one's body temperature rises, even for physiological reasons, we enter into danger and anything that interferes with physiological cooling, or adds to the internal heat load, exacerbates that danger. The wonder is, not that anyone gets hyperpyrexia, but that so few of us ever do.
>
> (p. 206)

This observation establishes a least two key principles to consider in understanding our interaction with the environment. First, given the range of ambient temperatures in which humans live, the capacity to regulate our temperature is an exceptional characteristic. Second, this characteristic must have provided a clear evolutionary advantage.

Previous chapters outlined the significance and advantages of bipedal locomotion, a characteristic unique to humans and apparently intimately tied to our thermoregulatory strategy (see Chapter 1). This is a key concept since thermoregulation is not just a physiological response to a given environmental challenge but an interactive survival strategy as evidenced by the varying ways in which animals are able to produce and offload heat (Angilletta et al. 2010) – for example, heterothermy, the ability of some animals to switch from having to depend on the environment to adjust their body temperature (poikilothermic) to being able to produce their own body heat (endothermic). Mammals and birds are normally described as having the capacity to maintain a constant temperature (homeotherms). This is undoubtedly an impressive capability which is dependent on the exchange of heat between the body and the environment as given by the equation:

$$S = M - W - E - Q$$

Where S is heat storage, M is metabolic rate of the body, W is the mechanical work produced, E is rate of total evaporative loss due to evaporation of sweat and Q is total rate of heat loss from the skin. Although homeotherms are able to maintain a relatively constant body temperature, it is now apparent that they are also able to vary their body temperature over the lifespan, with this variation likely to be relative to the latitude of their habitat (Angilletta et al. 2010)

To understand more fully why *Homo* adapted a particular thermoregulatory strategy, two key observations need to be considered. First, why mammals have "chosen" an approximate 37°C as a core temperature (T_c) about which thermal balance is regulated, and second, how the *Homo* strategy compares with that of our closest relatives and other mammals. This cannot be inconsequential and overemphasised since it is now clear that rising body temperature is associated with premature fatigue in both healthy and diseased populations (Marino 2004, 2009). Further to this is the relationship between human morphology and thermoregulation and how this relates to human performance (Havenith 2001; Marino et al. 2000).

There are other key issues that need to be considered to gain a more complete picture of the human thermoregulatory strategy. These include the role of the central nervous system, thirst and specific pathologies which provide insight into thermoregulatory health and behaviour. In this chapter we will extend the basic textbook understanding of temperature regulation to be inclusive of an evolutionary perspective and how this also plays a fundamental role in the development of fatigue.

The primordial soup to animal diversification

The typical textbook on the physiology of human performance or indeed human fatigue seldom considers the evolutionary forces that are thought to have contributed to our thermoregulatory strategy. Typically, consideration of human temperature regulation commences with the observation that there is a stable, resting T_c of ~37°C, and deviations from this temperature deploy a series of mechanisms which are geared towards defending the body from that deviation. What is also seldom considered or discussed is why humans and other mammals have chosen this particular T_c to defend. This stable T_c of ~37°C has for a long period been referred to as a set-point, analogous to a thermostat. From a practical point of view this terminology has served well in the general understanding that deviation from this T_c will turn on a number of physiological and behavioural responses in an attempt to maintain the thermal balance. However, this terminology is now thought to be imprecise since it refers to engineering principles rather than to the number of inputs that are required to defend the T_c, and since there is fluctuation within 0.2–0.5°C over the course of day (Benarroch 2007). To alleviate the imprecise terminology and arrive at a more complete conceptual model, the term 'balance point' has been suggested as it takes into account the variation and the number of inputs required to maintain thermal balance (Romanovsky 2007).

Regardless of the terminology used, a greater understanding of this particular problem requires consideration of how life on Earth began. Although there is no particular consensus about how life took hold, there is general consensus that early life was subjected to a hot environment (Van Kranendonk et al. 2018). In the 1920s, Oparin and Haldane (Miller et al. 1997) independently postulated that life on Earth began in a primordial soup. They suggested that the Earth's atmosphere was composed of certain elements, such as nitrogen, ammonia, methane and hydrogen. The addition of heat produced chemical reactions which eventually gave rise to molecules making their way to a water environment and creating a primordial soup largely composed of amino acids as the building blocks of life (Miller 1953). The key ingredient was heat, which assisted in the establishment of those building blocks. A reasonable conclusion would also be that primitive organisms would have a need to control their internal temperature since chemical reactions are necessary for metabolic function. If we also accept that organisms, regardless of how primitive they might be, were able to perform metabolic functions, they would also then be able to reproduce and move to accommodate their needs. A fundamental point in the evolution of organismic function is the ability to graduate from unicellular to multicellular organisms (Schopf 1978).

It is now thought that the major steps in the formation of life on Earth from 4.5 billion years ago included a stable hydrosphere, prebiotic chemistry, an environment which included ribonucleic acid (RNA) and the first forms of life which included deoxyribonucleic acid (DNA) and protein, eventually giving rise to a universal common ancestor approximately 3.6 billion years ago (Joyce 2002). Although we do not know what this specific universal common ancestor was, it was likely to have been a single-cell organism capable of reproducing (Woese et al. 1990). Eventually, an event commonly referred to as the Cambrian explosion occurred approximately 541 million years ago, lasting somewhere between 20 million and 25 million years. During this extraordinary period the fossil record indicates that this was a time when most of the animal diversification that we know of today occurred. Interestingly, mammals began to appear during the Cenozoic Era some 66 million years ago. There is still debate as to when the first primates appeared; however, recent evidence suggests that it is much earlier than previously thought, with the most complete primate skeleton dated at around the mid-Eocene Epoch some 40–47 million years ago (Franzen et al. 2009). Arguably, the appearance of mammals is perhaps the most important step in our own evolutionary history in addition to upright posture and bipedal locomotion.

The preferred temperature

Further evidence that temperature played a significant and determining factor in the evolution of life was demonstrated in the classic experiment by Mendelssohn (1895). It was demonstrated that a single-cell organism, such as paramecia, was able to adapt to the environmental temperature by dispersing and subsequently congregating to what eventually was a preferred temperature between 24°C and 28°C (Figure 7.1). What was also subsequently observed was that when paramecia were exposed to very high temperatures of up to 45°C, a drop of cold water on the microscope slide would promulgate an "avoidance reaction" to the high temperature, causing the paramecia to congregate beneath the new cooler region (Jennings 1906).

The behavioural response of these single-cell organisms is intriguing even more so since it lacks a neurological system, which would make sensing a change in the environmental temperature very challenging. However, the field of epigenetics proposes that there exists a non-neuronal system of cell memorisation enabling maintenance of functional and structural integrity and providing an evolutionary advantage as the environment alters (Ginsburg & Jablonka 2009). These observations on the most rudimentary organisms confirm the existence of a preferred temperature, and that organisms will alter their behaviour in order to achieve a preferred external medium and presumably maintain an internal environment.

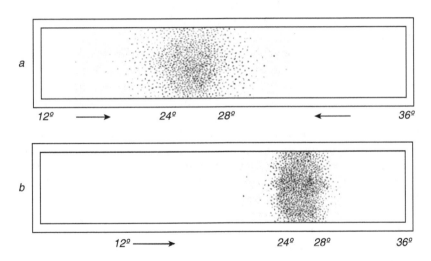

Figure 7.1 Congregation of single-cell paramecia at a 'preferred' temperature of 24–28°C. Note the avoidance of the extreme high (36°C) and low (12°C) temperatures and the preference for the moderate (24–28°C) temperatures.

Source: From Mendelssohn (1895). With kind permission of Springer Science and Business Media.

The temperature on much of the Earth's surface ranges from 0°C to 50°C. Therefore, it is not surprising that some animals, such as polar fish and other invertebrates, can survive in temperatures below 0°C, while some algae can also tolerate temperatures above 70°C (Schmidt-Nielsen 1995). Given our relatively long evolutionary path, it is difficult to pinpoint accurately what the prevailing environmental temperature might have been during the very early stages of hominid evolution. The ambient temperature range in which this occurred could provide the basis on which most animals (mammals and birds) chose a balance point T_c of ~37°C.

The basic premise relating the balance point temperature to mammalian functioning is that certain processes, such as denaturation of proteins, thermal coagulation and thermal inactivation of enzymes, and inadequate oxygen supply are likely to have been critical (Crompton et al. 1978; Portner 2004). The complexity of protein function is well beyond the scope of this text, but it is a key component to consider as to why homeotherms have in general opted for a stable body temperature normally well above the ambient temperature. Recall that heterothermy is the dependence of an organism on the environment to adjust and maintain its body temperature. This method would be cumbersome and disadvantageous for relatively larger animals since warming up to prepare for activity and prime metabolic functioning would carry a high risk of being underprepared for a predatory challenge. The maintenance of a high body temperature conceivably allows larger animals to be ready for a high rate and immediate physical exertion. Thus, organisms which require high body and tissue temperatures will also require protein function adapted for that higher rather than lower tissue temperature for catalytic action.

Although protein functionality is essential for processes which occur within a narrow temperature range, they do not provide an answer as to why the balance point chosen is 37°C and not some other temperature, such as 25°C or 45°C. To arrive at the common balance point of 37°C some assumptions must be made. Homeotherms evolved over a time span of ~60 million years when the ambient temperature was on average 25°C for long periods but interspersed with cooler fluctuating temperatures (Zachos et al. 2001) (see also www.scotese.com/climate.htm for an in-depth description). A further assumption relates to the law of *Arrhenius*, which states that heat production increases two- to three-fold with every 10°C increase. This is known as the Q_{10} effect so that each 1°C increase in T_c will increase heat production by $2.3^{0.1}$ (or 1.086). If we make these two reasonably reliable assumptions it is possible to arrive at the balance point T_c established by mammals by using the following equations (Gisolfi & Mora 2000). First, the temperature gradient between the T_c and the environment can be given as

$$T_c - 25°C$$

If there is a 1°C increase in core temperature this would result in

$$T_c + 1°C - 25°C = T_c - 24°C$$

Whereby the 1°C increase will alter the gradient between the environment and the core. Since maintenance of body temperature is highly dependent on heat loss, this will proceed according to the temperature gradient expressed as

$$(T_c - 24) / (T_c - 25) = 1.086$$

Solving for T_c results in 36.6°C or ~37°C. Although this mathematical model results in the stable T_c of homeotherms, its power suggests that ambient temperature where heat loss and heat gain mechanisms achieve their equilibrium is likely around 25°C. This model also shows that the ideal T_c would naturally be well above the ambient temperature so that heat loss can be an effective mechanism for heat transfer away from the body. The consequence is the higher threshold for the activation of the sweating response, which in turn results in reduced reliance on water.

There are also other possibilities for the maintenance of a high body temperature. One is that the thermodynamic properties of water, the universal medium for life, requires higher rather than lower temperatures to maintain thermal equilibrium (McGowan 1979). There is also the possibility that there exists a universal thermodynamic switch where balance between entropy and enthalpy allows for the basic biological processes of protein folding and self-assembly to occur (Chun 2005). This latter point cannot be underestimated, for any deviation from such a high temperature value or the universal thermodynamic switch becoming unavailable would be catastrophic.

The maintenance of a higher rather than lower T_c of 37°C can also be explained by several other possibilities and not just the prevailing conditions (Portner 2004). First, the fact that the human body is constituted largely by water (~60%), with major organs composed of differing amounts (Mitchell et al. 1945), indicates that evolutionary pressure must have accounted for the specific heat of water in its decision to have a high resting temperature. The specific heat of water is defined as the amount of heat required to raise its temperature 1°C, specifically 4.184 joules/gram/°C of heat. This is higher than most other known substances, making the human body incredibly resistant to heating. In fact, a breakdown of some of the organs indicates a high capacity for heat absorption, whereby the water content of the brain and heart is 73%, lungs 83%, skin 64% and muscles and kidneys 79% (Mitchell et al. 1945). This composition is a little appreciated but critical step in our evolutionary path since water is essentially the ingredient for life as we know it to exist.

Second, the maintenance of a higher body temperature means that a variety of habitats are available for shelter from the elements and there is a greater opportunity to survive compared with living in water, where the cooling potential by conduction would be too great (Portner 2004). Third, it appears that many species prefer an optimal performance temperature which is close to thermal limits of the organism (Angilletta et al. 2002). In Chapter 2, the evolutionary basis of trade-offs was discussed by illustrating that biological function is also determined and constrained by limited resources, space, energy availability and time so that increasing two traits at the same time is not possible (Taylor & Weibel 1981). This relationship and trade-off paradigm hold for respiration and circulation, which are also intimately dependent on body temperature. Since the affinity of haemoglobin for oxygen is reduced at higher temperatures the overall effect of increasing temperature leads to a more efficient unloading of haemoglobin so that free oxygen can enter the cells. As such this respiratory-circulatory-temperature relationship has an additional benefit. The capacity to unload oxygen more efficiently reduces the need for high mitochondrial densities but with maximal energy (ATP) production capacity, leaving cellular space for other functions, such as greater space for contractile proteins for muscular work (Portner 2004). Thus, a high balance point temperature has distinct physiological and functional advantages, particularly for aerobic performance.

Ultimately, the selection of a high rather than low balance point temperature provided *Homo* with the capacity for higher heat tolerance, greater possibilities for access to resources due to a larger roaming range and the immediate access to aerobic function.

Thermoregulation as a survival strategy

It is now well established that rising body temperature hampers performance and is associated with the onset of earlier fatigue in both health (Nielsen 1996; Nielsen et al. 1993) and disease (Marino 2009; White & Dressendorfer 2004). The reasons for this relationship are only beginning to be elucidated and point to the possibility that the central nervous system plays a major role (Nybo & Nybo 2007). Thus, the thermoregulatory system is now thought to be one of the limiting factors for human performance, but the question still remains as to what the casual mechanism might be. To elucidate this, the model presented in Figure 7.2 is an attempt to connect the known physiological responses occurring with the rise in body temperature during exercise.

The common misconception with the model presented in Figure 7.2 is that it applies to all homeotherms since body temperature is regulated around a similar balance point temperature of ~37°C. However, humans are the only hairless animals which possess more eccrine sweat glands, whereas other animals having a coat of hair will generally possess exocrine sweat glands. The difference between these sweat glands is also the difference between whether the skin surface is wet, as for humans, or sweat is secreted onto the hair follicle, as for other mammals. This alone indicates that different mammals operate with a different thermoregulatory strategy since evaporation for cooling is limited based on the type of sweat gland available (McGowan 1979).

The sprinter

To illustrate the difference in thermoregulatory performance it is useful to dichotomise performance into power versus endurance. Within the animal kingdom

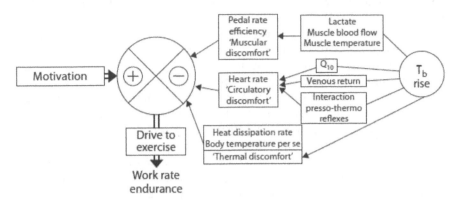

Figure 7.2 Physiological factors thought to be responsible for limiting endurance in the heat. The drive to exercise is influenced by signals generated by physiological systems on one side and by motivation on the other. Although not recognised at the time, motivation could be thought of as a central nervous system drive which we now understand to affect the motor output when hyperthermia is induced.

Source: From Brück and Olschewski (1987) with permission from NRC Research Press.

there are animals which will rely on their power for predatory behaviour and as a consequence survival. These include gazelles, hare and the large cats (family *felinae*). The African cheetah (*Acinonyx Jubatus*) is regarded as one of the fastest animals and has been reliably recorded to reach speeds of ~105 km/h (Sharp 1997), whereas the next fastest, the antelope, can reach speeds of ~80 km/h (Taylor & Lyman 1972). In contrast to these powerful animals are the fastest human sprinters, which are able to reach only 41–43 km/h over the 100 m according to the theoretical boundary of 9.3 s (Summers 1997). However, unlike the cheetah, which can maintain top speed for up to 300 m, human sprinters can achieve this for only up to 150 m. The reason for this short run distance is that the high speeds achieved for both cheetah and humans can be maintained for only as long as the energy for muscular contraction is available. Nevertheless, the extreme power and speed exhibited by the cheetah are related to the high preponderance of fast-twitch fibres in the *v. lateralis* muscle, which amount to approximately 83% of muscle fibres with only 2%–3.9% mitochondrial volume, representing the extreme range compared with trained sprinters, such as greyhounds and humans (Williams et al. 1997).

This muscle fibre composition, in part, also explains the rapid fatigue experienced by the cheetah and the reluctance for a subsequent predatory attempt within a short period of time. However, the classic view is that the cheetah abandons its predatory chase as a consequence of overheating (Taylor & Rowntree 1973). This inference is based largely on the observation that the cheetah under experimental conditions refused to run when its body temperature achieved 40.5–41°C (Taylor & Rowntree 1973). The critical observation leading to this conclusion was that heat storage was so rapid during running that even at a mere 17 km/h, almost 70% of heat produced was stored because the cheetah has not developed an effective evaporative cooling mechanism to maintain heat balance. The conclusion was that sprinters use heat storage as a strategy, but the consequence was that a repeat performance could not be attempted until body temperature was reduced. More contemporary observations suggest that overheating is not the primary cause for the cheetah to abandon its chase. When comparing between successful and unsuccessful hunts, subsequent peak body temperatures were higher for successful hunts (39.2 vs 38.7°C), which contradicts the overheating hypothesis (Hetem et al. 2013). It was also observed that the post-hunt increases in body temperature when the cheetah was successful are likely related to fear-induced hyperthermia due to high sympathetic nervous system activity, also exhibited in other animals, such as impala (Meyer et al. 2008). The reasons for this are not entirely clear but a stress-induced hyperthermia response has been suggested. Notably, the cheetah will not feed immediately after the kill, opting to survey the area and be vigilant, likely to avoid becoming prey (Hunter et al. 2006).

These observations suggest that body temperature is not likely to play a part in whether the cheetah abandons the chase. The question, however, is whether the cheetah will attempt a repeat maximal effort when its body temperature has increased to hyperthermic values. To date, this question has not been sufficiently answered, probably due to the number of variables that the free-ranging cheetah has to negotiate, such as habitat, cover, prey size, age and season (Eaton 1970). What is clear is that temperature is likely to play a key role in the cheetah's survival strategy.

In contrast to the cheetah, human sprinters do not seem to be adversely affected by high environmental temperatures with respect to single-sprint performance. An analysis of performances ranging from 100 m to the marathon shows that short distance events of 100–400 m have a positive change in performance – that is, faster times when ambient temperatures are greater than 25°C for both male and female athletes (Guy et al. 2014) (see Figure 7.3). The reasons for this are not entirely clear but are likely to include both biochemical and contractile responses to increased temperature, as outlined in Chapter 5.

Although a single explosive performance in the heat can be enhanced, a similar repeat performance is unlikely if recovery under these conditions is not sufficient. Under favourable ambient conditions there is almost complete recovery from an initial maximal sprint over the subsequent rest period of 60–300 s which is relative to the distance covered (Newman et al. 2004; Girard et al. 2011; Bogdanis et al. 1995). For example, Figure 7.4 shows that the percentage of the peak power resulting from a 30s cycle ergometer sprint was ~93% restored by 3 min but did not increase any further over the subsequent 3 min (at 6 min). Even though there is significant recovery for human sprinters, complete recovery is not evident within this timeframe even under normal ambient conditions.

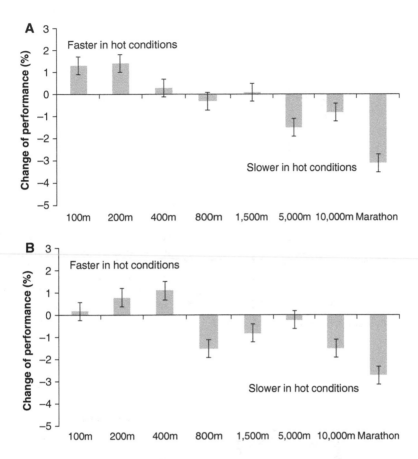

Figure 7.3 Comparative mean ± 95% confidence limits percentage change of performance in temperate (≤ 25°C) versus hot (≥ 25°C) conditions from International Association of Athletics Federation (IAAF) World Championship track events from 1999 to 2011 for males (a) and females (b). The positive percentage indicates faster performance, whereas negative percentage indicates slower performance in hot conditions.

Source: From Guy et al. (2014), reproduced with kind permission from Springer Nature.

However, recovery is apparently also dependent on body temperature, as shown in Figure 7.5 (Drust et al. 2005). The data in Figure 7.5 show that overall peak power for the repeated five sprints is reduced because of the individual consecutive decrements. What is evident is that recovery of peak power, and by extension repeated sprinting, is compromised to a greater extent when body temperature is elevated (Bishop & Maxwell 2009). The reduced power output in this repeated-sprint scenario was not attributed to the known metabolic fatigue

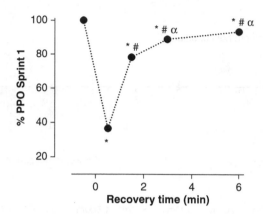

Figure 7.4 Peak power output (PPO) during recovery from a maximal 30s cycle ergometer sprint. The time course shows that by the end of the 30 s power was reduced to ~37% of peak. At 1.5 min there is an ~80% recovery and at 3 min there is ~89% recovery of the power exhibited in the initial 30s sprint. The values are mean ± SEM, N = 14. *P < 0.01 from sprint 1; #P < 0.01 from end of sprint 1; αP < 0.01 from 1.5 min.

Source: Redrawn from Bogdanis et al. (1995).

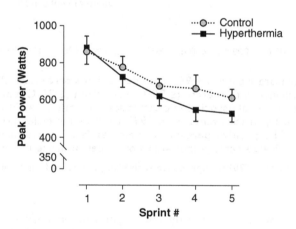

Figure 7.5 The peak power achieved at five consecutive maximal cycling sprints each lasting 15 s followed by 15 s of recovery. The ambient temperature for hyperthermia was 40°C versus 20°C for control. Core temperature in hyperthermia was measured via the oesophagus and reached 39 ± 0.2°C.

Source: Data redrawn from Drust et al. (2005).

agents, but the influence of the higher T_c on the central nervous system, irrespective of whether ambient temperature or passive heating was the cause for elevated body temperature (Drust et al. 2005).

The observation that animal and human sprinters are adversely affected by elevated body temperature when performing maximally and when recovering from these efforts is an indication that hyperthermia induces premature fatigue and increases the time needed for recovery. Since humans cannot reach speeds that come close to the cheetah, the capacity to remove heat that is generated due to high speeds is not as critical for humans. Heat storage can be a limiting factor for the cheetah since it will store about 70% of the heat produced when running at a mere ~11 km/h (Taylor & Rowntree 1973), whereas humans store relatively little heat (8%–12%) when running at 14 km/h (Marino et al. 2000). This discrepancy means that unlike the cheetah, humans are endowed with the capacity to avoid accumulating heat quickly, trading speed for endurance and utilising a different thermoregulatory strategy for survival.

The endurance athlete

A comparative analysis of the human endurance capability versus quadrupeds that trot suggests that endurance speeds for humans are relatively fast. Over short distances quadrupeds outrun humans, so surviving a chase by a lion is unlikely since any chance of accomplishing this particular feat would require reaching speeds above those of elite human sprinters, given the lion's top speed in the wild is 13–14 m/s (~50 km/h) (Elliott et al. 1977). However, human endurance speeds compare quite favourably with other cursorial mammals, as described by Bramble and Lieberman (2004). In their careful analysis of human endurance, they show that the range of human speeds for endurance running is 2.3–6.5 m/s, with elite athletes being in the upper range (Figure 7.6). Although these comparisons as given in Figure 7.6 are theoretical derivatives, they clearly show that humans possess exceptional endurance running capabilities which are not always appreciated.

As discussed in Chapter 3, the most unique human characteristic is habitual bipedal locomotion and the capability to walk and run long distances at reasonably fast speeds even in hot conditions. However, this does not imply that the heat of the day does not hamper our endurance; rather it implies that we are comparatively very able endurance runners even when environmental temperatures are relatively high. There is both experimental and field evidence that our endurance capacity is significantly reduced as ambient temperature rises. This is illustrated by the fundamental observation that time to exhaustion is relative to the ambient conditions so that performance appears to follow an inverted U-shaped relationship (Figure 7.7). Notably, the longest exercise time is achieved closer to ambient temperatures of 10.5°C, but interestingly, at lower ambient temperatures (3.6°C) exercise time is not prolonged any further compared with 20.6°C (Figure 7.7).

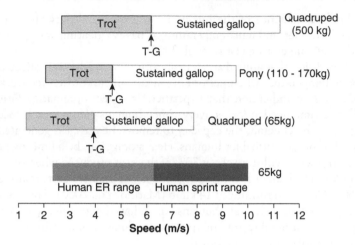

Figure 7.6 Comparative endurance running range (ER) in humans and quadrupeds of different sizes. Note the human ER to be comparable to quadrupeds adjusted for similar body mass (65 kg) when compared to trotting since bipedal running and trotting are biomechanically comparable. It is also notable that human ER speeds exceed the preferred trotting and trot-gallop transition (T-G) speeds of ponies and the preferred trotting speed predicted for large quadrupeds.

Source: Adapted from Bramble and Lieberman (2004) with kind permission from Springer Nature.

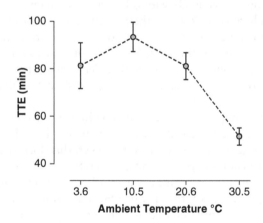

Figure 7.7 The time to exhaustion (TTE) for eight moderately trained non-acclimatised healthy males when cycling on a stationary ergometer at 70% maximal oxygen consumption at four different ambient temperatures with 70 ± 2% relative humidity and air velocity ~0.7 m/s. Exercise duration was shortest at 30.5°C and longest at 10.5°C.

Source: Data redrawn from Galloway and Maughan (1997).

The experimental observations reported in Figure 7.7 are also reproduced with highly trained runners during self-paced treadmill running at three different ambient temperatures (Figure 7.8). However, the main difference between the observations in the two studies is that in ambient temperatures of 15–25°C the running speed is not significantly different. The difference in running speed becomes apparent only when ambient temperatures rise above 25°C. Interestingly, the number of finishers in the Olympic Marathon over a period of 100 years correlates with the prevailing conditions where only ~54% of runners successfully complete the race when ambient temperatures are above 25°C, versus ~87% when ambient temperature is below 25°C (Marino 2004). These data also fit well with the observation that marathon times are progressively slower as ambient temperature rises above 10–12°C (Dennis & Noakes 1999) and that record times for races ranging from 5,000 m to 100 km are seldom set when ambient temperatures are above ~14°C (Marino 2004).

A further critical observation is that marathon running speeds for a range of participants are 4.3–5.2 m/s when ambient temperatures are 10–27.8°C with relative humidity (rh) no more than ~37%, but these speeds are drastically reduced to 3.3–3.6 m/s when rh is above 60% (Cheuvront & Haymes 2001). The effects of rh will be discussed in more detail subsequently; however, these observations indicate that ambient temperature alone is not the sole contributor to decreased performance in warm conditions.

Although there is no question that human endurance is hampered by high environmental temperatures, humans do have an impressive strategy to offload

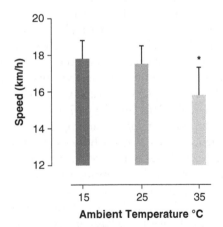

Figure 7.8 The running speed of 12 well-trained men at three different ambient temperatures during an 8km self-paced treadmill run. The mean ± SD run times were 27 ± 1.5, 27.4 ± 1.5 and 30.4 ± 2.9 min for 15, 25 and 35°C, respectively. *P < 0.05 compared with 15 and 25°C.

Source: Data from Marino et al. (2000).

endogenous heat. This capability must have evolved in order that persistence hunting was possible (see Chapter 1). Before outlining how *Homo* uses its thermoregulatory strategy during endurance running, it is useful to consider how other endurance animals deal with the heat. As we shall see, not all endotherms deploy the same strategy to deal with either endogenous or ambient heat load. One of the most impressive endurance athletes is the African hunting dog (*Lycaon pictus*). This species of the *Canidae* family has been observed to run at 56 km/h for 3–5 min and to be able to maintain an impressive 48 km/h over 5 km and can easily run 32 km/h for up to 8 km (Estes & Goddard 1967). In comparison, and as already noted, the best human endurance runners can average ~23 km/h over 5–10 km. The African hunting dog can outrun the best human endurance runner by ~9 km/h over comparable distances. This capability is even more impressive when considering this animal normally accomplishes this running feat in its habitat with ambient temperatures ranging between 25°C and 35°C during hunting (Creel et al. 2016).

The most widely cited study on the exercising African hunting dog shows that during a chase, this animal not only is able to run at higher T_c compared with the domestic dog but also can increase its T_c more rapidly in identical ambient conditions (Taylor et al. 1971). The key observation by these authors is that at rest, the African hunting dog is also able to raise its T_c above ambient temperature compared to the domestic dog, which maintains a constant T_c. These observations would seem at odds with the overwhelming evidence that high core temperatures lead to an early onset of exercise termination across a number of mammalian species (Caputa et al. 1986; Caputa et al. 1985; Walters et al. 2000; McConaghy et al. 2002). The African hunting dog is able to maintain an elevated core temperature and seemingly be unaffected because during running, it is able to reduce the evaporative cutaneous water loss while simultaneously increasing respiratory heat loss (Taylor et al. 1971). The ability to alter the heat dissipation mechanism has an overall effect of reducing reliance on water over long distances and between runs. In addition, this animal has evolved distinct morphological characteristics, such as slender, long legs and large vascularised ears, which assist in heat dissipation (Creel et al. 2016) (see Figure 7.9).

Although the African hunting dog has an impressive thermoregulatory strategy, recent field evidence shows that on hotter days, this animal hunted and killed more often, and the chases were shorter, suggesting that heat dissipation limits the escape of prey rather than limiting the African hunting dog's chase (Creel et al. 2016). As suggested by the authors, the key point is that temperature regulation with respect to the prevailing environmental conditions will essentially alter the interaction between predator and prey. As we shall see, an effective thermoregulatory strategy adopted by *Homo* provided the basis by which we were able to alter our interaction with prey for the procurement of food.

Human endurance in the heat is highly dependent on the potential heat exchange between the environment and the body surface. The first limitation for

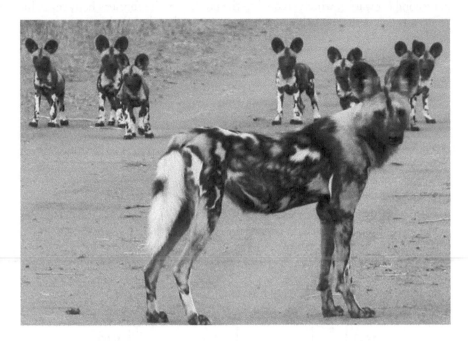

Figure 7.9 The African hunting dog. Note the long, slender legs and the large ears, which are highly vascularised (Creel et al. 2016). These features assist in the dissipation of heat and are the morphological adaptations which are thought to enhance thermoregulation. For a discussion on the relationship between morphology, efficiency and thermoregulation see Chapter 5.

Source: Photo with kind permission from Arathusa Safari Lodge.

heat exchange is related to the available gradient between the temperature at the skin surface and that of the environment. As these two temperatures come close to being equivalent, less heat is potentially offloaded from the body, and indeed as the environmental temperature rises above the skin surface temperature, heat can potentially be gained. Heat exchange potential is also heavily dependent on the percent relative humidity (% *rh*) of the ambient air whereby the vapour pressure gradient between skin and ambient air determines the amount of evaporation of sweat that can occur. These two physical properties – temperature and vapour pressure gradient – alter the skin surface temperature (Nielsen 1996). The overall aim of maintaining a gradient for offloading heat to the environment is to afford cooling the blood at the skin and returning it to the core. A simple calculation with some underlying assumptions demonstrates how critical this heat exchange potential can be. Heat production (*H*) during running can be calculated in joules per second (or watts), which is equal to the product of the runner's body mass, his or her running speed and the approximate 4 J produced per kilogram per metre run (Nielsen 1996):

$$H = \text{kilograms} \times \text{metres per second} \times 4 \text{ J/kg/min}$$

By calculating heat production and since the evaporation of 1 litre of sweat per hour dissipates ~625 J/s assuming all sweat is evaporated, then estimating the required evaporation (E_R) can show the effect of temperature and humidity on thermal balance. Figure 7.10 shows data from an 8km performance run in three different environments when *rh* was set at 60% and wind speed at 15 km/h when applying these assumptions and equations (Marino et al. 2000). What can be seen in Figure 7.10 is that runners produce less heat as ambient temperature rises from 15°C to 35°C because their speed is reduced, but the E_R climbs by virtue of the smaller temperature and vapour pressure gradients. This effectively means that at high ambient temperatures (35°C) when relative humidity > 60%, the runner will potentially store rather than offload heat.

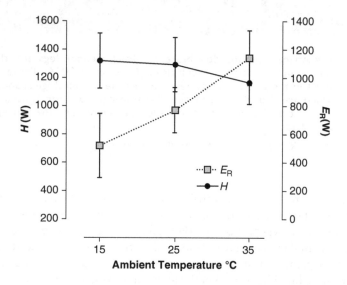

Figure 7.10 The heat production (*H*; left ordinate) and the required evaporation (E_R; right ordinate) in watts (W) when running an 8km performance run in three ambient temperatures (15, 25, 35°C and % relative humidity at 60%). Note that E_R would normally be expressed as a negative sign since this heat exchange parameter provides the main means of heat dissipation. The negative sign has been removed in order to show more clearly that E_R increases as heat and humidity also increase.

Source: Data redrawn from Marino et al. (2000).

Table 7.1 Evolutionary adaptations related to effective thermoregulation in humans.

Adaptation	Responses
Sweating – Eccrine glands: high density with distribution over body.	Secretion rates of 366–884 g/m²/h. Sweat rates during competitive sport can range from 2 to 4 l/h (Pugh et al. 1967; Armstrong et al. 1986).
Loss of fur – Humans are furless with vellus hair*.	This allows for the evaporation of sweat from the skin and improves air convection at the skin surface.
Head airflow – An external nose and obligate oro-nasal breathing.	Increased turbulent airflow during inhalation and possibly exhalation (Churchill et al. 2004). Humans are the only mammals that switch to oro-nasal breathing during heavy exercise (Wheatley et al. 1991).
Upright, slender body – Length of limbs will affect the volume-to-surface area relationship, altering the heat gain or loss from the limbs# (Tilkens et al. 2007).	Upright postural change with slender limbs provides for increased convective and evaporative heat loss and reduces surface area for solar radiation (Wheeler 1994).

Note: *Hair that grows from shallow follicles not connected to sebaceous glands. #For a discussion on limb length and morphology related to thermoregulation see Chapter 5.

Even though this example shows that we are at the mercy of the environment in maintaining thermal balance and preserving our endurance capabilities, humans are still at a relative advantage over most other mammals because we have particular adaptations. There are four key evolutionary adaptations which limit the extent of hyperthermia during physical activity. Table 7.1 lists the specific adaptations thought to provide humans with the capability to thermoregulate more effectively compared to other animals. This is an important distinction since any detriment in our endurance performance because of heat stress should be relatively less than that observed in other species if persistence hunting was a key to our survival (Liebenberg 2006, 2008). As we shall see, other animals and presumably those that early *Homo* hunted would have been less effective thermoregulators, giving *Homo* the advantage in the predatory stakes.

Morphology for effective endurance

Individual physical characteristics have been shown to be either an advantage or disadvantage in human performance (see Chapter 5 for discussion). This is also the case with respect to temperature regulation during physical exercise. The common observation is that distance runners have generally a smaller stature than sprinters or middle distance competitors. Data on height and mass of males winning the Boston Marathon suggest that these characteristics have remained relatively constant for over a century, with average height being 171.3 ± 5.4 cm and mass at 61.6 ± 5.1 kg (Norton & Olds 1996). Interestingly, these characteristics are in contrast to what seems to be the secular trend for the general population in many parts of the world, with stature increasing about 1 cm per decade for about six generations (Cole 2003). The relationship between maintenance of particular physical characteristics and maximising performance has been known for some time. However, the relationship between stature, mass and endurance requires further examination since endurance is also dependent on the interaction with the environment. Characteristics such as the ratio between body surface area (A_D) and mass (m, in kg) (A_D/m) can be important determinants of heat gain and loss (Epstein et al. 1983). In this case, heat loss can be maximised when the A_D/m ratio is large, but when this ratio is reduced heat can be gained from the environment (Epstein et al. 1983). These observations suggest that a greater degree of heat retention in larger, heavier runners could limit endurance performance. In fact, over 70 years ago it was shown that a large man (99 kg) could not maintain thermal balance compared with a smaller man (61 kg) during moderate exercise in warm conditions (31–33°C and 68%–74% rh), even with a larger surface area, which allowed for potentially greater evaporation of sweat (Robinson 1942). Other studies have also shown the rate of increase in T_{re} to be greater for individuals with high mesomorphy even when walking at 7 km/h in ambient temperatures of 30°C and 80% rh (Hayward et al. 1986).

Using heat exchange calculations (Kerslake 1972) and marathon runners as an example, it appears that lighter runners might be more advantaged than heavier runners when racing in warm, humid conditions (35°C, 60% rh) (Dennis & Noakes 1999). Heavier runners (75 kg) can maintain thermal balance in such conditions only with a maximum running speed of 12.2 km/h, whereas a 45kg runner could maintain thermal balance at 19.1 km/h – a clear body mass and speed advantage. These calculations suggest that body size (stature and mass) could be either an advantage or disadvantage for endurance in hot conditions. This relationship was evaluated with a group of well-trained (VO_{2max} of 64 ml/kg/min; 55–90 kg) runners in ambient temperatures of 15°C and 25°C, which showed that running speed was not compromised according to body mass (Marino et al. 2000). However, when the same group of runners attempted the performance in 35°C, mean running speed was significantly reduced as body mass increased (Figure 7.11).

In addition to these data are those comparing runners of different ancestry which show that African runners are usually at an advantage compared with their Caucasian counterparts because of the disparity in morphology (Marino et al. 2004). However, there is some evidence to suggest that differences in skeletal muscle and biochemical characteristics based on ancestry also potentially contribute to performance differences (Weston et al. 1999). The fact that when African runners are matched with Caucasian runners for both VO_{2max} (62.6 vs 64.3 ml/kg/min, respectively) and peak treadmill running speed (21.2 vs 20.8 km/h,

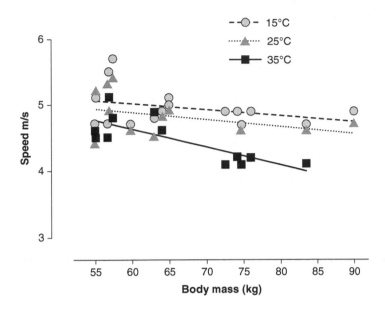

Figure 7.11 The relationship between body mass ranging from 55 to 90 kg versus the mean running speed during the 8km performance treadmill run in the three ambient conditions and relative humidity set at 60%. At 15°C and 25°C there was no significant correlation evident. A significant correlation was evident at 35°C ($y = 6.30 - 0.0265x$; $r = 0.77$, $P < 0.0004$).

Source: Reproduced from Marino et al. (2000), with kind permission from Springer Nature.

respectively) they can out-perform their Caucasian counterparts by running ~17% faster in the heat but not in the cooler condition indicates that smaller stature and mass are an advantage in the heat (Marino et al. 2004). Body morphology as it relates to stature and mass is key in the evolution of human endurance running, given that this capability is the basis for the persistence hunting hypothesis (Bramble & Lieberman 2004; Carrier et al. 1984). As outlined in Chapter 5 (Table 5.1), early species of *Homo* were relatively small, with heights ranging from 1.2 to 1.64 cm and mass of 50–65 kg. Since it is believed that endurance running originated ~2 million years ago (Bramble & Lieberman 2004), the morphology was likely well adapted to take advantage of the ambient conditions in which endurance running was used to compete for food. As we shall see, *Homo* has further adaptations which selected for endurance running capabilities and as a consequence persistence hunting in hot conditions became possible.

Homo as predator in the heat

We have seen that endurance in the heat is compromised to various degrees across a number of species. Persistence hunting has been proposed as a viable hypothesis that enabled *Homo* to advance as the dominant species even in hot conditions (Carrier et al. 1984; Bramble & Lieberman 2004; Liebenberg 2008). To be clear, the underlying premise of persistence hunting is that predation by early *Homo* required at least some biological advantage over their prey. To make this case the following observations are key (Carrier et al. 1984):

- Running can be a form of play in young cursorial mammals;
- Running for play can train and condition for running under other circumstances;
- In some instances, running is used for migration;
- Prey animals rely on speed and endurance to avoid predators;
- Running is used by predators to capture prey.

As already discussed many predators, such as the large cats, use speed to overtake their prey, while other animals, such as the African hunting dog, use endurance and hunting in packs to run down their prey. As already shown in Figure 7.6, the range of speeds for human endurance extends beyond the preferred running speeds of most mammals where the transition from trotting to sustained galloping occurs. However, the major problem for the larger cursorial animal is that being a quadruped reduces the possibility of panting while galloping, which in turn reduces the capacity for heat dissipation. A less appreciated consequence of being a quadruped versus a biped is the difference in the ratio of respiratory cycles and oscillations with respect to locomotion, where ventilation is thought to be principally a function of the kinetics of the neighbouring visceral mass (Carrier 1983). During sustained galloping the quadruped's viscera will be displaced back and forth, pushing into the diaphragm during each stride (Bramble & Jenkins 1993). This mechanical consequence of being on four legs reduces the ability to continuously gallop without being able to offload the heat generated by panting. Therefore, according to Figure 7.6, when pursued the animal has two choices: either sprint ahead at the fastest speed (gallop) and put distance between them and the predator, which might provide a rest period, or trot at the suboptimal speed and risk being captured. In the first scenario, the animal will effectively be required to exercise intermittently in the hope that the predator has given up the chase. If that does not occur, then intermittent activity will eventually lead to fatigue from hyperthermia since intermittent exercise reduces potential evaporative heat loss. A continuous gallop is limited by virtue of the lack of panting, eventually leading to hyperthermia. Thus, the most efficient runner with the capability of offloading heat while running would be at an advantage. Since bipedal running does not have the same mechanical consequences with the viscera pushing into the lungs, it is not a particular problem for healthy human runners to overcome.

To illustrate the difference between the effectiveness of panting versus sweating as a thermoregulatory strategy, a comparison between Thomson's gazelle (*Gazella Thomsonii*) and the eland (*Taurotragus oryx*) shows that when running at

15 km/h the gazelle's core temperature increases at a rate of 4°C/h, whereas the eland running at 25 km/h has a significantly lower rate of rise in core temperature of 3.5°C/h (Taylor & Lyman 1972). This difference is due to the profuse sweating exhibited by the eland, which is ~30% greater than that of the gazelle, which relies heavily on panting for heat dissipation. In contrast, humans can produce exceptional sweating rates of 2–4 l/h (see Table 7.1), which can be ~2–3.4 times that of the eland. The capacity to sustain high levels of exercise for long periods of time in the heat lies within the domain of those species that have high sweating capabilities, with the caveat that temperature and humidity permit the evaporation of sweat.

It is important to recognise that the persistence hunting hypothesis has been challenged on the basis that it could be viable only if early *Homo* had well-established tracking abilities and that modern-day hunter-gatherers do not particularly use endurance running (Pickering & Bunn 2007). This reasoning is underpinned by two key assertions. First, tracking is sophisticated and requires high-level reasoning skills and by implication large encephalisation. In fact, some have even argued that tracking can be regarded as the advent of scientific reasoning (Liebenberg 2013). The assumption is that tracking likely originated and evolved in conditions where it was easiest: sparse ground cover, or cold environments such as snow-covered ground for simple deductions rather than in woodland habitats (Liebenberg 1990; Pickering & Bunn 2007). The second assertion is that there was no need to adopt endurance running as a way of obtaining protein since scavenging and gathering were likely to yield the necessary food. This view is based on the observation that modern hunter-gatherers scavenge in woodland habitats where carcasses are less visible to other carnivores, and that butchery marks in meat-bearing sections of the limbs found at Plio-Pleistocene sites suggest successful acquisition and consumption of rich protein parts before other carnivorous competitors could make use of them (Pickering & Bunn 2007).

These counter-arguments to the persistence hunting hypothesis and more specifically that endurance running was a key component for establishing *Homo* as a dominant species have some merit. However, these counter-arguments also need to be balanced by the following observations. Animals with lesser encephalisation and cognitive abilities than early *Homo* track prey. In fact, animals engage in teaching their young by catch-and-release how to track and overcome prey (Caro 1995). Why this particular skill could not be utilised by early *Homo* to obtain food is not clear. A further observation from the fossil record shows that early *Homo* did not possess projectile weaponry until about 100,000–71,000 years ago (Marean 2015). Thus, without this kind of weapon, *Homo* must have found another method to exhaust or render the prey incapacitated before being able to approach at a distance to dispatch it safely. As we have seen, humans are exceptional distance runners able to run effectively in the heat compared to larger animals, which need to pant to offload heat. As shown in Figure 7.6, keeping the animal above its trotting speed increases its chances of developing hyperthermia, which eventually leads to exhaustion. The human capacity to sweat could not have been selected solely to run away from predators. Finally, we have discussed in detail in Chapters 3 and 5 that *Homo* opted for endurance rather than power and strength. As such engaging with other carnivores by scavenging would have been a dangerous activity since there are no comparably sized animals that we can compete with at close quarters using our strength and power. This, in addition to the lack of projectile weaponry, suggests that scavenging alone was unlikely to yield the nourishment required. Although both arguments for and against persistence hunting and the eventuality of endurance running as a selection pressure are difficult to establish, the morphology and physiology which make humans endurance specialists do suggest a distinct advantage.

Homo, non-human primates and the environment

As discussed earlier, the capacity to sweat is critical for humans, particularly so in higher ambient temperatures. It has also been argued that this physiological adaptation might have been selected when our ancestors moved from the forest patches to the warm, dry savanna, where persistence hunting and endurance running also evolved. However, it has also been argued that this is a difficult hypothesis to test. Nevertheless, data from non-human primates do provide some clues as to the viability of sweating as a key response in making *Homo* more resilient to surviving in a harsh, warm environment. Unfortunately, the data on sweating and more generally on thermoregulation in non-human primates is scarce. In comparing our closest living relatives, it has been shown that the chimpanzee sweats rapidly and reasonably profusely mainly around the axillae rather than the chest and back, as is the case in humans (Whitford 1976). Further to this was the observation that the chimpanzee has difficulty in maintaining a constant body temperature and is likely to suffer heat stroke when ambient temperatures approach 40°C (Whitford 1976). As noted earlier, this is not the case in humans. Notably, non-human primates increase their respiratory frequency in order to effectively increase their evaporative heat loss (Hiley 1976). However, thermoregulatory data for non-human primates when running in warm ambient conditions reveals that sweating is the main avenue for heat loss (Mahoney 1980). When considering the morphology and dark pelage of the chimpanzee, the capacity to tolerate radiation from the sun is limited and would result in increased heat loads within a short period of time (Kosheleff & Anderson 2009). Chimpanzees in the wild and in captivity thermoregulate behaviourally by using sun-avoidance strategies, seeking shade, moving to the ground and reducing their physical activity level (Kosheleff & Anderson 2009; Duncan & Pillay 2013). Since non-human primates are knuckle walkers, their exposure to the sun is increased because of their adopted stance, exposing large surface areas to the sun. Being bipedal reduces this exposure considerably and with the evaporative cooling makes *Homo* a better candidate for endurance running in the heat.

Selective brain cooling

In Table 7.1 four fundamental evolutionary adaptations are listed that are related to effective thermoregulation in humans. One adaptation that appears critical to some species is that of selective brain cooling (SBC). This suggests that the brain has a built-in mechanism to protect it from reaching high temperatures (Baker 1982). This has been shown to exist in a number of species, including mammals, birds and reptiles. But its existence in humans has been debated for at least 30 years (Cabanac 1993). A key component of SBC is that it can be more readily observed in animals which possess a developed carotid rete. The purpose of this structure is that it provides a counter-current in the head between the arterial and venous blood and respiration, assisting in evaporative and conductive heat loss between the warmer and cooler blood travelling through these vessels. A further observation, however, is that SBC has also been identified in species that do not have a developed carotid rete. For example, when the respiratory tract was bypassed by tracheotomy in the exercising horse there was an immediate reduction in the amount of SBC compared to that before tracheotomy (McConaghy et al. 1995). In this instance, SBC in the horse occurs via the cavernous sinus secondary to venous cooling within the upper respiratory tract. This is possible since the ratio of the respiratory tract surface area to brain mass is significant in the horse. Therefore, as blood flows into the cavernous sinus it is possible that cooling is augmented via this structure due to its relative size.

Although there is consensus that SBC exists in some species, there is no such consensus that humans possess a carotid rete. However, the lack of a carotid rete does not rule out SBC as there are many species in which this has been shown without the availability of this structure. Therefore, if SBC was a viable mechanism for thermoregulation and for protection of the brain from thermal injury, what structures would need to be available for this to occur? This has been addressed in a landmark paper detailing the concept of a 'radiator' for the human head (Zenker & Kubik 1996). The suggestion is that there are large vessels which penetrate the emissary foramina in the skull where an avenue for heat exchange between venous blood and heat loss through evaporation on the surface of the head can take place. These veins provide an avenue for conductive heat loss between the larger veins in the neck and the arteries entering the brain.

Evidence for SBC in humans comes from studies that show a direct effect of respiration on subdural temperature. For example, there is a negative correlation between the extent of nostril dilatation and tympanic temperature during exercise (White & Cabanac 1995), and following extubation there is a rapid reduction in cribriform plate temperature with increases in respiratory rate (Mariak et al. 1999). However, these data are in contrast to studies which show that middle cerebral artery blood velocity is reduced during hyperthermia by up to 26% so that convective heat removal from the brain is reduced by up to 20% (Nybo et al. 2002). Given the available evidence, it is difficult to say with any certainty that humans have been endowed with a mechanism for SBC.

Temperature, environment and pathology

Although healthy humans are well equipped to deal with high ambient and body temperatures, there are instances where tolerance is reduced to both exogenous and endogenous heat loads and can led to poor health outcomes. Heat intolerance beyond that caused by strenuous exercise is normally considered a pathology, and in some instances can be lethal (Jurkat-Rott et al. 2000). Some diseases which cause heat intolerance are a consequence of genetic mutations, but some are an outcome of other neurological disorders. For example, malignant hyperthermia is a condition in which there is a predisposition for individuals to respond with uncontrollable skeletal muscle hyper-metabolism when exposed to volatile anaesthetics or depolarising muscle relaxants (Denborough et al. 1970). The pathogenesis of this disease is related to the mutations in the ryanodine receptor RYR1, the calcium release channel of skeletal muscle (Jurkat-Rott et al. 2000). Since the etiology and the likely trigger for this disease are known, its treatment is also relatively effective (Kolb et al. 1982). A disease which is due to a genetic disorder, such as malignant hyperthermia, is quite different to one that causes heat intolerance due to heat exposure or physical exertion. For example, in certain neurological disorders heat intolerance and the eventuality of fatigue can be a hallmark of the disease. In Parkinson's disease there is usually autonomic dysfunction which can vary within the spectrum of the disease. For instance, the sweating response has been reported to be volatile so that in some Parkinson's patients it is increased while in others it is decreased. If sweating and vasodilation are compromised in this disease then it might also decrease heat elimination (De Marinis et al. 1991).

Multiple sclerosis (MS) is a neurodegenerative disease characterised by axonal loss and demyelination leading to debilitating symptoms related to motor dysfunction and muscle weakness (Smith & McDonald 1999). The pathology and related fatigue of this disease will be discussed in more detail in Chapter 10, but it is worth mentioning briefly that a particular symptom which seems to be a predominant outcome of MS is excessive fatigue (Bakshi et al. 2000). Fatigue as a symptom is of particular interest since it reduces the capacity to undertake activities of daily living and engagement in exercise. However, it appears that fatigue in this disease is precipitated by heat intolerance, which was documented and reported by Uhthoff (1890). Since this early report it is now thought that in neurological diseases, such as MS, there is heat reaction blockade of the action potentials in demyelinated neurons, termed frequency-dependant conduction block (Guthrie & Nelson 1995). Demyelination potentially slows the nerve conduction velocity, which can lead to conduction block whereby the affected axons are able transmit only single- or low-frequency impulses but not high-frequency trains (Rasminsky & Sears 1972), especially as body temperature increases (Schauf & Davis 1974). Thus, when there is demyelination it appears that only a small increase in temperature is able to completely block action potentials.

Exposure to high environmental heat and humidity can exacerbate the sensitivity of MS (Baker 2002). As discussed previously, it is well established that high core temperatures of ~39.5°C are associated with premature fatigue in healthy people, but this phenomenon has not been reported in people with MS since core temperatures of this magnitude are unlikely to be ever attained in this group. However, when patients with MS are precooled, exercise capacity is improved and symptomatic fatigue is ameliorated (White et al. 2000). Interestingly, before undertaking a fatiguing finger flexion and extension protocol, MS patients had greater activation in the areas of the brain such as the contralateral primary motor cortex, insula and cingulate gyrus than did healthy controls (White et al. 2009). After the fatiguing exercise was completed, MS patients did not show any further activation of these areas but actually decreased activity to the insula, whereas controls showed increased activation of the precentral gyrus and insula. The authors suggested that before fatiguing exercise, MS patients required more brain activation compared to controls, which is likely to be a functional adaptation to demyelination. As such the higher activation might reflect higher effort to perform even simple motor tasks, such as finger flexion and extension. The authors concluded that this functional alteration is likely to be a peripheral and central chronic adaptation of the disease. It is not entirely clear why heat exacerbates fatigue in MS; however, since precooling is known to alleviate the effect of heat in MS and can lead to increased exercise time without augmented perceived effort, it is possible that one function of attenuating rises in body temperature via precooling might be to maintain CNS activation rather than reduce it since in healthy individuals central activation of skeletal muscle is compromised with high core temperatures.

The evolutionary significance of heat intolerance in a disease such as MS is not clear. Nevertheless, our capability to withstand high heat loads sets us apart and perhaps when this is compromised because of the secondary consequences of disease, lowering the threshold for fatigue could be the assurance that overheating will not be possible so that overall organismic cellular integrity is not disrupted.

References

Angilletta, M.J., Jr, Niewiarowski, P.H. & Navas, C.A., 2002. The evolution of thermal physiology in ectotherms. *Journal of Thermal Biology*, 27(4), pp. 249–268.

Angilletta, M.J. et al., 2010. The evolution of thermal physiology in endotherms. *Frontiers in Bioscience (Elite Edition)*, 2, pp. 861–881.

Armstrong, L.E., Hubbard, R.W., Jones, B.H. & Daniels, J.T., 1986. Preparing Alberto Salazar for the Heat of the 1984 Olympic Marathon. *The Physician and Sports Medicine*, 14(3), pp. 73–81.

Baker, D., 2002. Multiple sclerosis and thermoregulatory dysfunction. *Journal of Applied Physiology*, 92, pp. 1779–1780.

Baker, M.A., 1982. Brain cooling in endotherms in heat and exercise. *Annual Review of Physiology*, 44, pp. 85–96.

Bakshi, R. et al., 2000. Fatigue in multiple sclerosis and its relationship to depression and neurologic disability. *Multiple Sclerosis*, 6, pp. 181–185.

Benarroch, E.E., 2007. Thermoregulation: recent concepts and remaining questions. *Neurology*, 69(12), pp. 1293–1297.

Bishop, D. & Maxwell, N.S., 2009. Effects of active warm up on thermoregulation and intermittent-sprint performance in hot conditions. *Journal of Science and Medicine in Sport*, 12(1), pp. 196–204.

Bogdanis, G.C. et al., 1995. Recovery of power output and muscle metabolites following 30 s of maximal sprint cycling in man. *Journal of Physiology*, 482(2), pp. 467–480.

Bramble, D.M. & Jenkins, F.A., 1993. Mammalian locomotor-respiratory integration: implications for diaphragmatic and pulmonary design. *Science*, 262(5131), pp. 235–240.

Bramble, D.M. & Lieberman, D.E., 2004. Endurance running and the evolution of *Homo*. *Nature*, 432, pp. 345–352.

Brück, K. & Olschewski, H., 1987. Body temperature related factors diminishing the drive to exercise. *Canadian Journal of Physiology and Pharmacology*, 65(6), pp. 1274–1280.

Cabanac, M., 1993. Selective brain cooling in humans: "fancy" or fact? *FASEB J*, 17, pp. 1143–1147.

Caputa, M., Feistkorn, G. & Jessen, C., 1986. Effects of brain and trunk temperatures on exercise performance in goats. *Pflügers Archives*, 406(2), pp. 184–189.

Caputa, M., Wasilewska, E. & Swiecka, E., 1985. Hyperthermia and exercise performance in guinea-pigs (Cavia porcellus). *Journal of Thermal Biology*, 10(4), pp. 217–220.

Caro, T.M.1995, 1995. Short-term costs and correlates of play in cheetahs. *Animal Behaviour*, 49, pp. 333–345.

Carrier, D.R., 1983. Running and breathing in mammals. *Science*, 219(4582), pp. 251–256.

Carrier, D.R. et al., 1984. The energetic paradox of human running and hominid evolution. *Current Anthropology*, 25, pp. 483–495.

Cheuvront, S.N. & Haymes, E.M., 2001. Thermoregulation and marathon running. *Sports Medicine*, 31(10), pp. 743–762.

Chun, P.W., 2005. Why does the human body maintain a constant 37-degree temperature? thermodynamic switch controls chemical equilibrium in biological systems. *Physica Scripta*, 2005(T118), p. 219.

Churchill, S.E., Shackelford, L.L., Georgi, J.N. & Black, M.T., 2004. Morphological variation and airflow dynamics in the human nose. *American Journal of Human Biology*, 16(6), pp. 625–638.

Cole, T.J., 2003. The secular trend in human physical growth: a biological view. *Economics & Human Biology*, 1(2), pp. 161–168.

Creel, S. et al., 2016. Hunting on a hot day: effects of temperature on interactions between African wild dogs and their prey. *Ecology*, 97(11), pp. 2910–2916.

Crompton, A.W., Taylor, C.R. & Jagger, J.A., 1978. Evolution of homeothermy in mammals. *Nature*, 272(5651), pp. 333–336.

De Marinis, M. et al., 1991. Alterations of thermoregulation in Parkinson's disease. *Functional Neurology*, 6(3), pp. 279–283.

Denborough, M.A. et al., 1970. Myopathy and malignant hyperpyrexia. *The Lancet*, 295(7657), pp. 1138–1140.

Dennis, S.C. & Noakes, T.D., 1999. Advantages of a smaller bodymass in humans when distance-running in warm, humid conditions. *European Journal of Applied Physiology*, 79(3), pp. 280–284.

Drust, B. et al., 2005. Elevations in core and muscle temperature impairs repeated sprint performance. *Acta Physiologica*, 183(2), pp. 181–190.

Duncan, L.M. & Pillay, N., 2013. Shade as a thermoregulatory resource for captive chimpanzees. *Journal of Thermal Biology*, 38(4), pp. 169–177.

Eaton, R.L., 1970. Hunting behavior of the cheetah. *Journal of Wildlife Management*, 34(1), p. 56.

Elliott, J.P. (null), M.C. & Holling, C.S., 1977. Prey capture by the African lion. *Canadian Journal of Zoology*, 55(11), pp. 1811–1828.

Epstein, Y. et al., 1983. Role of surface area-to-mass ratio and work efficiency in heat intolerance. *Journal of Applied Physiology*, 54(3), pp. 831–836.

Estes, R.D. & Goddard, J., 1967. Prey selection and hunting behavior of the African wild dog. *Journal of Wildlife Management*, 31(1), pp. 52–70.

Franzen, J.L. et al., 2009. Complete primate skeleton from the Middle Eocene of Messel in Germany: morphology and paleobiology J. Hawks, ed. *PLOS One*, 4(5), p. e5723.

Galloway, S.D. & Maughan, R.J., 1997. Effects of ambient temperature on the capacity to perform prolonged cycle exercise in man. *Medicine and Science in Sports & Exercise*, 29(9), pp. 1240–1249.

Ginsburg, S. & Jablonka, E., 2009. Epigenetic learning in non-neural organisms. *Journal of Biosciences*, 34(4), pp. 633–646.

Girard, O., Mendez-Villanueva, A. & Bishop, D., 2011. Repeated-sprint ability – Part I. *Sports Medicine*, 41(8), pp. 673–694.

Gisolfi, C.V. & Mora, F., 2000. *The hot brain: survival, temperature, and the human body*, Cambridge, MA: MIT Press.

Guthrie, T.C. & Nelson, D.A., 1995. Influence of temperature changes on multiple sclerosis: critical review of mechanisms and research potential. *Journal of the Neurological Sciences*, 129(1), pp. 1–8.

Guy, J.H. et al., 2014. Adaptation to hot environmental conditions: an exploration of the performance basis, procedures and future directions to optimise opportunities for elite athletes. *Sports Medicine*, 45(3), pp. 303–311.

Havenith, G., 2001. Human surface to mass ratio and body core temperature in exercise heat stress – a concept revisited. *Journal of Thermal Biology*, 26(4–5), pp. 387–393.

Hayward, J.S., Eckerson, J.D. & Dawson, B.T., 1986. Effect of mesomorphy on hyperthermia during exercise in a warm, humid environment. *American Journal of Physical Anthropology*, 70(1), pp. 11–17.

Hetem, R.S. et al., 2013. Cheetah do not abandon hunts because they overheat. *Biology Letters*, 9(5), pp. 20130472–20130472.

Hiley, P.G., 1976. The thermoregulatory responses of the galago (Galago crassicaudatus), the baboon (Papio cynocephalus) and the chimpanzee (Pan stayrus) to heat stress. *Journal of Physiology*, 254(3), pp. 657–671.

Hunter, J.S., Durant, S.M. & Caro, T.M., 2006. To flee or not to flee: predator avoidance by cheetahs at kills. *Behavioral Ecology and Sociobiology*, 61(7), pp. 1033–1042.

Jennings, H.S., 1906. *Behavior of the lower organisms*, London: Columbia University Press.

Joyce, G.F., 2002. The antiquity of RNA-based evolution. *Nature*, 418(6894), pp. 214–221.

Jurkat-Rott, K., McCarthy, T. & Lehmann-Horn, F., 2000. Genetics and pathogenesis of malignant hyperthermia. *Muscle & Nerve*, 23(1), pp. 4–17.

Kerslake, D.M., 1972. *The stress of hot environments*, Cambridge: Cambridge University Press.

Kolb, M.E., Horne, M.L. & Martz, R., 1982. Dantrolene in human malignant hyperthermia. *Anesthesiology*, 56(4), pp. 254–262.

Kosheleff, V.P. & Anderson, C.N.K., 2009. Temperature's influence on the activity budget, terrestriality, and sun exposure of chimpanzees in the Budongo Forest, Uganda. *American Journal of Physical Anthropology*, 139(2), pp. 172–181.

Ladell, W., 1957. Disorders due to heat. *Transactions of the Royal Society of Tropical Medicine and Hygiene*, 51(3), pp. 189–207.

Liebenberg, L., 1990. *The art of tracking: the origin of science*, Cape Town: David Philip Publishers.

Liebenberg, L., 2006. Persistence hunting by modern hunter-gatherers. *Current Anthropology*, 47(6), pp. 1017–1026.

Liebenberg, L., 2008. The relevance of persistence hunting to human evolution. *Journal of Human Evolution*, 55(6), pp. 1156–1159.

Liebenberg, L., 2013. *The origin of science*, Cape Town: CyberTracker.

Mahoney, S.A., 1980. Cost of locomotion and heat balance during rest and running from 0 to 55 degrees C in a patas monkey. *Journal of Applied Physiology*, 49(5), pp. 789–800.

Marean, C., 2015. The most invasive species of all. *Scientific American*, 313(2), pp. 23–29.

Mariak, Z. et al., 1999. Direct cooling of the human brain by heat loss from the upper respiratory tract. *Journal of Applied Physiology*, 87(5), pp. 1609–1613.

Marino, F.E., 2004. Anticipatory regulation and avoidance of catastrophe during exercise-induced hyperthermia. *Comparative Biochemistry and Physiology. Part B, Biochemistry & Molecular Biology*, 139(4), pp. 561–569.

Marino, F.E., 2009. Heat reactions in multiple sclerosis: an overlooked paradigm in the study of comparative fatigue. *International Journal of Hyperthermia*, 25, pp. 34–40.

Marino, F.E., Lambert, M.I. & Noakes, T.D., 2004. Superior performance of African runners in warm humid but not in cool environmental conditions. *Journal of Applied Physiology*, 96, pp. 124–130.

Marino, F.E. et al., 2000. Advantages of smaller body mass during distance running in warm, humid environments. *Pflügers Archives*, 441(2–3), pp. 359–367.

McConaghy, F.F. et al., 1995. Selective brain cooling in the horse during exercise and environmental heat stress. *Journal of Applied Physiology*, 79(6), pp. 1849–1854.

McConaghy, F.F. et al., 2002. Thermoregulatory-induced compromise of muscle blood flow in ponies during intense exercise in the heat: a contributor to the onset of fatigue? *Equine Veterinary Journal – Supplement*, 34(34), pp. 491–495.

McGowan, C., 1979. Selection pressure for high body temperatures: implications for dinosaurs. *Paleobiology*, 5(3), pp. 285–295.

Mendelssohn, M., 1895. Ueber den thermotropismus einzelliger organismen. *Pflügers Archives*, 60(1–2), pp. 1–27.

Meyer, L.C.R. et al., 2008. Hyperthermia in captured impala (Aepyceros melampus): a fright not flight response. *Journal of Wildlife Diseases*, 44(2), pp. 404–416.

Miller, S.L., 1953. A production of amino acids under possible primitive Earth conditions. *Science*, 117, pp. 528–529.

Miller, S.L., Schopf, J.W. & Lazcano, A., 1997. Oparin's 'Origin of Life': sixty years later. *Journal of Molecular Evolution*, 44, pp. 351–353.

Mitchell, H.H. et al., 1945. The chemical composition of the adult human body and its bearing on the biochemistry of growth. *Journal of Biological Chemistry*, 158, pp. 625–637.

Newman, M.A., Tarpenning, K.M. & Marino, F.E., 2004. Relationships between isokinetic knee strength, single-sprint performance, and repeated-sprint ability in football players. *Journal of Strength & Conditioning Research*, 18(4), pp. 867–872.

Nielsen, B., 1996. Olympics in Atlanta: a fight against physics. *Medicine and Science in Sports & Exercise*, 28(6), pp. 665–668.

Nielsen, B. et al., 1993. Human circulatory and thermoregulatory adaptations with heat acclimation and exercise in a hot, dry environment. *Journal of Physiology*, 460, pp. 467–485.

Norton, K. & Olds, T., 1996. *Anthropometrica: a textbook of body measurement for sports and health courses*, Sydney: UNSW Press.

Nybo, L. & Nybo, L., 2007. Exercise and heat stress: cerebral challenges and consequences. *Progress in Brain Research*, 162, pp. 29–43.

Nybo, L., Secher, N.H. & Nielsen, B., 2002. Inadequate heat release from the human brain during prolonged exercise with hyperthermia. *Journal of Physiology*, 545(2), pp. 667–704.

Pickering, T.R. & Bunn, H.T., 2007. The endurance running hypothesis and hunting and scavenging in savanna-woodlands. 53(4), pp. 434–438.

Portner, H.O., 2004. Climate variability and the energetic pathways of evolution: the origin of endothermy in mammals and birds. *Physiological and Biochemical Zoology: PBZ*, 77(6), pp. 959–981.

Pugh, L.G., Corbett, J.L. & Johnson, R.H., 1967. Rectal temperatures, weight losses, and sweat rates in marathon running. *Journal of Applied Physiology*, 23(3), pp. 347–352.

Rasminsky, M. & Sears, T.A., 1972. Internodal conduction in undissected demyelinated nerve fibres. *Journal of Physiology*, 227, pp. 323–350.

Robinson, S., 1942. The effect of body size upon energy exchange in work. *American Journal of Physiology*, 136, pp. 363–368.

Romanovsky, A.A., 2007. Thermoregulation: some concepts have changed. Functional architecture of the thermoregulatory system. *American Journal of Physiology: Regulatory, Integrative and Comparative Physiology*, 292(1), pp. R37–R46.

Schauf, C.L. & Davis, F.A., 1974. Impulse conduction in multiple sclerosis: a theoretical basis for modification by temperature and pharmacological agents. *Journal of Neurology Neurosurgery & Psychiatry*, 37(2), pp. 152–161.

Schmidt-Nielsen, K., 1995. *Animal physiology: adaptation and environment*, 4th ed., Cambridge: Cambridge University Press.

Schopf, J.W., 1978. The evolution of the earliest cells. *Scientific American*, 239(3), pp. 111–138.

Sharp, N., 1997. Timed running speed of a cheetah (Acinonyx jubatus). *Journal of Zoology (London)*, 241(3), pp. 493–494.

Smith, K.J. & McDonald, W.I., 1999. The pathophysiology of multiple sclerosis: the mechanisms underlying the production of symptoms and the natural history of the disease. *Philosophical Transactions of the Royal Society of London (Biological Sciences)*, 354(1390), pp. 1649–1673.

Summers, R.L., 1997. Physiology and biophysics of the 100-m sprint. *News in Physiological Sciences*, 12(3), pp. 131–136.

Taylor, C.R. & Lyman, C.P., 1972. Heat storage in running antelopes: independence of brain and body temperatures. *American Journal of Physiology*, 222(1), pp. 114–117.

Taylor, C.R. & Rowntree, V., 1973. Temperature regulation and heat balance in running cheetahs: a strategy for sprinters? *American Journal of Physiology*, 224(4), pp. 848–851.

Taylor, C.R. & Weibel, E.R., 1981. Design of the mammalian respiratory system. I: problem and strategy. *Respiration Physiology*, 44(1), pp. 1–10.

Tilkens, M.J., Wall-Scheffler, C., Weaver, T.D. & Steudel-Numbers, K., 2007. The effects of body proportions on thermoregulation: an experimental assessment of Allen's rule. *Journal of Human Evolution*, 53(3), pp. 286–291.

Taylor, C.R. et al., 1971. Effect of hyperthermia on heat balance during running in the African hunting dog. *American Journal of Physiology*, 220(3), pp. 823–827.

Uhthoff, W., 1890. Untersuchungen über bei multiplen Herdsklerose vorkommenden Augenstorungen. *Arch Psychiatr Nervenkrankh*, 21, pp. 55–106.

Van Kranendonk, M.J., Deamer, D.W. & Djokic, T., 2018. Life springs. *Scientific American*, 27(3), pp. 4–11.

Walters, T.J. et al., 2000. Exercise in the heat is limited by a critical internal temperature. *Journal of Applied Physiology*, 89(2), pp. 799–806.

Weston, A.R. et al., 1999. African runners exhibit greater fatigue resistance, lower lactate accumulation, and higher oxidative enzyme activity. *Journal of Applied Physiology*, 86(3), pp. 915–923.

Wheatley, J.R., Amis, T.C. & Engel, L.A., 1991. Oronasal partitioning of ventilation during exercise in humans. *Journal of Applied Physiology*, 71(2), pp. 546–551.

Wheeler, P.E., 1994. The thermoregulatory advantages of heat storage and shade-seeking behaviour to hominids foraging in equatorial savannah environments. *Journal of Human Evolution*, 26(4), pp. 339–350.

White, A.T. et al., 2000. Effect of precooling on physical performance in multiple sclerosis. *Multiple Sclerosis*, 6(3), pp. 176–180.

White, A.T. et al., 2009. Brain activation in multiple sclerosis: a BOLD fMRI study of the effects of fatiguing hand exercise. *Multiple Sclerosis*, 15(5), pp. 580–586.

White, L.J. & Dressendorfer, R.H., 2004. Exercise and multiple sclerosis. *Sports Medicine*, 24, pp. 1077–1100.

White, M.D. & Cabanac, M., 1995. Nasal mucosal vasodilatation in response to passive hyperthermia in humans. *European Journal of Applied Physiology*, 70(3), pp. 207–212.

Whitford, W.G., 1976. Sweating responses in the chimpanzee (Pan troglodytes). *Comparative Biochemistry and Physiology. A: Comparative Physiology*, 53(4), pp. 333–336.

Williams, T.M. et al., 1997. Skeletal muscle histology and biochemistry of an elite sprinter, the African cheetah. *Journal of Comparative Physiology B*, 167(8), pp. 527–535.

Woese, C.R., Kandler, O. & Wheelis, M.L., 1990. Towards a natural system of organisms: proposal for the domains Archaea, Bacteria, and Eucarya. *Proceedings of the National Academy of Sciences of the United States of America*, 87(12), pp. 4576–4579.

Zachos, J. et al., 2001. Trends, rhythms, and aberrations in global climate 65 Ma to present. *Science*, 292(5517), pp. 686–693.

Zenker, W. & Kubik, S., 1996. Brain cooling in humans – anatomical considerations. *Anatomy and Embryology*, 193(1), pp. 1–13.

Chapter 8

Energy in, energy out – and fatigue

And what is man without energy? Nothing – nothing at all.
— Mark Twain (1835–1910)

Introduction

Our current population's health profile and the prevalence of chronic conditions such as obesity, diabetes and cardiovascular disease are a consequence of our lifestyle and altered nutritional habits. These diseases not only have their own pathologies but also are associated with other comorbidities, such as cancer, neurological disorders and immune dysfunction. Each of these conditions and general ill health increase the incidence of people reporting symptoms of physical and mental fatigue, which in turn is costly and leads to low productivity. Therefore, it is no surprise that governments and healthcare organisations worldwide advocate physical activity as a preventative measure for improved health and better health outcomes for those who already suffer from chronic conditions. The link between sedentary life and preventable disease has been well known and is documented in both clinical and epidemiological studies. As a consequence, government health departments and other social organisations have developed guidelines in the hope that the population will take individual and collective action for their health. The Physical Activity and Sedentary Behaviour Guidelines (Australian Government Department of Health 2014) state the following:

1   Doing any physical activity is better than doing none. If you currently do no physical activity, start by doing some, and gradually build up to the recommended amount;
2   Be active on most, preferably all days every week;
3   Accumulate 150 to 300 minutes (2.5 to 5 hours) of moderate intensity physical activity or 75 to 150 minutes (1.25 to 2.5 hours) of vigorous intensity physical activity, or an equivalent combination of both moderate and vigorous activities, each week;
4   Do muscle strengthening activities on at least 2 days per week.

Notably these basic guidelines do not differ greatly among developed nations other than to be specific for different age groups (e.g., children, teenagers and young adults). However, physical activity guidelines need to be balanced by the reality of what populations might actually achieve or reportedly undertake. Other organisations which purport to have interest in the well-being of the population, such as the Australian Heart Association, report that the assessment of the actual community physical activity levels on 1,001 people over 18 years of age indicates that only about 7% undertake 30 minutes of vigorous physical activity 5 or more days per week (National Heart Foundation 2017). Thus, the minimum 2.5 hours (150 min) per week is seemingly a difficult target for the majority of the population to achieve. It is further stated that individuals with a body mass index (BMI) of 18.5–24.9 are more active than those with a BMI of >30, categorised as overweight/obese. These guidelines and assessments of this type make two distinct points about our health. First, many populations in developed countries do not achieve even the minimum recommended physical activity levels, and second, there is an underlying assumption that our body weight is intimately tied to physical activity level.

There are at least three implicit observations that arise from this assertion. One is that if we exercise enough, we could potentially reduce our body weight to acceptable levels. Two, it is easier to exercise if an individual is lighter to begin with. Stated differently, it is harder to achieve minimum physical activity levels if you are overweight/obese. This is a fundamental observation that seems to escape discussion when physical activity is touted as the primary method to achieve health by losing weight. The fundamental laws of physics are unlikely to be altered by desire alone in order to do away with the pesky problem of inertia. Stated simply, a heavier mass is a lot harder to move than a lighter one. The other observation is even more simplistic. If only a minimum 150 minutes per week is needed for long-term health benefits, why does the vast majority of the population avoid it? There could be many arguments for this, including busy schedules, poor access to facilities, illness, low motivation and a multitude of complex societal and personal issues which would require detailed analysis of their own. The third and less obvious implication related to the guidelines is that if we cannot find 150 minutes per week to expend the energy for better health, then we could reduce energy intake to achieve the same outcome for weight loss, notwithstanding the other many benefits of regular physical activity. Therefore, the fundamental underpinning of why we might engage in regular physical activity could have to do with energy and how we choose to distribute (consume and expend) it.

In Chapter 1 the cornerstone concept of evolution by natural selection, *adaptedness* or *adaptation*, was discussed. Recall that this concept implies that there is a shaping of a particular feature or features of an organism for a better fit with its physical environment. To achieve this the process relies on the multitude of individual differences within in a population so that all species, including humans, are variable in a number of their characteristics. The way in which energy is distributed by individuals is also not immune to this process. It is also the case that the use of energy is directed towards reproductive success; the number of offspring that can be produced and which eventually survive is costly in terms of energy. However, if natural selection favours characteristics and adaptations that are useful for reproductive success, it also follows that natural selection does not favour those characteristics and adaptations that might be *maladaptive*. That is, if there is energy which has become available because it has not been distributed either for reproduction, for growth or for the maintenance of life, then this excess energy might be spent on functions which are likely to yield a poor return and which might also be maladaptive (Lieberman 2015). This proposition is also bound by a caveat which needs to be carefully considered. Namely, favourable characteristics and adaptations are highly contextualised so that they are useful in some environments but perhaps not in others. When considering the use or even *misuse* of available energy for reproductive success, it seems abundantly clear that in our evolutionary past when there was less energy available, our adaptations were better equipped to deal with this scenario – perhaps not so much now.

Finally, in Chapter 7 the evidence for *Homo* being adapted for endurance rather than speed/power was discussed in detail. It seems more than paradoxical that we seemingly avoid or at least do not engage to any great extent as a population with the very activity that we are adapted to undertake. To understand this paradox this chapter will discuss how *Homo* has adapted to distribute the energy available for activities that sustain reproductive success and how this also potentially explains our lack of physical activity and the chronic ill health that is now so common.

Fundamental law

To understand the way in which humans distribute their energy, it is important to apply first principles to this concept since all matter within the known universe is governed by fundamental laws; humans are not an exception. Any discussion about the distribution or use of energy must entail the inviolate first law of thermodynamics as this governs the way energy is distributed within a system. The law simply states that energy cannot be created or destroyed – it can only be changed from one form to another. The equation that expresses this law is normally stated as:

$$\Delta U = Q - W$$

So that ΔU represents change in internal energy of the system, Q is the amount of heat and W is the amount of work. It is also useful to note that the sign convention is important in so far as knowing whether energy is going into versus going out of the system. However, for the purpose of illustrating this law's application to how we might use energy to explain our reproductive success, we will use the equation as stated earlier.

The equation also indicates that when more energy (Q) is put in to the system there will be an increase in the total internal energy, and likewise, when work (W) is performed energy is removed from the system and the total internal energy will have been reduced. When Q and W are matched, this is said to be energy balance. When we apply this concept to human energetics, and as extensively described, assuming that there is no problem with an individual's absorption of nutrients, storage of energy will increase only if energy intake exceeds energy expenditure (Spiegelman & Flier 2001). As such, the exercise sciences have appropriated this fundamental law to mean:

$$\Delta U = \text{energy in-energy out}$$

Which in simple terms is correct but is not the same as stating,

$$\Delta \text{Fat (energy store)} = \text{energy in-energy out}$$

The unit of measure for fat tissue is mass, whereas energy itself is a measure of heat. It is uncontroversial that increases in either energy consumption or expenditure will lead to either more or less energy in the system, respectively. Unfortunately, the first law of thermodynamics and its corresponding equation do not provide for what *causes* the increase or decrease in either Q or W; we can ascertain only the outcome, ΔU. When we apply this fundamental law to whether exercise can be a method for reductions in body weight for healthy outcomes, as suggested by the physical activity guidelines, we find the evidence to be less than compelling (Saris et al. 2003; Haskell et al. 2007). In fact, the consensus cannot be any clearer:

> The [physical activity level] PAL target for different objectives may in fact be very different. The optimal PAL for producing a weight loss by producing a negative energy balance may differ significantly from the optimal PAL for preventing weight gain across a general population. Additionally, the PAL necessary to maintain energy balance and keep body weight stable in a weight-reduced/obesity-prone individual or population may be substantially different from that for a population that is not prone to obesity or to maintain a healthy weight.
>
> (Saris et al. 2003, p. 109)

Therefore, if calories are a measure of heat going either into or out of the system whereby energy expenditure alone cannot account for the change in body weight, or if it makes little difference how much weight is either gained or lost, then the first law of thermodynamics is of no particular use if we wish to know the causation for why we either expend or take on more calories. This leads us back to what adaptations are likely to explain why we add or subtract more energy to our existence. That is, what physical activities are we adapted for to increase our energy expenditure versus those adaptations that reduce our energy expenditure? Understanding what these adaptations are could provide valuable clues as to why some of us are more prone than others to store more energy and increase our body weight, leading to less favourable health.

Energy utilisation

There are several ways to ascertain how humans expend energy, all of which come with methodological problems, restricting our interpretations. Nevertheless, the available data does shed some light on how we, as opposed to other animals, use energy for reproductive and survival purposes. To make sense of this relationship, we first need to consider which body tissues are more or less costly to maintain. Table 8.1 provides a breakdown of the various tissues and their metabolic rates (Ki) as kcal/kg/d and their estimated masses for men and women.

When the average mass of the brain is extrapolated as a percentage of total body mass, it represents only ~2%. However, what is remarkable about the brain is that for a small representation of total body mass, it requires somewhere between 20% and 30% of the metabolic turnover when at rest (Raichle & Gusnard 2002). An interesting aspect of this energy turnover is the remarkable constancy over time regardless of the level of motor function, including during intense physical activity (Nybo et al. 2002; Trangmar et al. 2014). Table 8.1 also shows that the heart and kidneys are even more expensive at ~18 kcal/kg/hr since they are continuously active. However, this does not explain why the brain should be so energetically expensive. Recent investigations suggest that brain tissue is expensive because it continuously propagates action potentials within axons and also transmits these signals between synapses (Raichle & Gusnard 2002). Beyond this continuous need to propagate signals, which accounts for

Table 8.1 The estimated metabolic rates and their respective masses of major organs and tissues for men and women.

Organ/tissue	Elia's Ki value (kcal/kg/d)	Mass (kg) males	Mass (kg) females
Liver	200	1.74 ± 0.31	1.58 ± 0.31
Brain	240	1.61 ± 0.10	1.45 ± 0.93
Heart	440	0.38 ± 0.73	0.306 ± 50.5
Kidneys	440	0.33 ± 58	0.30 ± 0.75
Skeletal muscle	13	32 ± 39	23.6 ± 5
Adipose tissue	4.5	18.9 ± 82	30.4 ± 13.9
Residual mass	12	–	–

Note: The mean mass ± SEE for males was 84.6 ± 13.4 kg and females 80.2 ± 20.8 kg.

Source: Elia's Ki (Elia 1992) value taken from Wang et al. (2010). Masses of individual organs and tissues taken from Müller et al. (2011) where sample was 330 volunteers (61% females) aged 17–78 years with a body mass index 15.9–47.8 kg/m².

about two-thirds of the energy requirement, the rest is dedicated to "housekeeping" or maintenance of cell health (Du et al. 2008). Unlike other body tissues and organs, such as the liver, skeletal muscle or even the kidneys, which are able to store fuel in the form of carbohydrates for immediate use, the brain is unable to store energy. This creates a further expense since it requires the circulatory system to continuously deliver glucose and oxygen. One of the curious observations is that exercise-induced hyperthermia reduces cerebral blood flow, but the cerebral metabolic rate is increased when this occurs (Nybo et al. 2002). When blood flow velocities from the internal, common carotid and middle cerebral arteries were measured during exercise to exhaustion in the heat and when dehydrated, there was a fast decline in cerebral perfusion with dehydration but this was accompanied by increased oxygen extraction (Trangmar et al. 2014). Therefore, cerebral circulatory strain even during intense exercise is compensated by an increase in oxygen extraction.

Neuronal maintenance and axonal conduction represent some but not all of the cost of fuelling the brain. One other less recognised cost is the function of the cerebrospinal fluid (CSF), which is produced in specialised areas of the brain known as the choroid plexus lining the ventricles. The functions of the CSF are to insulate the brain, provide a hydraulic effect and reduce the effective weight to ~50g, provide nourishment for brain cells and remove waste (Segal 2000; Pocock et al. 2013). This highly specialised function, which allows only the exchange of specific substances from blood to CSF, is expensive because of the constant pumping and active transport of substances requiring and consuming high levels of adenosine triphosphate. Added to this exchange and transport of substances are the turnover and synthesis of CSF, which amounts to ~500 ml per day in an average adult (Pocock et al. 2013). All of the processes related to neuronal maintenance and transmission, along with the active processes related to the CSF, are carried out within very small tolerances. For example, in children the synthesis rate of CSF is normally 0.35 ml/min so that any reduction in absorption which escalates the overproduction by three times (~1.05 ml/min) would result in pathology (Cutler et al. 1973).

The preceding discussion highlights that different body organs and tissues have a different energy expense, but the brain particularly so given its relative mass to the rest of the body. Some of the hidden processes indicate the brain is expensive to maintain so it is worth noting how this compares to other animals, in particular non-human primates. In Chapter 3 the endocranial volume (ECV) and its relationship with brain and body mass – encephalisation quotient (EQ) – were examined. As shown in Figure 3.7 for extant apes, extinct *Homo* and modern humans, as the ECV increases so too does the EQ. Although these are good estimates they are highly dependent on the regressions which are used to predict either measure. However, it is worth illustrating that when comparing the absolute brain mass with the body mass there is a further relationship which can be ascertained. Figure 8.1 shows that when brain and body mass are plotted, there is a close association, but this does not hold true for modern *Homo*.

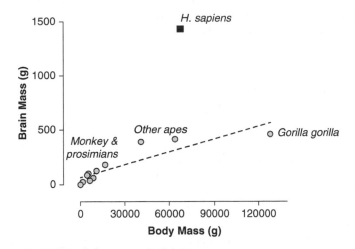

Figure 8.1 The absolute brain and body mass relationship for extant non-human primates (open circles) from Martin (1990). These species include apes (*Pan troglodytes, Gorilla gorilla, Pongo pygmaeus, Hylobates lar, H. syndactylus*), monkeys (*Macca, Anubis, Badius, Apella*) and prosimians (*Indri indri, Lemur mongoz*). The data for *H. sapiens* is a mean for both male and female. The regression equation which includes only extant non-human primates is $y = 0.003902 \cdot x + 64.77$, $R^2 = 0.78$, $P < 0.0001$.

What Figure 8.1 shows is that the brain-body mass relationship is quite tight for all extant non-human primates but not so for modern humans. It is an interesting observation that apes have brains about 3–4 times the mass of monkeys' and that humans have brains with a mass 3–4 times that of apes. The question to answer is, why did *H. sapiens* not follow the rule which is apparent for all other primates, as shown in Figure 8.1? The answer to this question is extraordinarily complicated, but the following are noted as being key features which can provide some clues as to the development of the human brain:

1   Humans tend to grow their brain for longer and faster than do other primates (Leigh 2004);
2   Body size takes longer to grow for humans so it makes sense that the relative size of brain to body will be larger (Walker et al. 2006);
3   The larger human brain will have a greater absolute number of neurons, which is about two times that of chimps (Haug 1987). This will also result in an absolute larger number of connections.

The purpose of describing the comparison between the brains of humans and our closest living relatives is to show that the option for the larger brain comes at a cost. Growing something faster and for longer to increase the amount of tissue requires access to more energy and for longer, more sustained periods. These outcomes, however, do not really shed light on what selection pressures lead humans to opt for a larger brain; they merely underscore the cost of feeding the brain.

Why more energy?

We have seen that the human brain is larger than expected for the body mass when compared to other extant primates and is metabolically more expensive. However, the expense does not in itself shed light on *why* humans have opted for a larger, more expensive brain. The reasons for this 'choice' are not readily apparent, and any hypothesis which attempts to answer this question is difficult to test. Nevertheless, there is evidence both in the fossil record and by comparison to existing primates that could help unravel this question.

The data provided in Table 8.2 shows that following our split from the last common ancestor, our very early ancestors were both tree climbers and bipedal to some degree while the brain mass was similar to that of chimps. This strongly indicates that brain expansion was achieved after erect posture was selected. Taking the data in Table 8.2 along with those depicted in Figure 8.2 confirms that brain expansion (by either mass or volume) was stable for long periods but was interspersed with dramatic jumps.

The apparent jump from *Australopiths* to *H. habilis* shows an increase of approximately one-third the brain volume, while the next jump from *H. erectus*

Table 8.2 The comparative data for average height, mass and brain mass of extant ape (*Pan troglodytes*), extinct species from the genus *Homo* and *H. sapiens* over time.

Species	Million years ago	Average height (m)	Average mass (kg)	Brain mass (kg)	Posture & locomotion
P. troglodytes[#]	5.0	1.2	41	0.391	TC & KW
Ard. ramidus[*]	4.4	1.20	50	0.300	TC & B
Aus. afarensis	3.9–2.9	1.51	42	0.453	TC & B
Aus. africanus	3.3–2.1	1.38	41	0.456	TC & B
H. habilis[#]	2.4–1.5	1.30	32	0.599	B + LA
H. erectus[#]	1.9–0.7	1.65	54	0.943	B + GD
H. Heidelbergensis	0.6–0.2	1.75	62	1.217	B
Neanderthals	0.4–0.3	1.64	65	1.432	B
H. sapiens	0.2 –	1.73	75	1.358	B

Note: [*]Female. [#]Based on current estimates but representing the split from last common ancestor (LCA) ~5 MYA. Posture: TC is tree climber; KW is knuckle walker; B is bipedal; LA is long arms; GD is ground-dwelling.

Source: Average height, mass and posture for extinct species taken from data provided by the Smithsonian Museum of Natural History: http://humanorigins.si.edu/evidence/human-fossils/species. Data for *H. sapiens* taken as an average for male from Walpole et al. (2012).

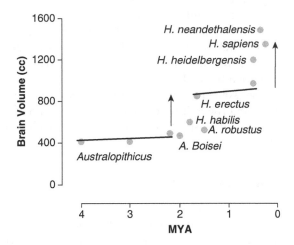

Figure 8.2 The transition in brain volume over time in million years ago (MYA) to present in extinct human species to *H. sapiens*. Note that brain volume is relatively stable for long time periods, with significant increases (arrows) over short periods.

Source: Redrawn and adapted from Lynch and Granger (2008) with kind permission from the authors.

to *Neanderthals* and *H. sapiens* shows a further staggering increase of two-thirds, 487–420 cc, respectively. Notably, by the time the brain almost doubled its size from *H. habilis* to *H. heidelbergensis*, the species was likely completely ground-dwelling and habitually bipedal. This timeline suggests that there was some trigger that permitted the expansion in brain size initially around 2 million years ago and again some 0.5 million years ago. It is now known that around 2–2.5 million years ago there was a shift in the habitat and available food supply when meat entered the diet (Pobiner 2016) (see Chapter 3, Figure 3.8 and associated text). The ability to procure high-quality protein at this time must have assisted greatly in fuelling the brain since we already have discussed that the bigger brain requires more energy. However, the ability to procure protein from animal sources must have come after the arrival of a larger brain, since there would otherwise be no apparent need for an extra energy requirement.

An enticing hypothesis explaining the larger human brain is that it arose in response to an erect posture and bipedality, which structurally altered the pelvis, enabling the delivery of large babies (Lynch & Granger 2008). The key observations that underpin this hypothesis are that humans give birth to relatively large babies compared with both chimps and gorillas; the larger baby has a larger head and brain. Locomotor adaptations are responsible for the changes in the lumbar and pelvic regions, allowing for the delivery of larger babies. However, this does not necessarily explain the second increase in brain size, which seems to have occurred within the last 0.5 million years. The hypothesis that bipedality was the main driver for brain expansion would seem to be limited since the genus *Homo* by this time was well adapted to walking for at least the previous 1.5 million years. However, if the larger baby with a big brain had already arrived by 2 million years ago, then the ability to use the large brain to conceive of better ways to procure energy would have been possible, including toolmaking, cooking, cognitive capability, and the ability to use endurance running for that purpose (Ruxton & Wilkinson 2013; Isler & van Schaik 2006; Dunbar & Shultz 2017; Byrne & Corp 2004).

The larger brain and fatigue

If the evolutionary timeline indicates that the larger human brain was essentially a side effect of the structural changes that came with an erect posture and habitual bipedality, it would also suggest that *Homo* selected endurance over power since bipedality is the prerequisite for successful endurance, and arguably the most proficient means for procuring the energy required to fuel the large brain. This is based on the fossil record, which indicates that meat entered the diet around 2.6 million years ago (Semaw et al. 2003) and subsequent evolution of endurance running with the genus *Homo* (*H. habilis*), who exploited their method for locomotion to enhance the prospect of hunting (Bramble & Lieberman 2004). However, an increased need for energy also requires a capacity to store fuel when there might have been reduced food availability and an appropriate distribution of that energy at all times. This leads us back to the fundamental application of the first law of thermodynamics, whereby energy balance is altered by either its input or usage with the potential to store energy (Spiegelman & Flier 2001). In this case, and as previously discussed, if natural selection favours characteristics and adaptations that are useful for reproductive success, then we should also consider what characteristics and adaptations might be maladaptive for life as we know it today.

In Chapter 3, it was mentioned that one widely accepted hypothesis for the larger brain was our trade-off for a smaller intestinal tract – the *expensive tissue hypothesis* (Aiello & Wheeler 1995). This hypothesis has been widely accepted since it also accounts for the comparatively longer intestinal tract in other primates which ingest a high-plant diet but with low energy yield. Thus, it makes sense that chimps have a highly metabolically active intestine. Conversely, as the *Homo* diet changed to include rich energy foods, such as protein and fat, the need for a large gut was abandoned, which led to a smaller abdominal cavity. There are two immediate problems with this proposition. First, it does not account for the fact that larger brains are also associated with altered body composition. Compared to other primates, it appears humans are 'under-muscled' but have relatively higher fatness (Leonard et al. 2003). This alone suggests that there may be a trade-off between having a large skeletal muscle mass versus a level of fatness favouring capacity for energy storage to fuel the brain by reducing the cost for the rest of the body. According to Table 8.1, skeletal muscle and adipose tissue masses constitute a large portion (~51 kg) but with low energy cost. Second, recent empirical evidence shows that when controlling for fat-free body mass, brain size is not negatively correlated with the mass of the digestive tract or any other expensive organ in mammals or non-human primates (Navarrete et al. 2011). These data raise questions as to whether the reduced size of the gut was indeed a trade-off for the larger brain. The most important point here is that if the larger brain required an energy store of fat in the event that energy availability was low, then this would be a potential maladaptation when energy availability was to become abundant and easily accessible for significant time periods.

Even if one accepts the possibility of the expensive tissue hypothesis, there is one further intriguing relationship that should be highlighted. Trading the amount of skeletal muscle would not have been useful since this would also have sacrificed our endurance and the little power we can exert to have enabled us to acquire the higher-quality food. However, Table 8.1 shows that the kidneys are also metabolically expensive at ~18 kcal/kg/h with a comparatively meagre mass of ~3 kg. Why would natural selection not act on reducing the metabolic cost of the kidneys or even reduce the need to one kidney? (See Chapter 3 on safety factors for a discussion on this latter point.) The inference we can draw from this observation is that reducing either the energy cost or number of kidneys would have resulted in the reduced capacity to excrete concentrated urine, leading to an inevitable higher daily water consumption and loss. This anatomical and physiological need confirms that early *H. sapiens* must have evolved in a dry environment when water was very likely less than freely available (Finlayson 2014, 2013).

The need for energy storage (e.g., fat) and conversely the capacity to deal with deficits (e.g., food, water) indicate that *Homo* was adapted to make concessions at various times. One of those concessions must have been to spare energy whenever it was in low supply. As discussed in Chapter 3, fatigue can result from several perturbations, including a lessening in one's response to or enthusiasm for something, caused by overexposure. This predicts that overexposure to long periods of low energy availability would potentially manifest as fatigue, precisely to avoid unnecessary energy expenditure. If we consider fatigue in this light, it would seem a reasonable suggestion that as energy availability became scarce, avoiding unnecessary physical exertion would be a useful adaptation. The converse of this proposition is that when energy availability is high, the need to conserve energy should be low. However, this does not seem to be the case since it is plainly obvious that a capacity to store energy in the form of fat seems to be much greater than our desire to expend it. As we shall see, the capability to expend energy may indeed be limited and maladapted. In essence, the adaptations required to meet the needs of our larger more expensive brain with high energy demands, fuelled mainly by storage of fat, may in effect be maladaptive in today's context.

Energy budgets – how do they compare?

Returning to the basic assumption that increases in physical activity can lead to a negative energy balance and result in weight loss for better health, it is important to underscore that this is based primarily on the first law of thermodynamics, as already discussed. We have also shown that applying this model of energy expenditure to weight loss for health does not yield the expected outcome. The reasons for this are not entirely clear, but there are now data which can shed light on this paradox. Figure 8.3 is a schematic representing what is expected to occur with increased physical activity (Pontzer et al. 2016; Pontzer 2015). That is, when we add physical activity the total energy expenditure is expected to increase, leading to a negative energy balance, assuming little or no change in energy input. This is in contrast to the constrained total energy expenditure model that accounts for the energy needed for such processes related to faecal and urine output and maintenance of temperature and homeostasis (Thomas & Heymsfield 2016). In simple terms, increasing the amount of physical activity cannot increase energy expenditure indefinitely or continue unabated.

In modern western populations the recommended energy intake per day for sedentary 31–50 year old males and females is ~2,366 and 1,912 kcal, respectively. However, when considering the energy expenditure with respect to physical activity, an unexpected picture emerges which does not seem to fit with the additive model of total energy expenditure as predicted in Figure 8.3. When hunter-gatherers were compared with western and farming populations there was no apparent difference in the total energy expenditure, even though the relative physical activity level was higher for the hunter-gatherers (Pontzer et al. 2012) (Figure 8.4).

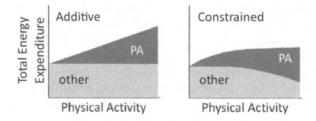

Figure 8.3 A schematic representation of additive total energy expenditure versus constrained total energy expenditure models. In the additive model the total energy expenditure is thought to be a linear function of the amount and variation in physical activity (PA) which determines the total energy expenditure. In the constrained model the body adapts to increased physical activity by reducing energy spent on other physiological activity, which maintains the energy expenditure within a narrow range.

Source: Reproduced from Pontzer et al. (2016) with kind permission from Elsevier.

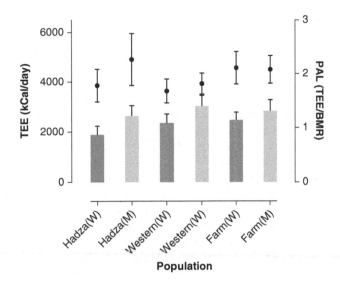

Figure 8.4 The total energy expenditure (TTE, bars; *left ordinate*) and the physical activity level (PAL, circles; *right ordinate*) for three different populations: Hadza hunter-gatherers, western (US and European adults) and farming (Bolivia) populations. The Hadza population were living in a savanna-woodland environment in Northern Tanzania. The TTE was measured using the doubly labelled water method; PAL was calculated as TEE/estimated basal metabolic rate (BMR). W is women, and M is men.

Data redrawn from Table 8.1 in Pontzer et al. (2012).

The data in Figure 8.4 are not easily reconciled with the model that adding physical activity leads to a liner increase in total energy expenditure. In fact, these data argue for a constrained total energy expenditure model that is tied to an evolved physiological trait and independent of the socio-cultural differences that might exist in relation to energy expenditure (Pontzer et al. 2012). The assumption that modern western lifestyles are geared to low energy expenditure resulting in positive energy balance and greater fat storage is not supported by these data. Added to this is the finding that adiposity was not correlated to either total energy expenditure or physical activity level. Notably, this lack of association has been identified several times across different ages (Goran et al. 1997; Westerterp 2010; Speakman & Westerterp 2010). One further observation is that exercise-induced increases in energy expenditure are found to also increase energy intake as compensation for the additional energy requirement (Westerterp 2010). Conversely, a reduction in physical activity towards a sedentary lifestyle does not have the opposite effect of reducing energy intake resulting in negative energy balance. The interesting aspect of this paradox is that obese individuals also tend to have high energy expenditure which is not associated with more physical activity but with a relative higher basal metabolic rate compared to controls or lean individuals (Westerterp 2010; Luke & Schoeller 1992; Dulloo & Jacquet 1998). If we take the data related to physical activity level from Figure 8.4 and assigning the respective % body fat for women and men (Pontzer et al. 2012) it suggests that basal metabolic rate is higher in obese individuals (Table 8.3). It is unclear why obese individuals demonstrate this characteristic basal metabolic rate even when energy intake is restricted. It is suggested, however, that obese individuals are likely to increase their energy intake to maintain their greater mass while moving less (Westerterp 2010). This observation fits with the first law of thermodynamics since a higher overall mass will require more energy input.

If adding physical activity does not linearly increase the total energy expenditure, then what effect does physical activity have on total energy expenditure? When total energy expenditure and physical activity are assessed using accelerometry, as expected there is an immediate energy cost for the increase in physical activity to a certain point (Pontzer et al. 2016). The basal metabolic rate is always constant at 1,540 kcal/d, so when adding physical activity, the total energy expenditure will increase to 2,336 kcal/d. However, total energy expenditure is then constrained to a constant 2,600 kcal/d with further physical activity. This suggests that total energy expenditure is adjusted and constrained. The reasons for this apparent constraint on energy expenditure are thought to be related to a compensatory effect on the energy expended for other activities, including reproduction and somatic maintenance (Pontzer et al. 2016).

The data in Figure 8.4 and Table 8.3 also show that both female and male hunter-gatherers are always closer to the margin of energy balance compared with western populations – the amount of physical activity versus their total energy expenditure. In addition to this, hunter-gatherers tend to be smaller and have a lower body mass and body fat percentage. Therefore, the stored energy available to these populations has to be balanced against physical activity necessity – for reproduction, maintenance and acquiring food and shelter. Arguably, any physical activity which we might consider to be therapeutic in today's context, as

Table 8.3 The basal metabolic rate (BMR) of women and men versus their percent body fat (%BF).

	Women			Men		
%BF	21_H	27_W	38_F	13_H	16_W	22_F
BMR (kCal/ day)	1054	1170	1397	1172	1372	1686

Note: BMR was recalculated from the physical activity level (PAL = total energy expenditure/BMR) data presented in Figure 8.4. Subscripts are for populations where H is hunter-gatherer, W is western and F is farming.

Source: Data from Pontzer et al. (2012).

that suggested by the physical activity guidelines, would be maladaptive in these populations (Lieberman 2015). When comparing the energy store as % body fat to other mammals, it is apparent that humans, regardless of population, tend to be fatter. Studies on adipose tissue indicate that there is an allometric relationship between adipocyte size and number (Pond 1987). Further to this is that the number of fat cells in humans tends to be about ten times that predicted in other mammals, although the size of the cells is smaller. When comparing humans and primates, increased fatness seems to be due to increasing the number of fat cells (Pond & Mattacks 1987), whereas in other mammals this is due to increasing the size of fat cells. Since fat is utilised for varied functions, such as insulation, energy reserve, visceral protection, buoyancy and hormone storage, it is difficult to ascertain which of these is the driving adaptation for human fatness. Nevertheless, it is not inconsequential that high levels of body fat increase the morbidity and escalating occurrence of chronic disease.

Energy storage and fatigue

Chapter 4 outlined some of the definitions and the methods used to measure fatigue. One definition is centred around the measurement of the decline in skeletal muscle force output since the magnitude of this change is measurable and observable. Energy availability for skeletal muscle metabolism is immediate and stored in the form of glycogen and converted to glucose for the replenishment of adenosine triphosphate. The classic understanding of skeletal muscle fatigue is that when energy utilisation is more than what can be supplied to maintain the rate and intensity of contraction a reduction in force output occurs. However, it is also known that skeletal muscle contraction is predominantly fuelled by aerobic glycolysis, with fat oxidation playing a minor role if at all under normal circumstances. In fact, fat as fuel is important for prolonged mild to moderate exercise, with lipid utilisation being a slow and complex process (Brooks et al. 2011). Blood-free fatty acid levels rise during exercise up to 50% of maximal oxygen consumption, but when intensity rises beyond this lipolysis is inhibited (Zinker et al. 1990).

If an abundance of energy availability potentially leads to positive energy balance in the form of excess fat, intuitively it would also suggest that larger, heavier individuals would be less inclined to be active. One reason for reduced physical activity is increased fatigue. This also seems paradoxical since heavier, obese individuals would not have limited energy availability. This is important since a host of comorbidities are associated with obesity, of which many also have fatigue as a symptom, making activities of daily living difficult to accomplish. When comparing the skeletal muscle strength and power of individuals that are either lean or obese, there is an apparent difference in the fatigue profile. Figure 8.5 shows the absolute quadriceps muscle power in lean and obese men corrected for body mass and fat-free mass (Maffiuletti et al. 2007). What is evident from these data is that absolute strength in obese individuals is significantly higher than

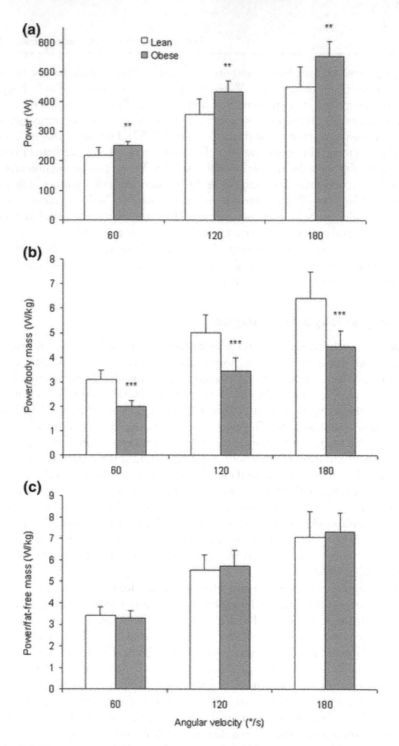

Figure 8.5 The power-velocity relation in absolute values (a), normalised to body mass (b) and to fat-free mass (c) in obese and lean subjects (mean ± SD). ** $P < 0.01$ and ** $P < 0.001$ obese different compared with lean.

Source: From Maffiuletti et al. (2007). Reproduced with kind permission from Springer Nature.

lean individuals. However, when this is normalised for body mass and fat-free mass, this advantage is respectively either reversed or negated. In addition, these researchers measured the loss in voluntary isometric torque over 50 maximal contractions with percutaneous stimulation (see Chapter 4 on measurement of voluntary muscular contractions) and showed that obese individuals fatigued faster when attempting a voluntary set of contractions but not when electrically stimulated. This indicates that obese individuals in this study demonstrated less fatigue resistance than lean individuals, although the central drive from the motor cortex remained intact. Since central activation was not likely to be the cause of the faster rate of fatigue, other factors must have contributed to the skeletal muscle fatigue observed in the obese.

The increased level of voluntary skeletal muscle fatigue observed in the obese could include but is not limited to such factors as a conscious decision to limit effort and minimise discomfort from exercise (James et al. 1995). However, there is also good evidence that skeletal muscle fibre type is correlated with body composition whereby obese individuals have a higher proportion of fast-twitch fibres (Wade et al. 1990; Kriketos et al. 1997). Specifically, there is an inverse relationship between fatness and the percentage of slow-twitch fibres. It is also interesting that a surrogate measure of adiposity, such as waist circumference, is positively associated with a greater proportion fast-twitch fibres (Kriketos et al. 1997). The mechanism responsible for altered skeletal muscle fibre type with adiposity, either as a high proportion of fast twitch or a low proportion of slow twitch, is not well understood. However, there is consistent reporting of reduced skeletal muscle cross-sectional area with ageing and a concomitant increase in fat mass (Cannon & Marino 2007). Although fibre type distribution is varied, a reduction in physical activity up to about 37 years of age is known to alter fibre type composition towards a greater proportion of fast-twitch fibres (Lexell et al. 1992). An important distinction would also be whether any increase in the proportion of muscle fibres type is due mainly to either fast Type 2a or 2b fibres. This distinction is important since there is a reduced capacity to use fat for continued energy turnover in fast Type 2b fibres (Kriketos et al. 1996) (see Chapter 5). Since increases in body fat are associated with a higher proportion of fast-twitch fibres, this would decrease the fatigue resistance in this population. Furthermore, the low capacity to use fat stores because of the higher proportion of fast-twitch fibres could also lead to further fat accumulation and lower levels of physical activity, which could further increase the proportion of fast-twitch fibres (Kriketos et al. 1997).

Finally, when excess fat is identified as predominantly visceral, there is a high degree of association with several other responses thought to cause fatigue. These include higher values of insulin resistance-producing inflammatory markers, such as tumour necrosis factor-α and interlukin-6, particularly in obese individuals who also suffer from sleep apnoea (Vgontzas et al. 2000). However, sleep apnoea in obesity is not of itself associated with heightened feelings of fatigue *per se*; rather the metabolic disturbances leading to insulin resistance and associated psychological factors predict the level of sleepiness and fatigue experienced in obesity (Vgontzas et al. 2006). It is also not inconsequential that an increasing body mass index (BMI) and waist circumference are associated with escalating feelings of fatigue and a reduced likelihood of achieving minimum recommended levels of physical activity (Resnick et al. 2006).

Energy, nutrition and diets

Having discussed how energy is apportioned and used, and how this relates to our evolutionary past, it is not possible to escape without dealing with the prickly issue of diet. The discourse dealing with diet has become a source of tension among health professionals. One reason for this tension is that there is really no argument about the merits of diet *per se* in achieving health; the tension is related to the supposed ideal composition of the diet. It is impossible to harness all of the available literature and the associated opinions into a consensus view amidst a worldwide debate. This debate seems divided between those advocating a diet which is significantly reduced in carbohydrate consumption compensated by increasing the fat intake and those who advocate this will not alter the long-term health status or body weight loss, instead advocating a caloric adjustment (www.sportsdietitians.com.au/factsheets/diets-intolerances/low-carbohydrate-diets). The argument for promoting a particular diet is not the same as promoting physical activity as a method for achieving health and well-being, since this debate has been had and for the large part won by those advocating physical activity, although some have suggested that exercise cannot overcome a "bad" diet (Malhotra & Phinney 2015). Notwithstanding the evidence that exercise is a relatively unreliable method to achieve weight loss, the consensus that exercise has a myriad of other health benefits is not in question. Since it is undeniable that diet plays a major role in achieving overall health, in this section the intention is not to reach a consensus as to the merits of one diet over another but to summarise the evidence related to how human diets might have evolved. As we shall see, referring to diets rather than a singular *diet* is much more useful since food consumption changed drastically over long periods for many reasons so that there is not one particular diet that is best suited for modern humans.

To understand the human diet, there are several critical aspects of eating that need to be considered. The first is anatomical and relates to the teeth. The characteristics which can provide a history of diets in this regard are tooth size, shape, enamel structure and dental microwear, together with jaw biomechanics (Teaford & Ungar 2000). However, considering the teeth in isolation provides only a partial picture for the evolution of diets. An additional aspect is the structure of the skull and mandible since these are the anchor points for the muscles required for mastication. A further critical aspect of diets is climate and seasonal variability, which determine the availability of specific foods. Mastication or chewing is a complex function dependent on tooth size and their respective shape and location. Figure 8.2 and Table 8.2 suggest that the *Australopithecines* were partially adapted for bipedality, but a striking feature of these hominids was the shape and bony features of the face and skull, which indicate adaptation for strong, powerful muscles for mastication. These structural features also came with relatively large molar teeth. The dental and cranial evidence suggests that *Australopthicines* were adapted primarily for a vegetarian diet mainly suited to breaking down hard, brittle foods, including fruits, nuts and flowers, but not well suited for meat (Teaford & Ungar 2000; Ungar & Sponheimer 2011). The relatively large, flat molars are a feature consistent with the need to crush food, whereas their thick enamel was well suited to withstand abrasion and fracture. This kind of eating suggests a diet consistent with an open environment, such as woodlands or grasslands (Sponheimer & Lee-Thorp 1999; van der Merwe et al. 2008). By the time *H. habilis* was on the scene, around 2.1 million years ago (see Figure 8.2 timeline), the capability to process tough foods changed since the teeth were very variable in size and thickness but not dissimilar to those of *Australopiths* (Puech et al. 1983). Dental microwear is thought to reflect diet, with the tendency for large microwear pits to be common in teeth used for hard objects versus teeth for tough food eaters, which exhibit more striations and smaller microwear features (Ungar et al. 2006). *H. habilis* likely did not specialise in eating particularly tough foods, suggesting that this species had an increasingly generalised and generally omnivorous diet (Ungar 2012). This also fits with the common view that *H. habilis* used stone tools for butchering meat that was scavenged from animal carcasses (Marean 1989).

Archaeological evidence of stone tool materials and their site placement suggest a switch from dense woodland to more open habitats, likely resulting in confrontational scavenging with other carnivores. This would have been a predation pressure driving morphological changes favouring a switch from *H. habilis* to *H. erectus* (Marean 1989). The transition to *H. erectus* also sees a further reduction in the postcanine dentition – smaller molars (Kaifu 2006). This means that consumption of tough food would have been substantially reduced since the smaller molars have less capacity to manage the breakdown of a large range of foods. To compensate, *H. erectus* would have been chewing comparatively higher-quality foods than that of its predecessors. Evidence from archaeological sites also suggests that *H. erectus* scavenged carcasses and butchered many different bones from both large and small animals, including choice bones from which the meat was likely eaten first by other carnivores (Pobiner 2016).

The lineage from *H. erectus* to *H. heidelbergensis* has been the subject of much debate, but in general *Heidelbergensis* had a larger jaw and smaller teeth compared to humans, although Neanderthals may have had a uniquely derived dental morphology (Bailey 2002; Buck & Stringer 2014). Given the differences in dentition there are two hypothesised lineages from *H. erectus* to *H. sapiens*: in one lineage modern humans are closely related to Neanderthals, but in the other, humans are directly related to *H. erectus* (Buck & Stringer 2014).

A further consideration beyond the morphology of teeth is the structure and function of the key masticatory muscles. Although this function is extremely complex because it involves the interrelationships of the shape of the face, mandible and angles of musculature insertion, when considered in unison this function provides an interesting observation with respect to chewing capacity. As Figure 8.6 shows, there is an apparent reduction of ~20% in the ration of bite force/molar area in modern humans compared with archaic *Homo* (Lieberman 2011).

The reduction in this ratio is likely due to the reduction in cranial size, including a smaller face, but it also indicates that modern humans are adapted to chew comparatively softer foods. Recent studies have shown that by adding meat so that it composed about one-third of the diet, chewing cycles per year would have been reduced by ~2 million and masticatory force by about 15% (Zink & Lieberman 2016). Importantly, these studies also showed that slicing and pounding would have improved chewing meat into smaller particles by 41%. The selection of softer foods was also made possible by cooking, which renders most foods tender, thereby reducing the need to generate greater load on the teeth. Although it is not settled when cooking was first used, it is possible that *H. erectus* used fire to cook, but this was probably more common by about 0.5 million years ago if not later (Shimelmitz et al. 2014) (see Figure 8.7 for timeline). An additional benefit of cooking is that it increases the energy value of food by reducing the energy cost of digestion for cooked versus raw food, and it reduces the energetic costs of detoxification and defence against pathogens, resulting in a rise in energy availability (Carmody & Wrangham 2009).

In summary, our evolutionary path involved a shift in diets and the energy that new foods provided. Although dentition and cranial structure played a

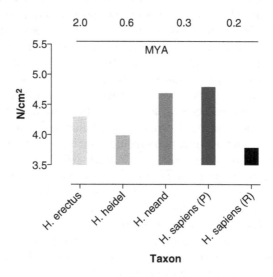

Figure 8.6 The estimates of maximum bite force/molar area (N/cm²) in *Homo*. MYA is millions of years ago, P is Pleistocene and R is recent.

Source: Data redrawn from Lieberman (2011) from Table 13.6.

significant role in determining the selection of foods we ate, other factors, such as cooking, tracking, running, tool making and social cohesion and cooperation among other behaviours, would have added to the co-evolution of diets. Modern humans evolved from a lineage of hunter-gatherers, but it is fallacious to consider that one specific hunter-gatherer diet exists which includes a set of specific foods. In reality, there is likely to be many versions of this kind of subsistence, highly dependent on seasonality and climate. The only certainty is that selection pressures favoured high-energy foods, in particular animal protein and associated fat.

References

Aiello, L.C. & Wheeler, P., 1995. The expensive-tissue hypothesis: the brain and the digestive system in human and primate evolution. *Current Anthropology*, 36(2), pp. 199–221.

Australian Government, Department of Health, 2014. Fact sheet: adults (18–64 years). pp. 1–2. Available at: http://health.gov.au/internet/main/publishing.nsf/content/health-pubhlth-strateg-phys-act-guidelines.

Bailey, S.E., 2002. A closer look at Neanderthal postcanine dental morphology: the mandibular dentition. *The Anatomical Record*, 269(3), pp. 148–156.

Bramble, D.M. & Lieberman, D.E., 2004. Endurance running and the evolution of *Homo*. *Nature*, 432, pp. 345–352.

Brooks, G.A. et al., 2011. *Exercise physiology: human bioenergetics and its applications*, 4th ed., Dubuque, IA: McGraw-Hill.

Buck, L.T. & Stringer, C.B., 2014. Homo heidelbergensis. *Current Biology*, 24(6), pp. R214–R215.

Byrne, R.W. & Corp, N., 2004. Neocortex size predicts deception rate in primates. *Proceedings of the Royal Society B: Biological Sciences*, 271(1549), pp. 1693–1699.

Cannon, J. & Marino, F.E., 2007. Comparative effects of resistance training on peak isometric torque, muscle hypertrophy, voluntary activation and surface EMG between young and elderly women. *Clinical Physiology and Functional Imaging*, 27(2), pp. 91–100.

Carmody, R.N. & Wrangham, R.W., 2009. The energetic significance of cooking. *Journal of Human Evolution*, 57(4), pp. 379–391.

Cutler, R.W., Murray, J.E. & Moody, R.A., 1973. Overproduction of cerebrospinal fluid in communicating hydrocephalus. A case report. *Neurology*, 23(1), pp. 1–5.

Du, F. et al., 2008. Tightly coupled brain activity and cerebral ATP metabolic rate. *Proceedings of the National Academy of Sciences*, 105(17), pp. 6409–6414.

Dulloo, A.G. & Jacquet, J., 1998. Adaptive reduction in basal metabolic rate in response to food deprivation in humans: a role for feedback signals from fat stores. *American Journal of Clinical Nutrition*, 68(3), pp. 599–606.

Dunbar, R.I.M. & Shultz, S., 2017. Why are there so many explanations for primate brain evolution? *Philosophical Transactions of the Royal Society of London (Biological Sciences)*, 372(1727), pp. 20160244.

Elia M., 1992. Organ and tissue contribution to metabolic rate. In: J.M. Kinney & H.N. Tucker, eds. *Energy metabolism: tissue determinants and cellular corollaries*. New York, NY: Raven Press, pp. 61–80.

Finlayson, C., 2013. The water optimisation hypothesis and the human occupation of the mid-latitude belt in the Pleistocene. *Quaternary International*, 300, pp. 22–31.

Finlayson, C., 2014. *The improbable primate: how water shaped human evolution*, Oxford: Oxford University Press.

Goran, M.I. et al., 1997. Physical activity related energy expenditure and fat mass in young children. *International Journal of Obesity and Related Metabolic Disorders*, 21(3), pp. 171–178.

Haskell, W.L. et al., 2007. Physical activity and public health: updated recommendation for adults from the American College of Sports Medicine and the American Heart Association. *Circulation*, 116(9), pp. 1081–1093.

Haug, H., 1987. Brain sizes, surfaces, and neuronal sizes of the cortex cerebri: a stereological investigation of man and his variability and a comparison with some mammals (primates, whales, marsupials, insectivores, and one elephant). *American Journal of Anatomy*, 180(2), pp. 126–142.

Isler, K. & van Schaik, C.P., 2006. Metabolic costs of brain size evolution. *Biology Letters*, 2(4), pp. 557–560.

James, C., Sacco, P. & Jones, D.A., 1995. Loss of power during fatigue of human leg muscles. *Journal of Physiology*, 484(Pt 1), pp. 237–246.

Kaifu, Y., 2006. Advanced dental reduction in Javanese Homo erectus. *Anthropological Science*, 114(1), pp. 35–43.

Kriketos, A.D. et al., 1996. Interrelationships between muscle morphology, insulin action, and adiposity. *American Journal of Physiology*, 270(6 Pt 2), pp. R1332–R1339.

Kriketos, A.D. et al., 1997. Muscle fibre type composition in infant and adult populations and relationships with obesity. *International Journal of Obesity and Related Metabolic Disorders*, 21(9), pp. 796–801.

Leigh, S.R., 2004. Brain growth, life history, and cognition in primate and human evolution. *American Journal of Primatology*, 62(3), pp. 139–164.

Leonard, W.R. et al., 2003. Metabolic correlates of hominid brain evolution. *Comparative Biochemistry and Physiology – Part A: Molecular & Integrative Physiology*, 136(1), pp. 5–15.

Lexell, J. et al., 1992. Growth and development of human muscle: a quantitative morphological study of whole *vastus lateralis* from childhood to adult age. *Muscle & Nerve*, 15(3), pp. 404–409.

Lieberman, D.E., 2011. *The evolution of the human head*, Cambridge, MA: Harvard University Press.

Lieberman, D.E., 2015. Is exercise really medicine? An evolutionary perspective. *Current Sports Medicine Reports*, 14(4), pp. 313–319.

Luke, A. & Schoeller, D.A., 1992. Basal metabolic rate, fat-free mass, and body cell mass during energy restriction. *Metabolism Clinical and Experimental*, 41(4), pp. 450–456.

Lynch, G. & Granger, R., 2008. *Big brain: the origins and future of human intelligence*, New York: Palgrave Macmillan.

Maffiuletti, N.A. et al., 2007. Differences in quadriceps muscle strength and fatigue between lean and obese subjects. *European Journal of Applied Physiology*, 101(1), pp. 51–59.

Malhotra, A. & Phinney, S., 2015. It is time to bust the myth of physical inactivity and obesity: you cannot outrun a bad diet. *British Journal of Sports Medicine*, 49(15), pp. 967–968.

Marean, C.W., 1989. Sabertooth cats and their relevance for early hominid diet and evolution. *Journal of Human Evolution*, 18(6), pp. 559–582.

Müller, M.J. et al., 2011. Effect of constitution on mass of individual organs and their association with metabolic rate in humans – A detailed view on allometric scaling. *PLoS ONE*, 6(7): e22732–e22739.

National Heart Foundation, 2017. National physical activity plan. pp. 1–26. Available at: www.health.gov.au/internet/main/publishing.nsf/content/health-pubhlth-strateg-phys-act-guidelines.

Navarrete, A., van Schaik, C.P. & Isler, K., 2011. Energetics and the evolution of human brain size. *Nature*, 480(7375), pp. 91–93.

Nybo, L. et al., 2002. Effects of hyperthermia on cerebral blood flow and metabolism during prolonged exercise in humans. *Journal of Applied Physiology*, 93(1), pp. 58–64.

Pobiner, B., 2016. Meat-eating among the earliest humans. *American Scientist*, 3, pp. 1–8.

Pocock, G., Richards, C.D. & Richards, D., 2013. *Human physiology*, 4th ed., Oxford: Oxford University Press.

Pond, C.M., 1987. Fat and figures. *New Scientist*, 114(1563), pp. 62–66.

Pond, C.M. & Mattacks, C.A., 1987. The anatomy of adipose tissue in captive Macaca monkeys and its implications for human biology. *Folia Primatologica*, 48(3–4), pp. 164–185.

Pontzer, H., 2015. Constrained total energy expenditure and the evolutionary biology of energy balance. *Exercise and Sport Sciences Reviews*, 43(3), pp. 110–116.

Pontzer, H. et al., 2012. Hunter-Gatherer energetics and human obesity. *PLOS One*, 7(7), pp. e40503–e40508.

Pontzer, H. et al., 2016. Constrained total energy expenditure and metabolic adaptation to physical activity in adult humans. *Current Biology*, 26(3), pp. 410–417.

Puech, P-F., Albertini, H. & Serratrice, C., 1983. Tooth microwear and dietary patterns in early hominids from Laetoli, Hadar and Olduvai. *Journal of Human Evolution*, 12(8), pp. 721–729.

Raichle, M.E. & Gusnard, D.A., 2002. Appraising the brain's energy budget. *Proceedings of the National Academy of Sciences*, 99(16), pp. 10237–10239.

Resnick, H.E. et al., 2006. Cross-sectional relationship of reported fatigue to obesity, diet, and physical activity: results from the third national health and nutrition examination survey. *Journal of Clinical Sleep Medicine*, 2(2), pp. 163–169.

Ruxton, G.D. & Wilkinson, D.M., 2013. Endurance running and its relevance to scavenging by early hominins. *Evolution*, 67(3), pp. 861–867.

Saris, W.H.M. et al., 2003. How much physical activity is enough to prevent unhealthy weight gain? Outcome of the IASO 1st Stock Conference and consensus statement. *Obesity Reviews*, 4(2), pp. 101–114.

Segal, M.B., 2000. The Choroid Plexuses and the barriers between the blood and the cerebrospinal fluid. *Cellular and Molecular Neurobiology*, 20(2), pp. 183–196.

Semaw, S. et al., 2003. 2.6-Million-year-old stone tools and associated bones from OGS-6 and OGS-7, Gona, Afar, Ethiopia. *Journal of Human Evolution*, 45(2), pp. 169–177.

Shimelmitz, R. et al., 2014. 'Fire at will': the emergence of habitual fire use 350,000 years ago. *Journal of Human Evolution*, 77(C), pp. 196–203.

Speakman, J.R. & Westerterp, K.R., 2010. Associations between energy demands, physical activity, and body composition in adult humans between 18 and 96 y of age. *American Journal of Clinical Nutrition*, 92(4), pp. 826–834.

Spiegelman, B.M. & Flier, J.S., 2001. Obesity and the regulation of energy balance. *Cell*, 104(4), pp. 531–543.

Sponheimer, M. & Lee-Thorp, J.A., 1999. Isotopic evidence for the diet of an early hominid, *Australopithecus africanus*. *Science*, 283(5400), pp. 368–370.

Teaford, M.F. & Ungar, P.S., 2000. Diet and the evolution of the earliest human ancestors. *Proceedings of the National Academy of Sciences of the United States of America*, 97(25), pp. 13506–13511.

Thomas, D.M. & Heymsfield, S.B., 2016. Exercise: is more always better? *Current Biology*, 26(3), pp. R102–R104.

Trangmar, S.J. et al., 2014. Dehydration affects cerebral blood flow but not its metabolic rate for oxygen during maximal exercise in trained humans. *Journal of Physiology*, 592(14), pp. 3143–3160.

Ungar, P.S., 2012. Dental evidence for the reconstruction of diet in African Early *Homo*. *Current Anthropology*, 53(S6), pp. S318–S329.

Ungar, P.S. & Sponheimer, M., 2011. The diets of early hominins. *Science*, 334(6053), pp. 190–193.

Ungar, P.S. et al., 2006. Dental microwear and diets of African early Homo. *Journal of Human Evolution*, 50(1), pp. 78–95.

van der Merwe, N.J., Masao, F.T. & Bamford, M.K., 2008. Isotopic evidence for contrasting diets of early hominins Homo habilis and Australopithecus boisei of Tanzania. *South African Journal of Science*, 104(3–4), pp. 153–155.

Vgontzas, A.N. et al., 2000. Sleep apnea and daytime sleepiness and fatigue: relation to visceral obesity, insulin resistance, and hypercytokinemia. *Journal of Clinical Endocrinology and Metabolism*, 85(3), pp. 1151–1158.

Vgontzas, A.N., Bixler, E.O. & Chrousos, G.P., 2006. Obesity-related sleepiness and fatigue: the role of the stress system and Cytokines. *Annals of the New York Academy of Sciences*, 1083(1), pp. 329–344.

Wade, A.J., Marbut, M.M. & Round, J.M., 1990. Muscle fibre type and aetiology of obesity. *The Lancet*, 335(8693), pp. 805–808.

Walker, R. et al., 2006. Life in the slow lane revisited: ontogenetic separation between Chimpanzees and humans. *American Journal of Physical Anthropology*, 129(4), pp. 577–583.

Walpole, S.C., Prieto-Merino, D., Edwards, P., Cleland, J., Stevens, G. & Roberts, I., 2012. The weight of nations: an estimation of adult human biomass. *BMC Public Health*, 12(1), p. 439.

Wang, Z. et al., 2010. Specific metabolic rates of major organs and tissues across adulthood: evaluation by mechanistic model of resting energy expenditure. *American Journal of Clinical Nutrition*, 92(6), pp. 1369–1377.

Westerterp, K.R., 2010. Physical activity, food intake, and body weight regulation: insights from doubly labeled water studies. *Nutrition reviews*, 68(3), pp. 148–154.

Zink, K.D. & Lieberman, D.E., 2016. Impact of meat and Lower Palaeolithic food processing techniques on chewing in humans. *Nature*, 531(7595), pp. 500–503.

Zinker, B.A., Britz, K. & Brooks, G.A., 1990. Effects of a 36-hour fast on human endurance and substrate utilization. *Journal of Applied Physiology*, 69(5), pp. 1849–1855.

Chapter 9

Power versus endurance

Endurance pierces marble.

– Moroccan proverb

Introduction

Why did *Homo* choose endurance and as a consequence higher fatigue resistance compared to other primates and many other mammals? The answer to this question is no doubt complex, but our observations should provide a basis for this claim. Some of these observations have been outlined in the previous chapter but are summarised here.

First, the key concept is that our features fit with the environment so that we have been able to maximise our survival through reproductive success over a long evolutionary period; specifically, that there was shaping of our features which when under pressure at various times were selected and passed on to offspring. Second, when we consider our closest living relatives, chimpanzees, knuckle walking is energetically more costly than bipedal locomotion by almost 75% (Sockol et al. 2007). It is at least intuitive to select for a method which costs less, so that appropriate energy can be directed to reproductive success. Third, bipedal locomotion came with trade-offs. Although there is a myriad of these trade-offs, the essential ones are our skeleton and neuromuscular adaptations that favour endurance and fatigue resistance. Fourth, a comparatively larger and more expensive brain altered the energy requirements and how that energy is apportioned. Our capacity to store energy in the form of fat does not seem to parallel with our ability to expend it. Current evidence indicates that our energy budget seems to favour conservation of energy over expending it. Fifth, the long, slow change in the climate must have favoured the adaptation of profuse sweating with high physical activity loads. The power of the evaporation of sweat as the mechanism for continued physical activity in the heat accounts to a great extent for favouring endurance over speed/power since this response is relatively only invoked as body temperature rises.

In this chapter we will explore the key concepts and models related to endurance and power and how these have and continue to shape our understanding of human fatigue.

What is endurance?

The classic understanding of endurance with respect to physical performance is based on the relationship between energy systems and time. Typically, textbooks on the subject will categorise maximal physical activity that can last up to 3 seconds as power, 4–50 seconds as speed and anything more than 2 minutes of continuous activity as endurance (Brooks et al. 2005). Figure 9.1 depicts this relationship as three different energy sources that can be potentially used for the replenishment of adenosine triphosphate.

The critical point is the switching from one energy system to another, particularly from glycolysis to aerobic (Figure 9.1). An important point to consider is that glycolysis, the breakdown of glucose, and glycogenolysis, the breakdown of glycogen (stored in muscle as carbohydrate), can occur by non-oxidative processes (without oxygen or anaerobically). Conversely, the breakdown of these substrates also occurs through oxidative or aerobic glycolysis. In the latter, the energy yield is much greater but occurs at a much slower rate than by non-oxidative pathways. However, other available substrates, such as fats and certain amino acids, can be catabolised only through aerobic processes even though in terms of per unit of weight stored, the energy yield is potentially even greater than aerobic glycolysis. From an evolutionary perspective, it is intriguing that the preferred energy source for physical exercise is carbohydrate in the form of glucose and glycogen, but the abundance of energy stored as fat is not mobilised immediately. There are, of course, good reasons for this physiological and biochemical difference, one being that carbohydrates are more efficient to store and hydrolyse, although their total storage is limited.

From an empirical point of view, when trained and untrained individuals have fasted for 12 hours, lipid oxidation is enhanced during exercise at low to

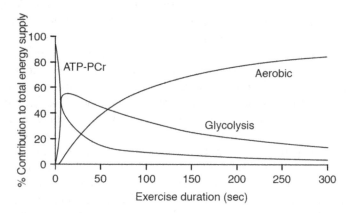

Figure 9.1 The relative energy system contribution to total energy supply for a given duration of maximal exercise.

Source: Reproduced from Gastin (2001) with kind permission from Springer Nature.

moderate intensities, but when these individuals are fed only 3 hours before exercise, carbohydrate oxidation increases, whereas lipid oxidation decreases (Bergman & Brooks 1999). Interestingly, when obese individuals have restricted carbohydrate intake, the result is an increase in fat oxidation both at rest and during exercise regardless of whether this restriction is combined with exercise (Sartor et al. 2010). These observations indicate that carbohydrate is the preferred energy substrate, whereas fat is the preferred form of energy storage which is accessed when carbohydrate availability is limited. The trade-off here is that a mechanism for fuel storage was selected because of the pressure of having expensive organs to fuel in the event that energy availability might have been low or not freely available.

Measuring endurance

Our modern-day fascination with human endurance likely stems from our capacity to explore our biological limitations. The classic story that recounts both human endurance and ultimate fatigue is that of the ancient Greek courier Pheidippides (530–490 BC), who over 2 days supposedly ran about 240 km to ask for help from the Spartans when the Persians landed at Marathon. As legend would have it, he then ran 40 km from Marathon to Athens to announce victory over Persia, before dying from exhaustion (Martin et al. 1977). In modern times our fascination with endurance can in part be attributed to the pedestrian or 'the go as you please' races of the mid-1870s and the feat of American Edward Payson Weston, who walked 713 km from Boston to Washington DC to attend the inauguration of President Abraham Lincoln (Osler & Dodd 1977). Over the following decade these races became so popular that significant monetary rewards were available, with events also held indoors, where contestants would walk around a track for up to 6 days. These events were typically contrived to measure endurance in some way – for example, 'the one that goes the farthest' (see Figure 9.2).

As the understanding of the workings of muscular contraction and respiration grew, it was then shown that the level of oxygen consumption was indeed a key determinant of endurance. The basis for this understanding can be traced back to the classic experiments of Hill and Lupton, of which the key findings are shown in Figure 9.3. In explaining their observations, these authors wrote (Hill & Lupton 1923),

> [S]o far we have discussed a genuine steady state of exercise in which the lactic acid concentration of the muscle attains a constant value and the subject would be able . . . to continue the exercise almost indefinitely. This was almost certainly the case in the experiments recorded in the three lower curves of Fig. 2 [Figure 9.3]. In the highest curve, at a speed of about 10 miles per hour, it was quite certainly not the case for the subject of our experiments . . . he would manifestly have been unable to continue at this speed for more than 10 min, if so long. In such severe exercise the lactic acid is continuously

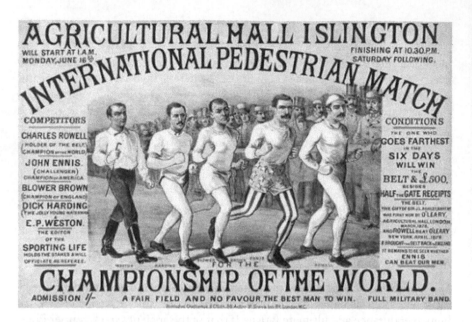

Figure 9.2 Advertisement for an international pedestrian race for the world championship. Note the start time of 1 a.m. Monday and end time of 10:30 p.m. on Saturday, featuring known competitors. The prize money was also significant, with the winner rewarded with half the gate receipts.

Source: Reprinted with kind permission from London Borough of Islington/Islington Local History Centre.

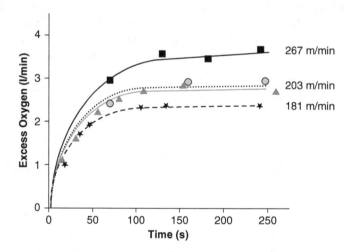

Figure 9.3 The Hill and Lupton (1923) measurement of oxygen consumption measured during running at three different constant speeds. The data show what the authors assumed was the attainment of 'steady state.' Note that the rate of oxygen intake is measured in excess of that measured during standing. The lower three curves (181 and 203 m/min) represent a genuine steady state, whereas the uppermost curve represents an apparent steady state when oxygen intake is assumed to be at its maximum and the oxygen debt is increasing rapidly.

Source: Redrawn from Hill and Lupton (1923).

accumulating in the muscles, the maximum oxygen intake (depending upon the capacity of the heart and lungs) being inadequate to maintain the recovery at a high level enough to cope with the production of lactic acid . . . considering the case of running, there is clearly some critical speed for each individual, below which there is a genuine dynamic equilibrium, break-down being balanced by restoration, above which, however, the maximum oxygen intake is inadequate, lactic acid accumulating, a continuously increasing oxygen debt being incurred, fatigue and exhaustion setting in.

(pp. 150–151)

These observations and the accompanying explanation are critical given that they have shaped the thinking and understanding in the field of exercise physiology and fatigue for the major part of 70 years. Notable, however, is that Hill and Lupton 'confirmed' the concept that when ATP usage cannot be matched by the requirement for ATP re-synthesis, muscular exercise cannot be maintained because the by-product of this, lactic acid, accumulates and muscular fatigue ensues. This concept of energy usage outstripping supply gave way to the more general concept that the skeletal muscle is a slave to the heart since the pumping action of the heart determined the availability of oxygen to fuel exercise, a view that is still widely held (Joyner & Coyle 2008; Levine 2008). However, the concept of what limits or more importantly what regulates exercise performance has evolved over the last 20 years (Noakes 1997, 2008a, 2008b; Noakes & Spedding 2012; Noakes 2000). A major aspect of the debate on what limits exercise performance and the measurement of endurance, and ultimately fatigue, is whether the heart is actually the organ which is limiting. This is key, as a limiting cardiac output limits the supply of oxygen to the working skeletal muscle but is also the limiting factor for the heart's own oxygen supply. Although this aspect is only partially addressed by proponents of the classical understanding, it is worth reiterating that a truly maximal cardiac output is never reached (Zhou et al. 2001) because should this occur, there would be a restriction in cardiac blood flow and myocardial ischemia would ensue (Noakes & St Clair Gibson 2004). Attempts to show that cardiac output limits exercise capacity have not been overly successful. For example, cardiac output, heart rate and stroke volume were all the same during exercise at both 100% and 120% of VO_{2max} when maximum blood pressure was in fact significantly lower at 100% VO_{2max} (Brink-Elfegoun et al. 2007). This indicates that the heart worked harder at 120% than at 100% VO_{2max} or that the heart worked sub-maximally at an apparent 100% VO_{2max} (Noakes & Marino 2009). Either way, the appropriate and logical question is what limits the pumping action of heart before a dangerous plateau in cardiac output occurs which will cause a lower saturation of the arterial blood and risk tissue damage? Interestingly, this apparent flaw was considered by Hill et al. (1924) and was a critical part of explaining the limitations of their observations during severe exercise. They wrote,

[I]t would clearly be useless for the heart to make an excessive effort if by so doing it merely produced a far lower degree of saturation of the arterial blood; and we suggest that, in the body (either in the heart muscle itself or in the nervous system), there is some mechanism which causes a slowing of the circulation as soon as a serious degree of unsaturation occurs, and vice versa. This mechanism would tend . . . to act as a "governor," maintaining a high degree of saturation of the blood.

(pp. 161–162)

This concept, having been ignored until it was reasserted as a potential explanation for why the heart is unlikely to be the sole factor limiting severe exercise and precipitating fatigue (Noakes 1998), has fuelled a debate in the exercise sciences centred around the paradigm commonly referred to as the 'central governor model' (CGM) (Noakes & Marino 2008; Shephard 2009; Noakes 2011; Marino 2010; Marcora 2008; Inzlicht & Marcora 2016; St Clair Gibson et al. 2018). The CGM, as with all other models, makes certain assumptions but was and remains an attempt at introducing an alternative mechanism which could explain why the heart is not the limiting factor in severe exercise but in fact is an organ in a system which has redundancy and controls so that it never reaches a dangerous level of desaturation. As its central tenet, the CGM proposed that "the ultimate control of exercise performance resides in the brain's ability to vary the work rate and metabolic demand by altering the number of skeletal muscle motor units recruited during exercise" (Noakes & St Clair Gibson 2004, p. 513). This implies that the brain regulates rather than limits the number of motor units recruited in the exercising limbs. In simplistic terms, if one wishes to limit the work undertaken by the pump (heart), it is not necessary to turn off the pump; it is far more efficient to regulate the work (skeletal muscle) that the pump needs to accommodate.

Of course, there is continued resistance to this alternative model of exercise physiology since it challenges the inconsistency that is apparent in the classic understanding (Shephard 2009; Noakes 2011). In addition, others have proposed yet another alternative understanding of what regulates endurance performance (Marcora 2008). In this alternative model, motivational intensity theory is proposed to explain task disengagement (i.e., exhaustion) that occurs when the effort required is equal to the maximum effort that an individual is willing to exert to succeed, or when there is belief that a true maximal effort has been given and continuation of exercise is perceived to be impossible. In a study which induced mental fatigue by subjecting individuals to a cognitive demanding task versus an emotionally neutral task before attempting to exercise to exhaustion at 80% of peak power, subjects who were mentally fatigued disengaged and terminated exercise ~1.9 min earlier (Marcora et al. 2009). Importantly, these authors found that neither cardiorespiratory nor musculo-energetic responses were different between conditions but that mental fatigue resulted in similar high ratings of perceived exertion much earlier (~2 min) during exercise compared with the control condition. Therefore, these authors suggested their findings provide experimental evidence that mental fatigue limits exercise tolerance in humans through higher perception of effort rather than physiological mechanisms *per se*.

The purpose of the preceding discussion was to highlight the different schools of thought that dominate the understanding of what determines physical and to an extent psychological endurance (Chapter 6 discusses in detail the mental aspects of fatigue). If one model is more correct than the other, further experimentation and scholarly debate will determine their individual merits. However, the critical aspect is that each of these understandings will also determine how endurance is measured and what component of endurance is most important: heart, lungs, muscle, brain, motivation and so on.

While these models of endurance continue to be debated, the traditional method used to determine endurance is still the VO_{2max} test, whereby an individual either runs on a treadmill or cycles on a stationary ergometer, commencing with a low speed or power output with progressive increments until voluntary termination or exhaustion. The prediction of the classic understanding of exercise limitation is that oxygen consumption during increasing intensity should level off since the delivery (cardiac output) and the usage (skeletal muscle) of oxygen for the generation of ATP through oxidative processes should be at their limit. An early description suggested that when exercise is at its limit – at exhaustion – oxygen consumption should plateau (Taylor et al. 1955). This is an essential outcome if the model predicts that exercise terminates because there is hypoxia-induced failure of mitochondrial ATP production which leads to fatigue. It is also an essential outcome because training studies show that improvements in VO_{2max} are a result of either enhanced delivery of oxygen to the tissues or increased capillarisation and mitochondrial capacity (Daussin et al. 2007). As is shown in Figure 9.4, when oxygen consumption is continuously sampled and is then plotted against increasing work rate, oxygen consumption increases somewhat linearly early on and then slows as exercise intensity increases. What is also evident from the top panel is that oxygen consumption for a particular individual shows an asymptote rather than a true plateau, whereas in the bottom panel a plateau for a different individual is never attained. The data shown in Figure 9.4 are redrawn and based primarily on those provided in the classic study of Wyndham et al. (1959). When these authors assessed these data, they suggested that the VO_{2max} value should be based on the mean of three values falling on the asymptote, with the caveat being that these points should not differ more than 0.15 l/min. The issue here is that the plateau in oxygen consumption during maximal incremental exercise is as common as it is elusive. In fact, the literature dealing with this topic is littered with studies that show a plateau in oxygen consumption is identified in only a fraction of the population studied. For example, see Cumming and Borysyk (1972) and Myers et al. (1989).

Therefore, if a plateau in oxygen consumption, however defined, represents the limits of cardiac output and skeletal muscle oxygen utilisation, the critical question is, what does the lack of an observable plateau in oxygen consumption represent? The logical answer to this question is that other factors cause the

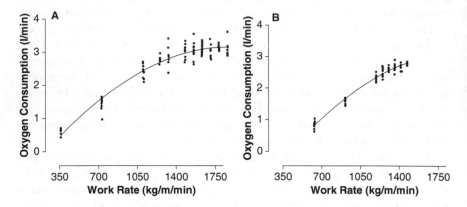

Figure 9.4 Data points represent sampling of oxygen consumption during incremental exercise to exhaustion. In the top panel (A) the individual shows an apparent asymptote for oxygen consumption towards the end of the trial, while in the bottom panel (B) a different individual shows no sign of an asymptote.

Source: Data adapted, redrawn and reanalysed from those provided by Wyndham et al. (1959); they represent typical VO_{2max} data from continuous sampling.

termination of exercise rather than a limiting cardiac output and the eventual onset and development of skeletal muscle anaerobiosis. For a full description of these concepts and debate see Bassett and Howley (1997) and Noakes (1998). When considering the plateau phenomenon others have found that when comparing world-class athletes to sedentary controls, a plateau during incremental maximal testing was observed in only 47% of athletes and 24% of sedentary controls (Lucia et al. 2006). These authors unequivocally concluded that "in a good number of highly trained humans, the main factor limiting maximal endurance might not necessarily be oxygen-dependent, i.e. levelling off in oxygen delivery to (or extraction by) muscles" (p. 990). The reasons given for this observation were two-fold and provide a pivotal insight into human endurance. First, it may be possible that there is a physiological difference between those achieving versus not achieving a plateau. This, the authors suggest, might be due to a tendency to have a higher skeletal muscle buffering capacity in those achieving a plateau, which would allow increments in workload near exhaustion (Lucia et al. 2006). This was posited because the relative buffering capacity (calculated from power output, ventilatory threshold and respiratory compensation point) tended to be higher in those achieving a plateau.

The second possibility is more enticing and suggests that those not achieving a plateau may not have pushed to a 'true maximum level' and is perhaps determined by individual motivation. As there is now evidence for task disengagement during exercise to exhaustion (Marcora et al. 2009), this possibility seems a good candidate. It is reasonable to expect that sedentary individuals would likely disengage earlier during incremental exercise compared with trained individuals, which the data provided by Lucia et al. (2006) now confirm (e.g., 24% versus 47% of individuals achieving a plateau).

In an attempt to further elucidate whether the cardiovascular system is truly the limiting factor in severe exercise, a novel approach was used whereby trained athletes were subjected to repeated bouts of VO_{2max} testing (Beltrami et al. 2012). In these series of tests, one group of athletes (control) undertook incremental running tests to exhaustion on four separate occasions so that the VO_{2max} could be reproduced and verified with the usual criteria. In contrast, the experimental group completed similar testing, but one of those four tests was a reverse test, whereby they commenced the test at a higher speed than that achieved during VO_{2max} verification. Rather than the speed being incremental to exhaustion, the speed was then reduced at regular intervals. The authors reasoned that if the cardiovascular system was truly limiting then when commencing the test at a higher speed than when the VO_{2max} was achieved and reducing the speed from that point, there should be no difference in the VO_{2max} achieved by these athletes. The authors confirmed quite the opposite. As shown in Figure 9.5, in the control condition, where the athletes undertook the conventional incremental running tests to exhaustion, the VO_{2max} was no different across the trials. However, when completing the reverse test, an approximate 4.4% higher VO_{2max} was achieved.

There are three crucial findings from this study which suggest that the cardiovascular system is not the sole limiting factor in severe exercise. First, the additional VO_2 (2.7 ml/kg/min) achieved in the reverse attempt was of the magnitude that should have allowed for an additional stage to be completed during the conventional incremental test. Therefore, these athletes terminated the conventional test with cardiorespiratory reserve and prior to achieving absolute limitation of oxygen delivery or usage. Second, these authors also found that the additional VO_2 was achieved with the same heart rate, respiratory rate and ventilation across all tests, which together strongly indicate that the outcome was not due to additional mechanical work of the heart or the respiratory muscles. Third and most intriguing is that the additional VO_2 achieved during the reverse test was actually retained for the final conventional incremental test (see Figure 9.5). The reasons for this are not entirely clear, but the authors suggest that this might be due to retaining the adaptation that caused the additional VO_2 to be attained. This, they speculate, could be due to altered recruitment of different skeletal muscle fibre types as a consequence of the reverse test. However, the causative mechanism for this proposed skeletal muscle recruitment adaptation is not definitive, but evidence suggests that skeletal muscle fatigue is the event that initiates the increase in VO_2 during the intense phase of exercise (Cannon et al. 2011). Thus, if there is additional or different motor unit recruitment required during the reverse test, then it is possible that this was retained for the subsequent incremental test.

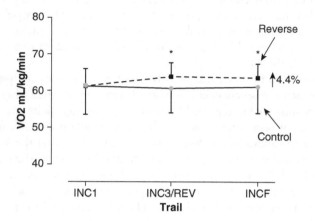

Figure 9.5 The VO$_{2max}$ achieved during consecutive conventional incremental (INC) running tests to exhaustion (control) versus an experimental trial where a reverse (REV) running test was performed. In REV, the speed commenced one stage above that achieved in the INC and was reduced every 30 s up to 120 s by 0.5 km/h. INC1 is the initial conventional incremental test, INC3 is the third conventional incremental test and INCF is the final conventional incremental test. Note the 4.4% increase in the VO$_{2max}$ value at the completion of REV, which was also retained in the INCF. *$P < 0.05$ compared with control.

Source: Data redrawn from Beltrami et al. (2012).

Finally, if endurance as measured by the VO$_{2max}$ test cannot definitively identify the putative cause of exercise termination, it suggests that the basis of human fatigue is not entirely explicable based on the traditional understanding that there is one limiting factor. Rather, it seems plausible that there are redundancy and controls yet to be definitively identified which limit the fatigue experienced even during the most severe exercise. This makes evolutionary sense since adaptability by having multiple controls that could be accessed to regulate endurance seems very desirable.

What is power?

From the point of view of definition, power would seem an easier proposition since there are only a few variables to consider. However, this would negate the reality that power is an outcome of complex relationships which are dependent on both biomechanical and physiological systems. In Chapter 3 the relationship between the skeletal and muscular mechanics was discussed, with emphasis on the differences between humans, chimpanzees and some of our extinct relatives. Not unlike endurance, the definition of power can be restricted to its relationship with energy expenditure, as shown in Figure 9.1. However, power is derived from several concepts which are not easily measured. These are force, strength and work. Just like gravity, force is not easily observed since we see only the outcome or the effect of a force. In simple terms, if a force is acting on an object we will be able to observe the movement, provided there is no equally opposing force to that movement. The object will continue to move and even accelerate if the force continues to act. Although not easily observed, force can be measured in newtons (N), a unit which by convention is the force require to accelerate 1 kg by 1 m/s^2. This is based on the fact that all objects fall towards the Earth at 9.81 m/s^2 so that all force acting on a body is 9.81 x mass (kg), which is conventionally termed weight. Although strength is what is required to generate the force, we use the outcome as a measure of strength.

If a force is applied to an object with a given mass and it moves a given distance, this will equate to the amount of work that has been completed so that work = force × distance in newton metres (Nm or joule, which represents the energy transferred to the mass). If we then divide the work completed by the time it took to complete, we are able to derive the power (P = work/time) in which the unit of measure is joules/s or watts. These derived units of measure allow for the comparison of power between individuals, groups and even species. As a simple example, an 80kg individual travelling 50 m will undertake work calculated as 80 kg × 9.81 N = 784.8 N or joules × 50 m, which is equivalent to 39,240 Nm or joules of work. If it takes this individual 10 s to travel this distance, then 39,240 joules/10 s = 3,924 J/s or watts. If we compare this to a 70 kg individual completing the same task in 8 s then power would be 4,905 J/s or watts. As such the smaller, lighter individual having completed the same task faster would by definition be more powerful by 20%.

In Chapter 3 a comparative analysis of biomechanical and functional differences was presented with respect to chimpanzees and humans which account to a large extent for the disparity in power between the two. However, the magnitude of the difference was not discussed. Here, by using the foregoing calculations it can be seen that in terms of strength alone chimps are well endowed. Figure 9.6 shows a comparative analysis of the weights and pulling forces of male and female chimps compared with male humans. It is noteworthy that in terms of absolute strength male chimps and male humans are quite similar. However, in terms of this particular comparison, chimp body weight is ~26.7% lighter for male and ~35.4% for female chimps than humans. When the strength is correct for body weight it is apparent that male chimps are ~26% stronger than male humans, who in turn exhibit comparatively similar strength to female chimps. These comparisons show definitively that our closest living relatives can produce larger force outputs.

The absolute strength can account for a significant portion of the power produced if strength is exerted over a given time period. Therefore, the assumption is that humans are less powerful than chimps simply because of the strength (force) produced as a ratio of body weight. However, power is difficult to measure in

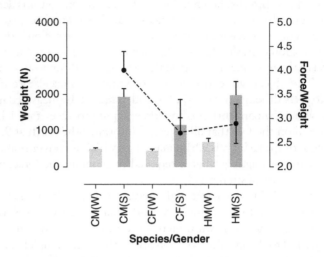

Figure 9.6 The body weight (W, *solid bars*) and strength (S; *open bars*) of both male (CM) and female (CF) chimpanzees compared with male humans (HM) (*left ordinate*). The ratio of force produced to body weight (*right ordinate; solid circles*).

Source: Data redrawn from table 9.1 in Finch (1943). Original data given in *lb* converted in present figure to SI units.

chimps because we never know whether chimps are motivated to produce maximal efforts during a given activity, let alone during an activity that compares to humans. Nevertheless, there are some data which have provided some insights. In a carefully executed comparison of vertical jumping in bonobo and humans, it was shown that bonobo skeletal muscle performs superiorly to human muscle, translating to a higher power output (Scholz et al. 2006). These authors compared a smaller bonobo (34 kg) to a human (61 kg) trained jumper and found that the bonobo hind limb was able to produce 792 W/kg compared to the human 314 W/kg, a difference of 478 W/kg (60%).

The strength and power disparity between human and extant non-human primates is confirmation that humans are adapted for endurance rather than power. The reasons for this apparent difference are complex and, as already discussed (see Chapter 3, Table 3.1), the muscle architecture plays a significant role. For example, the skeletal muscle fascicle length in humans is comparatively short when expressed as a ratio of body mass even though the human lower limb is a component of a higher percentage of total mass. Since fascicle length determines the number of sarcomeres where the contractile elements are located, the number of sarcomeres plays an important role in muscle shortening and force production. This suggests that power generation in the lower limbs of chimps is likely to be a function of the muscle, neurological and skeletal architecture, not muscle mass *per se*. In essence, to understand the physical power differential that exists between humans and other living primates it is necessary to consider in detail the following characteristics (Walker 2009): body mass distribution, moment arm differences, motor control of limb muscles and the quantity of white and grey matter within different areas of the nervous system.

Beyond the apparent architecture of skeletal muscle and biomechanical advantages, which account for strength and power differential, there are other selection pressures and the role of sexual dimorphism which also need consideration. It is clear that limb length (lever) is an important characteristic which can have a significant effect on skeletal muscle force production, and therefore power. In general terms it has been thought that a shorter limb length is an advantage for arboreal living since shorter hind limbs can improve stability by reducing the height of the centre of mass and can also facilitate climbing broad trees (Jungers 1978). There is little doubt that shorter limbs are a specialisation for climbing; however, recent studies on sexual dimorphism on extant apes show very distinctly that the males of the species (including orangutan, chimpanzee and gorilla) have shorter relative hind limb lengths compared with females, but this relationship does not hold for forelimbs (Carrier 2007). As a consequence, it is thought that selection for hind and forelimb length is determined by different pressures. One potential selection pressure for shorter hind limbs is thought to be in response to male-male aggression since a characteristic which improves bipedal stance also potentially improves fighting performance, whereby short legs might be indicative of persistent selection for high levels of aggression (Carrier 2007). An interesting point to consider in this light is whether leg length transitioned from shorter to longer lengths from early to more recent *Homo* respectively in response to a reduction in male-male aggression. The fact that shorter hind limbs might be more advantageous for arboreal living is not in dispute. However, when one considers that our distant relatives, the australopiths, were adapted for both bipedal locomotion and arboreal living because their hind limbs were intermediate between chimps and humans (McHenry & Berger 1998), it is possible that the retention of shorter legs might also have served the need for high levels of aggression (Carrier 2007). As a consequence, the selection of strength and power over endurance might also be related to whether aggression and fighting prowess were a dominant factor in the social structure of the time.

Measuring power

Not unlike endurance, the ability to accurately measure power comes with its own limitations and methodological constraints. For the purpose of this discussion, the concept of power will be limited to the maximum amount of muscular force that can be produced within the shortest amount of time. To understand these limitations, let us consider the usual representation of skeletal muscle shortening, remembering that power is time dependent.

In basic terms, muscular power is the product of the force produced by the muscular contraction and the velocity of muscle shortening. As shown in Figure 9.7,

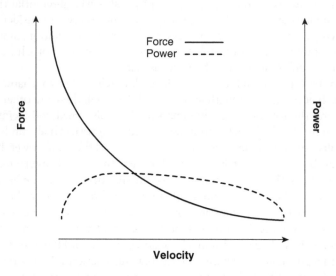

Figure 9.7 The typical representation of the relationships among skeletal muscle shortening, the velocity of shortening and muscle power.

maximum muscle power occurs at about one-third of the maximum velocity and maximum force that can be produced. The first limitation is that neither muscular force nor the speed at which the muscle shortening occurs can be directly measured in humans. As such, the relationship depicted in Figure 9.7 is actually a measure of the rate of torque (force × perpendicular distance) development and the angular velocity occurring at the joint. This means that power in reality is related to the strength and how fast the movement of the limb (lever) occurs. The second aspect of the force-velocity-power relationship that can be seen is that as muscle shortening continues the force that can be developed falls as the velocity increases. Third, no force can be developed at maximal shortening velocity.

Although the relationships shown in Figure 9.7 are broadly accepted, one further limitation when measuring strength and power *in vivo* is that isolation of the muscle under study is not entirely possible and the result depicted in Figure 9.7 cannot exclude assistance from synergistic muscles. The alternative is to study these relationships *in situ* so that individual muscle response can be reasonably isolated. Electrical stimulation of skeletal muscle *in situ* has been studied in a range of species with similar results being observed. The parameters to consider with this kind of methodology are the frequency of electrical of stimulation (Hz), the amplitude of the stimulus (millivolts, mv) and the width of stimulation pulse (micro seconds, μs). Although there are many limitations even with this type of methodology (e.g., signal strength, electrode placement, risks of exceeding fatigue thresholds), it is recognised that each of these parameters will have a bearing on the response of the muscle. Stimulation frequency will determine the relationship of the force response to the stimulation so that at low frequency the muscle will respond to a one-to-one relationship since there is sufficient recovery time between stimuli. However, as the frequency increases to higher values, and the muscle has little or no time to relax, higher continuous forces result. The stimulation amplitude will directly affect the overall force that is generated because as amplitude rises, the force develops quickly from a threshold and reaches a maximum. Therefore, the maximum force that is observed for a given amplitude varies inversely with the width (time) of stimulation pulse.

The relationships shown in Figure 9.8 are for different stimulation frequencies for both force (strength)–velocity and power-velocity in a rat muscle (de Haan 1998). The curves show that increasing stimulation frequency from 80 Hz to 120 Hz increases peak power by 25%, while further increasing stimulation to 400 Hz increases peak power by 45%. However, this power increase is also accompanied by a shift in the velocity from where power peaked at 50 mm/s for low-frequency stimulation to peaking at 100 mm/s for the high-frequency stimulation. It is also notable that at the highest velocity of 250 mm/s, the force and power produced at the higher frequency were also increased compared to the low-frequency stimulation. Therefore, shortening velocity is highly dependent on the stimulation frequency, or at very high shortening velocities high-frequency stimulation is required to maintain the higher muscle force and power output.

The relationship between stimulation frequency and muscle fatigue is a key aspect of human performance and how muscle power can be measured. Stimulus

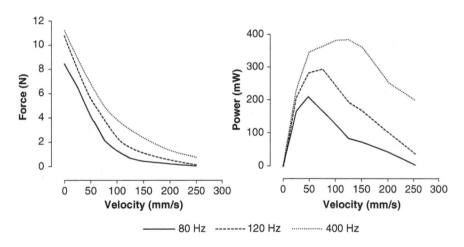

Figure 9.8 Force-velocity (top panel) and power-velocity (bottom panel) relationships of rat medial gastrocnemius muscles at three different stimulation frequencies.

Source: Data redrawn and adapted from de Haan (1998).

intensity, which is a combination of frequency and pulse width, can have very different effects on muscle fatigue. For example, when comparing low-frequency stimulation (11.5 Hz) coupled with a long pulse width (600 µs) versus quite different stimulus intensities (30 Hz and 150 µs versus 60 Hz and 131 µs), muscle fatigue was less pronounced when the pulse width was longest (600 µs) (Kesar & Binder-Macleod 2006). The authors reasoned that the lower stimulation frequency with a longer duration resulted in less force produced per individual muscle fibre but matched the overall force produced as that of the higher stimulus intensities. This, they speculate, was due to less ATP utilisation and lower metabolic demand per muscle fibre because of the longer stimulation pulse, resulting in less pronounced whole muscle fatigue.

In terms of relative fatigue profiles, a direct comparison of strength and power production using electrical muscle stimulation between humans and extant apes has not been reported. Nevertheless, using existing anatomical and morphological comparisons some reasonable assumptions can be made. First, compared with slow-twitch muscle fibres, fast-twitch fibres produce high force with faster speed of contraction. This difference is due to the neural input which determines the muscle fibre characteristics; larger myelinated neurons innervate fast-twitch fibres. However, the cost of this neuronal arrangement is greater fatigability for the fast-twitch fibre. Second, humans have substantially less myelinated spinal cord axons than do chimpanzees, which in turn have comparatively lower numbers of slow-twitch fibres (MacLarnon 1995, 1996). These general characteristics of fast- and slow-twitch fibres mean that when subjected to stimulation they will exhibit different force responses. When stimulated at 1 Hz with similar pulse width, fast-twitch fibres will react faster but will also exhibit a faster relaxation time so that the muscle fibre can be ready for the next stimulation. This particular characteristic has the advantage of developing high force output, but when stimulated at higher frequencies, such as 10–20 Hz, the slow-twitch fibre does not have time to reach baseline relaxation, which means the next impulse will be superimposed. As the stimulating frequency increases, the individual twitches fuse or summate until the muscle produces a smooth force (Figure 9.9).

The curves in Figure 9.9 provide at least four distinct elements in relation to force production and power. These are shape of the actual twitch, relaxation time, frequency at which force summation occurs and fatigability. The rate of fatigue that is exhibited by either fibre type is a critical element in considering the difference between endurance and power. This is commonly referred to as the "fatigue index," which relates the declining tension over time when muscle is repeatedly stimulated. However, even this requires careful delineation because fatigue of the muscle fibre is not the same as the fatigue that develops related to the nerve or the neuromuscular junction. For instance, there is an apparent increasing failure of neuromuscular transmission whereby tension declines more rapidly when there is direct stimulation of the nerve versus the actual muscle (Johnson & Sieck 1993). Regardless, the fatigue index in all respects is distinct between fast- and slow-twitch fibres. As shown in Figure 9.10, when stimulated

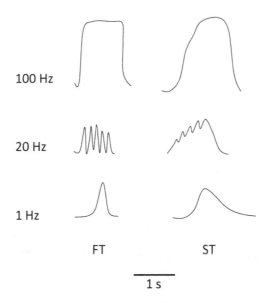

100 Hz

20 Hz

1 Hz

FT   ST

1 s

Figure 9.9 Responses of fast-twitch (FT) and slow-twitch (ST) muscle fibres to stimulation at different frequencies but similar pulse widths. Figures are examples of stimulation curves redrawn from experimental trials conducted in the author's laboratory and broadly accepted as representing the response of distinct skeletal muscle fibres.

continuously to reach maximum attention over a similar time period, not only will muscle fibres will exhibit different twitch-tension curves but also the decreasing tension will exhibit a decline distinctive to the muscle fibre type (Burke et al. 1971, 1973). The cause of the rapid development of fatigue is multifactorial, and as already mentioned is relative to whether the actual muscle fibre or the nerve is stimulated. However, one element to consider is that of neurotransmitters' substance availability and recycling (see Chapter 2 for a discussion on skeletal muscle safety factor and neuromuscular junction and transmitter substance release and recycling). Although complete depletion seldom occurs due to the safety factor of transmitter quanta, it is now thought that the quantal content of neurotransmitter substance is substantially greater in fast-twitch fibres but is expended to a greater extent than for slow-twitch fibres (Reid et al. 1999). As such, the end-plate terminals associated with the different fibres are adapted to their individual activity patterns.

The relevance of endurance versus power

The intent of this chapter was to contrast and compare the basis for endurance and power and how these two distinct aspects of physical activity are related to

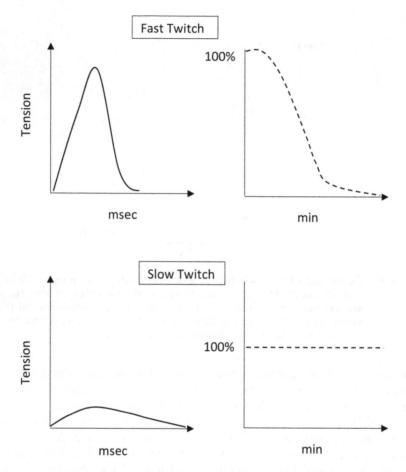

Figure 9.10 A schematic representation of the typical fatigue index for fast- (top panel) and slow- (lower-panel) twitch muscle fibres. The fast-twitch fibres are innervated by large myelinated neurons and respond to stimulation with a higher tension development but fatigue more rapidly under continued stimulation. In contrast, the smaller neurons that innervate the slow-twitch fibres develop low tension but can sustain this for a longer period under continued stimulation. The curves have been redrawn from the work of Burke et al. (1971) on cat gastrocnemius muscle. Note that the original work identified an intermediate fast fatigue-resistant muscle fibre, which has been omitted here for clarity.

why humans are adapted for endurance. In making this comparison it is not possible to avoid the characteristics of other mammals, in particular our closest living relatives. A further unavoidable comparison is the relationship between muscle fibre types and physical capabilities across species. In the most simplistic terms, and as already outlined in detail, fast-twitch fibres reach peak force more rapidly, have shorter relaxation time, require higher stimulation frequency to reach a smooth contraction but fatigue more rapidly. Since our closest living relatives have a higher preponderance of myelinated axons and fast-twitch fibres, we can safely assume that they have a distinct advantage in strength and power production, but the trade-off might be greater fatigability. However, because there are no data available for direct comparison of muscle fatigability of human and chimpanzee, we can only speculate that due to their higher preponderance of myelination and fast-twitch fibres, the threshold for fatigue could be substantially higher in chimps than in humans. On the one hand, *Homo* is adapted for endurance, but why did the divergence from the last common ancestor leave our closest living relatives with the adaptation for strength and power?

It is recognised that chimpanzees and perhaps other primates spend a significant amount of time, possibly up to ten times more energy per day, on terrestrial walking than they do on vertical climbing (Pontzer & Wrangham 2004). If this is the case, it would seem paradoxical that this species selected power over endurance if terrestrial locomotion is so important. Even so, chimpanzees usually travel terrestrially only about 2.5 km per day (Wrangham et al. 1993), whereas *Homo* is thought to have a large range per day and indeed pursue prey over several days if needed (Carrier et al. 1984). This observation should also be balanced with the fact that chimpanzees, whether using quadrupedal or bipedal locomotion, expend about the same amount of energy (Rowntree 1973). More importantly, because chimpanzees are adapted primarily for arboreal living, it would not be useful if vertical climbing was energetically costly, and as shown, human bipedal locomotion is about 75% less costly than quadrupedal and bipedal walking in chimpanzees (Sockol et al. 2007). Therefore, if living well above the ground is important, then strength and power would be advantageous since maintaining balance and posture, swinging from tree limbs and reducing the likelihood of falls from the canopy would be a key selection pressure for strength and power. In fact, the risk of trauma from falls for chimpanzees is significant (Jurmain 1997) and explains to a great extent why muscular strength and power would be one useful energetic adaptation complementing the anatomical and biomechanical differences.

Inherent training for endurance and power

There is abundant evidence that physical training for humans and animals results in improved capacity for both power and endurance (Gallaugher et al. 2001; Gibala & McGee 2008; Jacobs et al. 2013; Zhang et al. 2015). Although there is no doubt about the outcomes of 'self-imposed' or planned physical training for humans and in some contexts animals, the broader question is whether animals in their natural environment actually exercise to maintain their fitness. Although this would be a difficult question to answer, it is thought that exercising for fitness by animals is likely a function of their ecology (Halsey 2016). It has been shown that should access to wheel running be available, rats will spontaneously utilise the wheel and run, resulting in increased fitness (Lambert & Noakes 1990). In this particular study, the researchers found that there were rats which performed either high, moderate or low levels of spontaneous running but their VO_{2max} was not different to control rats after 8 weeks of this kind of training. However, they did find that submaximal VO_2 was indeed reduced across the spontaneous runners versus the controls, which suggested that a training effect did occur in those running a minimum distance over the training period.

In a subsequent study (Lambert et al. 1996), which separated rats of similar genetic stock into a sedentary control versus a spontaneous exercise group, it was found that after 8 weeks the average spontaneous running distance was ~29.7 km/wk but ranged from 1.4 to 71.1 km/wk. The interesting finding was that none of the running performance or oxygen consumption measurements conducted at the start of the experiment were related to subsequent average spontaneous running distance. However, peak force generated by electrically stimulating the gastrocnemius/plantaris muscles was greater in the spontaneous running group than in the sedentary one, but this difference was not related to running distance. These authors concluded that spontaneous running in rats cannot be predicted by the measures of running performance taken before the experiment so that low levels of spontaneous running in some rats are not explained by skeletal muscular and cardiovascular factors thought to determine running capacity. As might be expected, spontaneous running over 8 weeks altered muscle oxidative enzymes but not the contractile properties of the muscles. These findings suggest that in the captive laboratory animal model of exercise training, there are likely to be animals that will exercise more so than others and these animals may be more inclined to do so because of innate muscular characteristics.

In addition to the captive laboratory conditions, similar observations of spontaneous exercise training are reported if running wheels are made available in a natural environment whereby voluntary training is briefly undertaken (Meijer & Robbers 2014). The reasons for this are not entirely clear but the following have been suggested to explain this phenomenon (Halsey 2016). First, and as outlined in Chapter 8, all animals need to consider their rates of energy expenditure. Therefore, enhancing athletic ability requires the apportionment of energy for spontaneous exercise to either maintain or enhance fitness for the purpose of chasing, fleeing, searching or fighting. Second, improved athletic capacity can enhance an animal's capability for increased physical demands that come with changes in the ecology, including caring for infants and other group dynamics. However, physical training after these demands are identified and then needed to be deployed clearly would be useless, which could explain why spontaneous exercise in both captive and natural environments occurs. Third, there is a clear trade-off between avoiding starvation and predation so that energy reserves in the form of fat are reduced in favour of leanness when animals are regularly preyed upon in order to improve their fitness (Halsey 2016; MacLeod et al. 2007). Fourth, the energy trade-off which reduces energy stores in favour of leanness and fitness also occurs in females lactating so that spontaneous exercise is reduced in favour for maintaining reproduction.

In contrast to the apparent spontaneous exercise that is undertaken by animals in both laboratory and natural environments, humans seemingly do not undertake this kind of spontaneous activity. The promotion and maintenance of our athleticism need constant exercise and are usually either strength- or endurance-based but sometimes both. The reasons why we do not necessarily engage in regular spontaneous exercise are unclear, but an evolutionary perspective could provide valuable insights. One such evolutionary hypothesis is based on the altered risk of predation that has occurred since our divergence from our last common ancestor (Speakman 2007). It is suggested that we were released from the predation risks which were experienced by *Australopithicus*, who were under heavy predation from specialist predators (Speakman 2014). However, when *H. erectus* appeared some 2 million years ago socialisation, weaponry and fire likely reduced predation. Therefore, if spontaneous or even regular exercise was a function of predation, then any reduction in the need to avoid predation would be offset by reducing the need for increased physical fitness. Of course, the change in the predation dynamics has likely had other effects on energy consumption and conservation. However, the important point in the context discussed here is whether predation altered the human need for regular exercise to maintain fitness. Testing this hypothesis in humans will be difficult given the complex social structure and the abundance of energy available in modern and developed industrialised countries.

A final consideration as to whether exercise training for fitness is inherent in humans, or even other animals, is whether the development of endurance or power is most important. Assuming that training for fitness and survival is important for the organism, what does it choose to train for? Endurance, power or both? This question is likely to be very dependent on the individual needs and, as already suggested, dependent on the ecology. However, one further aspect to consider is what the fatigue profile shows when comparing endurance- and power-trained individuals. This is a difficult comparison to make in animals; however, we have sufficient data to make this comparison for humans. When sprint-trained cyclists were compared with endurance-trained cyclists for power output during a maximal Wingate cycling test, the sprint athletes achieved higher power output only for the initial 10 of the 27.5 seconds, after which endurance athletes were able to generate the same power for the remainder of the test (Calbet et al. 2003). In fact, these authors found that endurance-trained athletes had a higher VO_2 during the final 15 s of the test, which indicates that their power was derived from aerobic sources. However, when comparing the fatigability of individuals with low and moderate VO_{2max} values but matched for power performance, decrements in power output were smaller for those with a moderate VO_{2max} (Bishop & Edge 2006).

Overall these findings indicate that endurance can have a significant effect in maintaining greater fatigue resistance even when the activity is power-based. Therefore, if humans were to engage in spontaneous physical exercise, anything that would enhance endurance will also enhance fatigability even when power would be required. As already outlined in Chapter 2, improved running economy in short-endurance exercise (5 km) following explosive strength training is thought to be in large part due to changes in neuromuscular characteristics and not improvements in aerobic capacity *per se* (Paavolainen et al. 1999). This improvement is usually attributed to more synchronous motor unit recruitment for any given movement leading to greater efficiency in force production (Carroll et al. 2001). Given these general findings, on balance, if spontaneous exercise was an inherent characteristic for *Homo*, then efficiency would also dictate that endurance training would be preferred if improved fatigability was the selection pressure.

References

Bassett, D.R.J. & Howley, E.T., 1997. Maximal oxygen uptake: "classical" versus "contemporary" viewpoints. *Medicine and Science in Sports & Exercise*, 29(5), pp. 591–603.

Beltrami, F.G. et al., 2012. Conventional testing methods produce submaximal values of maximum oxygen consumption. *British Journal of Sports Medicine*, 46(1), pp. 23–29.

Bergman, B.C. & Brooks, G.A., 1999. Respiratory gas-exchange ratios during graded exercise in fed and fasted trained and untrained men. *Journal of Applied Physiology*, 86(2), pp. 479–487.

Bishop, D. & Edge, J., 2006. Determinants of repeated-sprint ability in females matched for single-sprint performance. *European Journal of Applied Physiology*, 97(4), pp. 373–379.

Brink-Elfegoun, T. et al., 2007. Maximal oxygen uptake is not limited by a central nervous system governor. *Journal of Applied Physiology*, 102(2), pp. 781–786.

Brooks, G.A., Fahey, T.D. & Baldwin, K.M., 2005. *Exercise physiology: human bioenergetics and its applications*, 4th ed., New York: McGraw-Hill.

Burke, R.E. et al., 1971. Mammalian motor units: physiological-histochemical correlation in three types in cat gastrocnemius. *Science*, 174(4010), pp. 709–712.

Burke, R.E. et al., 1973. Physiological types and histochemical profiles in motor units of the cat gastrocnemius. *Journal of Physiology*, 234(3), pp. 723–748.

Calbet, J.A.L. et al., 2003. Anaerobic energy provision does not limit Wingate exercise performance in endurance-trained cyclists. *Journal of Applied Physiology*, 94(2), pp. 668–676.

Cannon, D.T. et al., 2011. Skeletal muscle fatigue precedes the slow component of oxygen uptake kinetics during exercise in humans. *Journal of Physiology*, 589(3), pp. 727–739.

Carrier, D.R., 2007. The short legs of great apes: evidence for aggressive behavior in australopiths. *Evolution*, 61(3), pp. 596–605.

Carrier, D.R. et al., 1984. The energetic paradox of human running and hominid evolution. *Current Anthropology*, 25, pp. 483–495.

Carroll, T.J., Riek, S. & Carson, R.G., 2001. Neural adaptations to resistance training. *Sports Medicine*, 31(12), pp. 829–840.

Cumming, G.R. & Borysyk, L.M., 1972. Criteria for maximum oxygen uptake in men over 40 in a population survey. *Medicine and Science in Sports*, 4(1), pp. 18–22.

Daussin, F.N. et al., 2007. Improvement of VO_{2max} by cardiac output and oxygen extraction adaptation during intermittent versus continuous endurance training. *European Journal of Applied Physiology*, 101(3), pp. 377–383.

de Haan, A., 1998. The influence of stimulation frequency on force-velocity characteristics of in situ rat medial gastrocnemius muscle. *Experimental Physiology*, 83(1), pp. 77–84.

Finch, G., 1943. The bodily strength of chimpanzees. *Journal of Mammology*, 24(2), pp. 224–228.

Gallaugher, P.E. et al., 2001. Effects of high-intensity exercise training on cardiovascular function, oxygen uptake, internal oxygen transport and osmotic balance in chinook salmon (Oncorhynchus tshawytscha) during critical speed swimming. *Journal of Experimental Biology*, 204(16), pp. 2861–2872.

Gastin, P.B., 2001. Energy system interaction and relative contribution during maximal exercise. *Sports Medicine*, 31(10), pp. 725–741.

Gibala, M.J. & McGee, S.L., 2008. Metabolic adaptations to short-term high-intensity interval training: a little pain for a lot of gain? *Exercise and Sport Sciences Reviews*, 36(2), pp. 58 63.

Halsey, L.G., 2016. Do animals exercise to keep fit? *Journal of Animal Ecology*, 85(3), pp. 614–620.

Hill, A.V. & Lupton, H., 1923. Muscular exercise, lactic acid, and the supply and utilization of oxygen. *Quarterly Journal of Medicine* (62), p. 135.

Hill, A.V., Long, C.N.H. & Lupton, H., 1924. Muscular exercise, lactic acid and the supply and utilisation of oxygen. – Parts VII – VIII. *Proceedings of the Royal Society B: Biological Sciences*, 97(682), pp. 155–176.

Inzlicht, M. & Marcora, S.M., 2016. The Central Governor Model of exercise regulation teaches us precious little about the nature of mental fatigue and self-control failure. *Frontiers in Psychology*, 7(967), p. 313.

Jacobs, R.A. et al., 2013. Improvements in exercise performance with high-intensity interval training coincide with an increase in skeletal muscle mitochondrial content and function. *Journal of Applied Physiology*, 115(6), pp. 785–793.

Johnson, B.D. & Sieck, G.C., 1993. Differential susceptibility of diaphragm muscle fibers to neuromuscular transmission failure. *Journal of Applied Physiology*, 75(1), pp. 341–348.

Joyner, M.J. & Coyle, E.F., 2008. Endurance exercise performance: the physiology of champions. *Journal of Physiology*, 586(1), pp. 35–44.

Jungers, W.L., 1978. The functional significance of skeletal allometry in Megaladapis in comparison to living prosimians. *American Journal of Physical Anthropology*, 49(3), pp. 303–314.

Jurmain, R., 1997. Skeletal evidence of trauma in African apes, with special reference to the Gombe chimpanzees. *Primates*, 38(1), pp. 1–14.

Kesar, T. & Binder-Macleod, S., 2006. Effect of frequency and pulse duration on human muscle fatigue during repetitive electrical stimulation. *Experimental Physiology*, 91(6), pp. 967–976.

Lambert, M.I. & Noakes, T.D., 1990. Spontaneous running increases VO2max and running performance in rats. *Journal of Applied Physiology*, 68(1), pp. 400–403.

Lambert, M.I. et al., 1996. Tests of running performance do not predict subsequent spontaneous running in rats. *Physiology & Behavior*, 60(1), pp. 171–176.

Levine, B.D., 2008. VO$_{2max}$: what do we know, and what do we still need to know? *Journal of Physiology*, 586(1), pp. 25–34.

Lucia, A. et al., 2006. Frequency of the VO2max plateau phenomenon in world-class cyclists. *International Journal of Sports Medicine*, 27(12), pp. 984–992.

MacLarnon, A., 1995. The distribution of spinal cord tissues and locomotor adaptation in primates. *Journal of Human Evolution*, 29(5), pp. 463–482.

MacLarnon, A., 1996. The scaling of gross dimensions of the spinal cord in primates and other species. *Journal of Human Evolution*, 30(1), pp. 71–87.

MacLeod, R. et al., 2007. Mass-dependent predation risk and lethal dolphin-porpoise interactions. *Proceedings of the Royal Society B: Biological Sciences*, 274(1625), pp. 2587–2593.

Marcora, S.M., 2008. Do we really need a central governor to explain brain regulation of exercise performance? *European Journal of Applied Physiology*, 104(5), pp. 929–931.

Marcora, S.M., Staiano, W. & Manning, V., 2009. Mental fatigue impairs physical performance in humans. *Journal of Applied Physiology*, 106(3), pp. 857–864.

Marino, F.E., 2010. Is it time to retire the "Central Governor?" A philosophical and evolutionary perspective. *Sports Medicine*, 40(3), pp. 265–270.

Martin, D.E., Benario, H.W. & Gynn, R.W.H., 1977. Development of the marathon from Pheidippides to the present, with statistics of significant races. *Annals of the New York Academy of Sciences*, 301(1), pp. 820–852.

McHenry, H.M. & Berger, L.R., 1998. Body proportions of Australopithecus afarensis and A. africanus and the origin of the genus Homo. *Journal of Human Evolution*, 35(1), pp. 1–22.

Meijer, J.H. & Robbers, Y., 2014. Wheel running in the wild. *Proceedings. Biological Sciences*, 281(1786), pp. 1–5.

Myers, J. et al., 1989. Can maximal cardiopulmonary capacity be recognized by a plateau in oxygen uptake? *Chest*, 96(6), pp. 1312–1316.

Noakes, T.D., 1997. Challenging beliefs: ex Africa semper aliquid novi. *Medicine and Science in Sports & Exercise*, 29(5), pp. 571–590.

Noakes, T.D., 1998. Maximal oxygen uptake: "classical" versus "contemporary" viewpoints: a rebuttal. *Medicine and Science in Sports & Exercise*, 30(9).

Noakes, T.D., 2000. Physiological models to understand exercise fatigue and the adaptations that predict or enhance athletic performance. *Scandinavian Journal of Medicine & Science in Sports*, 10(3), pp. 123–145.

Noakes, T.D., 2008a. How did AV Hill understand the VO2max and the "plateau phenomenon?" Still no clarity? *British Journal of Sports Medicine*, 42(7), p. 574.

Noakes, T.D., 2008b. Testing for maximum oxygen consumption has produced a brainless model of human exercise performance. *British Journal of Sports Medicine*, 42(7), pp. 551–555.

Noakes, T.D., 2011. Is it time to retire the A.V. Hill model? *Sports Medicine*, 41(4), pp. 263–277.

Noakes, T.D. & Marino, F.E., 2008. Does a central governor regulate maximal exercise during combined arm and leg exercise? A rebuttal. *European Journal of Applied Physiology*, 104(4), pp. 757–759.

Noakes, T.D. & Marino, F.E., 2009. Point: counterpoint: maximal oxygen uptake is/is not limited by a central nervous system governor. *Journal of Applied Physiology*, 106(1), pp. 338–339.

Noakes, T.D. & Spedding, M., 2012. Olympics: run for your life. *Nature*, 487(7407), pp. 295–296.

Noakes, T.D. & St Clair Gibson, A., 2004. Logical limitations to the "catastrophe" models of fatigue during exercise in humans. *British Journal of Sports Medicine*, 38(5), pp. 648–649.

Osler, T.J. & Dodd, E.L., 1977. Six-day pedestrian races. *Annals of the New York Academy of Sciences*, 301(1), pp. 853–857.

Paavolainen, L. et al., 1999. Explosive-strength training improves 5-km running time by improving running economy and muscle power. *Journal of Applied Physiology*, 86(5), pp. 1527–1533.

Pontzer, H. & Wrangham, R.W., 2004. Climbing and the daily energy cost of locomotion in wild chimpanzees: implications for hominoid locomotor evolution. *Journal of Human Evolution*, 46(3), pp. 315–333.

Reid, B., Slater, C.R. & Bewick, G.S., 1999. Synaptic vesicle dynamics in rat fast and slow motor nerve terminals. *The Journal of Neuroscience*, 19(7), pp. 2511–2521.

Rowntree, V.J., 1973. Running on two or on four legs: which consumes more energy? *Science*, 179(4069), pp. 186–187.

Sartor, F. et al., 2010. High-intensity exercise and carbohydrate-reduced energy-restricted diet in obese individuals. *European Journal of Applied Physiology*, 110(5), pp. 893–903.

Scholz, M.N. et al., 2006. Vertical jumping performance of bonobo (Pan paniscus) suggests superior muscle properties. *Proceedings of the Royal Society B: Biological Sciences*, 273(1598), pp. 2177–2184.

Shephard, R.J., 2009. Is it time to retire the 'central governor'? *Sports Medicine*, 39(9), pp. 709–721.

Sockol, M.D., Raichlen, D.A. & Pontzer, H., 2007. Chimpanzee locomotor energetics and the origin of human bipedalism. *Proceedings of the National Academy of Sciences*, 104(30), pp. 12265–12269.

Speakman, J.R., 2007. A nonadaptive scenario explaining the genetic predisposition to obesity: the "predation release" hypothesis. *Cell Metabolism*, 6(1), pp. 5–12.

Speakman, J.R., 2014. If Body Fatness is under physiological regulation, then how come we have an obesity epidemic? *Physiology*, 29(2), pp. 88–98.

St Clair Gibson, A., Swart, J. & Tucker, R., 2018. The interaction of psychological and physiological homeostatic drives and role of general control principles in the regulation of physiological systems, exercise and the fatigue process – the integrative governor theory. *European Journal of Sport Science*, 18(1), pp. 25–36.

Taylor, H.L., Buskirk, E. & Henschel, A., 1955. Maximal oxygen intake as an objective measure of cardio-respiratory performance. *Journal of Applied Physiology*, 8(1), pp. 73–80.

Walker, A., 2009. The strength of Great Apes and the speed of humans. *Current Anthropology*, 50(2), pp. 229–234.

Wrangham, R.W., Gittleman, J.L. & Chapman, C.A., 1993. Constraints on group size in primates and carnivores: population density and day-range as assays of exploitation competition. *Behavioral Ecology and Sociobiology*, 32(3), pp. 199–209.

Wyndham, C. et al., 1959. Maximum oxygen intake and maximum heart rate during strenuous work. *Journal of Applied Physiology*, 14(6), pp. 927–936.

Zhang, Y. et al., 2015. Cross-training in birds: cold and exercise training produce similar changes in maximal metabolic output, muscle masses and myostatin expression in house sparrows (Passer domesticus). *Journal of Experimental Biology*, 218(Pt 14), pp. 2190–2200.

Zhou, B. et al., 2001. Stroke volume does not plateau during graded exercise in elite male distance runners. *Medicine and Science in Sports & Exercise*, 33(11), pp. 1849–1854.

Chapter 10

Fatigue in disease

Sickness is felt, but health not at all.

– Thomas Fuller (1608–1661)

Introduction

Individuals that fall victim to pathology which develops into a disease state will normally report they have difficulty carrying out activities of daily living because of the inherent fatigue they experience. These individuals typically describe the need to increase their effort to accomplish a given task or activity. In many instances this will be an activity such as rising from a chair, bathing, grooming, getting in and out of a car and many other simple tasks which many of us seemingly undertake with little effort. There is a myriad of diseases which promote physical fatigue whereby either muscular force production is significantly compromised or sensations and feelings associated with fatigue are heightened, compromising the capacity to resist fatigue. However, when individuals with pathology report that they experience significant fatigue, it is typically assumed that this is a feeling, emotion or some subjective assessment rather than an objective estimate of the reduced capacity to undertake a given task. As discussed in detail in Chapter 4, unravelling how fatigue is manifested is complex and based on the context and the definition used to assess it.

Recall that fatigue as a response can also be thought of as a regulated process along a 'chain' of overlapping biological structures, which extend from the corticospinal interneurons arising from the motor cortex, descending to the spinal cord and eventually innervating the skeletal muscles, which generate force via the contractile apparatus (see Figure 4.3). Thus, the fatigue process is dependent on a series of interconnections which can either individually or collectively develop incapacity to produce a target force; fatigue can be a consequence of failure at any one point in the system. In addition to this chain of structures is the generation of perception of effort, which is dependent on central and local cues (Figure 6.3). These two interconnected aspects of fatigue – biological structures involved in transmission from the central nervous system to the muscle and the generation of perception from multiple cues – are important distinctions as fatigue that results from physical exertion serves to halt or regulate the exertion, whereas a heightened perception of the cues leading to fatigue may diminish the drive for exertion before it even begins. Therefore, when dealing with fatigue as related to pathology, the differentiation as to biology or perception is critical as people suffering from a particular disease often complain that fatigue is the most distressing and debilitating symptom of their condition. This would explain to an extent that in pathology, fatigue could represent either difficulty sustaining voluntary activity or even difficulty initiating movement (Chaudhuri & Behan 2004).

In this chapter the difference between maintaining voluntary activity versus initiating movement will be the central tenet of fatigue as related to disease. To illustrate this, two distinct pathologies will be discussed: multiple sclerosis (MS) and myasthenia gravis (MG). The reason for this choice is that each has distinct central and peripheral derangements which provide clues as to how fatigue is manifested.

Generalised fatigue in multiple sclerosis

Multiple sclerosis (MS) is a neurodegenerative disease which affects over 2.5 million people worldwide and is usually more prevalent in women than in men by approximately 3 to 1, according to the Australian MS Society (www.msaustralia. org.au/what-ms). The main characteristics of the disease are the loss of axons and demyelination, which result in motor dysfunction and muscle weakness (Smith & McDonald 1999; Noseworthy et al. 2000). Individuals afflicted with MS can exhibit a range of symptoms, including depression, poor balance, elimination dysfunction and ventilatory muscle weakness (White & Dressendorfer 2004), although a predominant symptom regularly reported is excessive fatigue (Bakshi et al. 2000). Beyond the degenerative symptoms and consequences associated with this disease, excessive fatigue is an additional problem because it reduces the capacity to undertake activities of daily living and limits opportunities in relation to long-term employment and recreation, thereby reducing the potential for quality of life. In addition, excessive fatigue can lead to the development of secondary morbidities associated with sedentary lifestyle, such as obesity and cardiovascular disease (Lambert et al. 2002; Slawta et al. 2002). In sedentary but symptom-free individuals, prescribed exercise can significantly increase the capacity to resist fatigue. In contrast, in conditions such as MS, improving the tolerance to fatigue presents difficulties. Since demyelination is the primary characteristic of the disease, which slows the axonal conduction velocity, it is difficult to distinguish whether the ability to complete a task is diminished because of this compromised neuronal transmission or whether the heightened feeling of fatigue itself is the predominant cause. Further, skeletal muscle atrophy is a consequence of MS because of reduced physical activity, which also leads to premature fatigue for any given task.

An additional consideration is that the disease is characterised by the changes in axonal structure and function which are primarily peripheral in nature and cannot fully explain the observation that fatigue in this disease is of central origin (Garner & Widrick 2003; Ng et al. 2004). However, an intriguing symptom of MS is the heightened heat sensitivity that is commonly reported and also thought to hasten fatigue (Baker 2002). This is not unlike the observation in normal, healthy individuals in which thermal strain also induces premature fatigue versus when physical activity is undertaken in cooler or normal conditions (Nielsen & Nielsen 1962; Nybo & Nielsen 2001; Marino 2004). In this latter case, it is thought that thermoregulatory strain either through exercise or by passively heating the body reduces central nervous system drive to skeletal muscle (Nybo & Nielsen 2001; Morrison et al. 2004; Saboisky et al. 2003). Whether this mechanism also exists to the same extent in MS is yet to be investigated.

Skeletal muscle fatigue in multiple sclerosis

In healthy humans, fatigue is usually assessed by quantifying the reduction in force output which occurs as a consequence of changes along the neuromuscular pathway. Thus, the cause of fatigue is not always definitive whereby the origin is either central or peripheral or a combination of these (see Chapter 4). In MS, there are decreases in maximal motor unit firing rates and recruitment (Rice et al. 1992; Sharma et al. 1995). However, when the electromyographic (EMG) changes are compared to healthy controls as force output increases from 10% to 70% of maximal voluntary contraction, the EMG response rises more sharply compared with healthy controls (Ng et al. 1997). This distinct relationship suggests that a relatively greater central motor drive was necessary for the MS group to achieve the same relative force as healthy control subjects. In addition, it appears that the muscle weakness typically observed in MS is not related to reductions in the cross-sectional area or in peripheral muscle function (Ng et al. 2004). This was concluded after assessing the central activation, symptomatic fatigue and the fat-free cross-sectional area along with the peripheral muscle function of the dorsi-flexor. In contrast, in healthy controls the maximal voluntary contraction was related to how much muscle could be recruited rather than how much muscle was actually available. Interestingly, when comparing the central activation and the compound muscle action potential (M-wave) between MS and healthy controls, there were no differences at baseline (Sheean et al. 1997). That force output had decreased ~55% in MS but not in controls, so that the M-wave remained unchanged, suggested that the reduction in force output following fatiguing exercise in the MS group was likely due to a reduction in central drive and not due to peripheral changes.

One of the difficulties in assessing the origin of fatigue in MS is that the disease has a number of facets in relation to the severity. For instance, there are those with MS who do not exhibit weakness and therefore have normal motor function versus those that display significant weakness. However, even when this difference is observed it seems that muscular fatigue is still very much a central phenomenon. By using transcranial magnetic stimulation (TMS) and assessing the effects of the fatiguing exercise on maximum grip strength in healthy controls versus MS subjects with and without apparent motor function, the fatiguing exercise resulted in a prolonged motor conduction time with MS (Petajan & White 2000). The most important finding these authors report is that neither in controls nor in MS was a difference observed in phosphocreatine (PCr) depletion and re-synthesis. Further to this was that cortical excitability was reduced for the non-fatigued contralateral muscle for MS, suggesting that there was impaired conduction in the corpus callosum. This study provides strong evidence that skeletal muscle fatigue in MS is likely to be centrally mediated.

Although MS is a neurodegenerative disease characterised by demyelination, the issue as to whether there is a differential loss of either Type I or Type II muscle fibres remains a fertile area of research. However, muscle biopsy analysis of MS versus healthy tibialis anterior muscle showed that there were fewer Type I fibres (66 ± 6 vs $76 \pm 6\%$), and that all fibre types were smaller and had lower oxidative enzyme activity, suggesting that in MS, skeletal muscle is smaller and relies more on anaerobic rather than aerobic-oxidative energy supply than does muscle of healthy individuals (Kent-Braun et al. 1997). This was also confirmed with observations that during a series of repeated contractions, there are greater decrements in isometric force and in the maximal rate of rise in force in MS (by $31.3 \pm 10.3\%$ and $50.1 \pm 10.0\%$) than in control subjects ($23.8 \pm 6.6\%$ and $39.0 \pm 8.1\%$) likely due to diminished oxidative capacity (de Haan et al. 2000). However, progressive resistance exercise in MS patients has been found to induce compensatory increases in muscle fibre size (Dalgas et al. 2010). Figure 10.1 shows the results of changes in cross-sectional area (CSA) of the different fibre types following progressive resistance exercise undertaken twice per week over 12 weeks in MS patients. In the top panel, after 12 weeks of normal physical activity the healthy controls did not display any changes in any of the fibre types studied. In contrast, the MS group had changes throughout the Type II fibres only. Although at pre-training there was a higher Type II and Type IIa CSA, the MS patients further increased the CSA with progressive training. This also resulted in overall isokinetic strength gains for the MS patients. An interesting result from this study was that progressive resistance training did not alter percentage distribution of muscle fibre types, which remained relatively unchanged between controls and MS patients. The authors suggested that the training stimulus was not sufficient to evoke a substantial fibre type transformation in these middle-aged MS patients.

The fact that MS patients exhibit heightened symptoms of fatigue points to the physical deconditioning which accompanies this disease. In particular there is some consensus that the disease has a central origin since there is evidence of reduced motor drive. However, the observation that resistance training increases the CSA of Type II fibres and as a consequence also improves strength does not mean that the symptoms of fatigue are ameliorated to any great extent since these fibres have low fatigue resistance. Conversely, fatigue severity could be improved

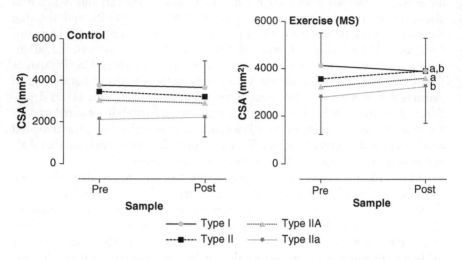

Figure 10.1 The changes in cross-sectional area (CSA) of different skeletal muscle fibre types in healthy controls over 12 weeks undertaking a normal physical activity routine (top panel) versus progressive resistance training (exercise) for multiple sclerosis (MS) patients (bottom panel) pre- and post-12 weeks (2 x per week). There was a significant change pre to post in MS compared with the control pre to post for Type II and Type IIa[a] and a significant difference compared with pre-trial value within group for Type II and Type IIx[b].

Source: Data redrawn from table 10.4 in Dalgas et al. (2010).

if the CSA of Type I fibres were either maintained or increased. Early studies in this area found that 15 weeks of aerobic conditioning in MS and controls improved cardiorespiratory responses, lipid profile and body composition similarly in both groups but this did not improve fatigue severity (Petajan et al. 1996). This relationship between aerobic training and improvements in maximal work capacity and peak oxygen uptake has been consistently reported, but notably these positive changes do not seem to improve symptomatic fatigue to any great extent (Rampello et al. 2007). However, more recent studies in this area have shown that maximal aerobic capacity and lung function were not changed by either training or non-training in MS patients (Mostert & Kesselring 2016). The authors suggested that this might have been related to low overall compliance to the training (65%) by the less severely affected patients.

Heat reactions in MS

In many MS patients, sensitivity to heat can be just as debilitating as all other symptoms. This particular symptom can to be traced back to the reports of Uhthoff (1890) (Guthrie & Nelson 1995), who described changes in the visual acuity during heating. In fact, the early observation was that not only visual acuity but also colour perception and other neurological signs were altered specifically following exercise, suggesting that exercise-induced increases in body temperature were the cause for these neurological changes. However, it is now known that heat exposure alone regardless of exercise can induce neurological signs in patients with MS (Guthrie & Nelson 1995). The current understanding for this observation is that there is a heat reaction blockade of the action potential in demyelinated neurons which is termed 'frequency dependent conduction block' (FDCB). Essentially, this suggests that nerve conduction velocity is slowed due to demyelination so that the axon is able to transmit only single or low-frequency impulses rather than high-frequency trains (Rasminsky & Sears 1972), which is especially the case with demyelinated axons exposed to increasing temperature (Schauf & Davis 1974). As a consequence, even a small increase in temperature might be able to completely block action potentials (Guthrie & Nelson 1995).

It is apparent that elevated environmental temperature, humidity and exercise exacerbate the sensitivity to heat in MS (Baker 2002). In healthy individuals, exercise-induced hyperthermia can hasten fatigue with the mechanism thought to be related to mediated reduction in motor drive (Nybo & Nielsen 2001). An interesting observation is that in healthy individuals, termination of exercise usually coincides with a core temperature of ~39.5°C. This particular phenomenon has not been reported in people with MS, even though heat sensitivity reduces exercise tolerance time in these patients (White et al. 2000). It is still unknown whether the severity of MS contributes in any to exacerbating heat sensitivity or even the appearance of neurological signs with rising body temperature due to the inconsistency of these observations among this group of patients (Ponichtera-mulcare 1993). However, what is clear is that the rate of rise in core temperature is less pronounced in patients with MS than in healthy controls, even though the terminal temperature is substantially less (Marino 2009). The reasons for this are likely to be related to autonomic dysfunction affecting such responses as sweating capacity, skin temperature and shifts in thermoregulatory control due to lesions within the central nervous system. First, it has been shown that the adaptive sweating responses following 15 weeks of aerobic training in MS found that sweat rate and sweat gland output were significantly less than in healthy controls (Davis et al. 2005). Further to this there is the possibility that in MS there is an upward shift in the thermoregulatory balance point whereby the threshold for invoking effector mechanisms for heat dissipation would be delayed. It has also been reported that in about 80% of MS patients paradoxical heat sensation is apparent when cooling skin (Hansen et al. 1996). A further consideration is the location of lesions within the central nervous system, which could affect temperature control by the hypothalamus, although the relationship between lesion load and location in MS is not well understood.

Fatigue in myasthenia gravis

Myasthenia gravis (MG) is a disease characterised by abnormally elevated fatigue and weakness which fluctuates between bouts of activity and rest. The hallmark of this disease is that weakness develops quickly after only brief physical exertion, but a period of rest will seemingly allow the muscles to return to normal capability. The disease usually involves all muscles, but primarily facial muscles are affected, whereby speech and swallowing are compromised, with respiratory muscles also being affected, and can lead to some distress. As with MS, this disease is also more prevalent in women than in men, although its occurrence increases in older men from the age of 60 years (http://brainfoundation.org.au/disorders/myas thenia-gravis). MG is an autoimmune disease whereby the immune system mistakenly attacks itself so that antibodies interfere with the normal transmission of nerve impulses to the muscles. This prevents the skeletal muscle from initiating and completing a normal contraction. This is essentially due to the disease targeting the neuromuscular junction, although it is still not definitive as to whether this involves the pre- or post-synaptic membrane. In addition, the disease can be in the form of either acquired or congenital, in which case the neurotransmitter acetylcholine (Ach) plays a different role in its capacity for neurotransmission (Keesey 2004). For example, if the pre-synaptic membrane is involved there will be defective Ach synthesis and release, whereas in post-synaptic involvement there will be decreased response to Ach. Of particular interest are the antibodies against the nicotinic Ach receptors on the post-synaptic membrane of the neuromuscular junction which reduces the number of Ach receptors (Fambrough et al. 1973; Fambrough 1979). One would expect that a reduced number of post-synaptic receptors would result in reduced Ach quanta; however, this does not seem to be the case, although the amplitude of the end-plate potentials is reduced, which can block nerve impulses (Lambert et al. 1976; Engel et al. 1976). A common observation in people with this disease is the "jittering" of skeletal muscle action, which is thought to be caused by variability in the firing of different muscle fibres within the same motor unit, eventually causing significant muscle weakness. An additional aspect is that MG patients not only complain of physical fatigue but also report that fatigue produces mild to moderate effects on cognitive and social function (Paul et al. 2000, 2002). Thus, MG produces physical fatigue which is manifested by the pathology related to the neuromuscular junction, but cognitive fatigue is also an important symptom of the disease.

Skeletal muscle fatigue in MG

In general terms the skeletal muscle force produced by patients with MG is lower and varies substantially across individuals. In fact, muscle weakness fluctuates from day to day or hour by hour and progresses through the day (Keesey 2004). However, the long-term consequence of the disease is the muscle atrophy and the particular loss of Type II fibres (Brooke & Engel 1969; Ringqvist 1971). As such, the loss of these muscle fibres will have a dramatic effect on the development and sustainability of power. Although there are only a few studies that have compared the muscle strength of MG patients to healthy controls, the typical observation is that in this disease there is a tendency for fatigability to be independent of muscle strength (Nicklin et al. 1987) and that force declines are greater in MG than in healthy controls (Secher & Petersen 1984).

Disease severity is thought to potentiate the muscle force and fatigue that MG patients exhibit and report. However, when patients are exposed to repetitive stimulation, muscular force can be either decrementing or non-decrementing. For example, Figure 10.2 shows the maximum voluntary isometric force that can be produced by patients with either decrementing (MG-D) or non-decrementing (ND-MG) disease versus healthy controls and their subsequent recovery from fatiguing muscular contractions of the shoulder abductors (Symonette et al. 2010). What is immediately observed is that ND-MG patients are unable to produce maximal force output to either D-MG or controls, although the D-MG patients also have reduced maximal force output compared with controls. In addition, during the fatiguing contractions, the decline in force output was steeper for both controls and ND-MG compared with D-MG. The reasons for this are not clear, although it is possible that the inability to reach high levels of maximum force output may have attenuated the decline that is normally possible. Following the fatiguing contractions, the recovery over the initial 0.5 min was faster for the D-MG than in D-MG and controls, with the recovery at 15 min being almost complete for both MG groups but not controls. This confirms that one aspect

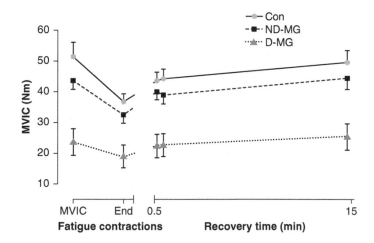

Figure 10.2 The force output as maximum voluntary isometric contraction (MVIC) followed by 12 x fatiguing contractions and recovery from this for up to 15 min (recovery time) for controls (con), myasthenia gravis that is classified as non-decrementing (ND-MG) and decrementing (D-MG) as assessed by repetitive neural stimulation.

Source: Data redrawn from figures 10.2 and 10.3 from Symonette et al. (2010).

of this disease is that rest reverses the muscular fatigue quickly (Nicolle 2002). However, the most salient finding in this study is that patients with MG reported greater fatigue than healthy controls but higher levels of fatigue in MG were associated with reduced muscle strength but no difference in muscle fatigue. Unfortunately, a measure of perceived exertion was not reported but these findings do suggest that MG patients are likely to report higher levels of fatigue regardless of muscle strength.

Heat reaction in MG

Not unlike MS, patients with MG are commonly heat sensitive and are affected by both rising body and ambient temperature (Borenstein & Desmedt 1974; Gutmann 1980). The reason for this sensitivity in MG is that increases in temperature affect the physiology at the neuromuscular junction in contrasting ways. First, an increase in temperature can improve the replenishment of Ach in the pre-synaptic terminals, whereas this might also reduce Ach release by way of the diminished calcium availability at the nerve terminal (Rutkove 2001). However, one observation in MG is the muscle jitter that occurs as the muscle temperature is altered. When assessing the single fibre electromyography of healthy controls versus that of MG patients, there is a distinct change in the jitter response (Sener & Yaman 2008). When temperature was increased from resting 37°C to 42°C the jitter was decreased significantly in controls, but the same temperature change in MG patients resulted in the opposite – an increase in muscle jitter. In clinical terms, the change of jitter with temperature in opposite directions in MG and healthy controls could be helpful to detect neuromuscular dysfunction (Sener & Yaman 2008). In addition, when applying an icepack to the eye of MG patients, the ptosis (droop) improves dramatically (Sethi et al. 1987) even when compared with rest (Kubis et al. 2000). In total, these findings indicate that in neurological disorders such as MG, temperature changes can have a dramatic effect on normal function and can potentially alter the capacity to undertake the most basic of activities. As such, temperature stability is a critical aspect of maintaining low levels of generalised fatigue.

Central or peripheral fatigue in disease?

The aim of this chapter was to highlight the effects of pathology on fatigue and in doing so it was also critical to evaluate the known mechanism as either central or peripheral in nature. There is wide consensus that in MS the fatigue that is reported is likely to be of central origin since a number of studies show that cortical excitability is reduced. On the other hand, the organic nature of MG is that this is known to be a disease which affects the neuromuscular junction, which, depending on whether the impairment is pre- or post-synaptic, will determine the overall effect on muscle performance. However, regardless of whether the disease is functionally manifested centrally or peripherally, patients with these neurological pathologies report a heightened sense of fatigue. Studies which attempt to interrogate the psychological component of these pathologies are scarce, but further understanding of the psychological effect and the impairment that this might cause in terms superimposing on the actual functional aspect would be critical in elucidating how fatigue is interpreted.

Evolutionary basis of pathology and fatigue

Finally, if humans opted for endurance and fatigue resistance over strength and power, of what benefit would this be in relation to the kinds of diseases just highlighted? This is a difficult question and any answer would be speculative at best. However, MS and MG are rarely identified in non-human primates, although some models exist (Brok et al. 2001).

An enticing but speculative hypothesis is that diet is a significant factor in the development of neurological pathology. For example, since MS seems to develop exclusively in humans it is hypothesised that non-human primates are resistant against MS but susceptible to the MS animal model, known as experimental autoimmune encephalomyelitis (EAE) ('t Hart 2016). These authors suggest that an important difference between human and non-human primates is that humans are unable to synthesise the sialic acid N-glycolylneuraminic acid (Neu5Gc). As such they propose that long-term ingestion of red meat increases the foreign Neu5Gc, which is introduced into vital regions of the central nervous system, such as the blood-brain barrier (BBB) and the axon-myelin unit. This potentiates binding of de novo synthesised heterophilic anti-NeuGc antibodies, causing blood-brain barrier leakage and destabilisation of axon-myelin coupling, which could initiate the characteristic pathological features of MS. This hypothesis does not auger well if we accept that *Homo* developed a propensity for meat eating as a way to fuel the development and maintenance of the large brain. In addition, the fact that these pathologies restrict the development of high muscular forces suggests that at a systemic level fatigue might have been much more debilitating if strength and power were selected because larger myelinated fibres are less fatigue resistant.

The relationship between evolutionary biology and pathology requires further research and empirical testing but could provide very useful information for further understanding fatigue as a human condition.

References

Baker, D., 2002. Multiple sclerosis and thermoregulatory dysfunction. *Journal of Applied Physiology*, 92, pp. 1779–1780.

Bakshi, R. et al., 2000. Fatigue in multiple sclerosis and its relationship to depression and neurologic disability. *Multiple Sclerosis*, 6, pp. 181–185.

Borenstein, S. & Desmedt, J., 1974. Temperature and weather correlates of myasthenic fatigue. *The Lancet*, 304(7872), pp. 63–66.

Brok, H.P. et al., 2001. Non-human primate models of multiple sclerosis. *Immunological Reviews*, 183, pp. 173–185.

Brooke, M.H. & Engel, W.K., 1969. The histographic analysis of human muscle biopsies with regard to fiber types. 3: myotonias, myasthenia gravis, and hypokalemic periodic paralysis. *Neurology*, 19(5), pp. 469–477.

Chaudhuri, A. & Behan, P.O., 2004. Fatigue in neurological disorders. *Lancet*, 363, pp. 978–988.

Dalgas, U. et al., 2010. Muscle fiber size increases following resistance training in multiple sclerosis. *Multiple Sclerosis*, 16(11), pp. 1367–1376.

Davis, S.L. et al., 2005. Pilocarpine-induced sweat gland function in individuals with multiple sclerosis. *Journal of Applied Physiology*, 98(5), pp. 1740–1744.

de Haan, A. et al., 2000. Contractile properties and fatigue of quadriceps muscles in multiple sclerosis. *Muscle & Nerve*, 23(10), pp. 1534–1541.

Engel, A.G. et al., 1976. Experimental autoimmune myasthenia gravis: a sequential and quantitative study of the neuromuscular junction ultrastructure and electrophysiologic correlations. *Journal of Neuropathology & Experimental Neurology*, 35(5), pp. 569–587.

Fambrough, D.M., 1979. Control of acetylcholine receptors in skeletal muscle. *Physiological Reviews*, 59(1), pp. 165–227.

Fambrough, D.M., Drachman, D.B. & Satyamurti, S., 1973. Neuromuscular junction in myasthenia gravis: decreased acetylcholine receptors. *Science*, 182(4109), pp. 293–295.

Garner, D.J.P. & Widrick, J.J., 2003. Cross-bridge mechanisms of muscle weakness in multiple sclerosis. *Muscle & Nerve*, 27(4), pp. 456–464.

Guthrie, T.C. & Nelson, D.A., 1995. Influence of temperature changes on multiple sclerosis: critical review of mechanisms and research potential. *Journal of the Neurological Sciences*, 129(1), pp. 1–8.

Gutmann, L., 1980. Heat-induced myasthenic crisis. *Archives of Neurology*, 37(10), pp. 671–672.

Hansen, C., Hopf, H.C. & Treede, R.D., 1996. Paradoxical heat sensation in patients with multiple sclerosis: evidence for a supraspinal integration of temperature sensation. *Brain*, 119 (Pt 5), pp. 1729–1736.

Keesey, J.C., 2004. Clinical evaluation and management of myasthenia gravis. *Muscle & Nerve*, 29(4), pp. 484–505.

Kent-Braun, J.A. et al., 1997. Strength, skeletal muscle composition, and enzyme activity in multiple sclerosis. *Journal of Applied Physiology*, 83(6), pp. 1998–2004.

Kubis, K.C. et al., 2000. The ice test versus the rest test in myasthenia gravis. *Ophthalmology*, 107(11), pp. 1995–1998.

Lambert, C.P., Lee Archer, R. & Evans, W.J., 2002. Body composition in ambulatory women with multiple sclerosis. *Archives of Physical Medicine & Rehabilitation*, 83(11), pp. 1559–1561.

Lambert, E.H., Lindstrom, J.M. & Lennon, V.A., 1976. End-plate potentials in experimental autoimmune myasthenia gravis in rats. *Annals of the New York Academy of Sciences*, 274(1), pp. 300–318.

Marino, F.E., 2004. Anticipatory regulation and avoidance of catastrophe during exercise-induced hyperthermia. *Comparative Biochemistry and Physiology. Part B, Biochemistry & Molecular Biology*, 139(4), pp. 561–569.

Marino, F.E., 2009. Heat reactions in multiple sclerosis: an overlooked paradigm in the study of comparative fatigue. *International Journal of Hyperthermia*, 25, pp. 34–40.

Morrison, S., Sleivert, G.G. & Cheung, S.S., 2004. Passive hyperthermia reduces voluntary activation and isometric force production. *European Journal of Applied Physiology*, 91(5–6), pp. 729–736.

Mostert, S. & Kesselring, J., 2016. Effects of a short-term exercise training program on aerobic fitness, fatigue, health perception and activity level of subjects with multiple sclerosis. *Multiple Sclerosis*, 8(2), pp. 161–168.

Ng, A.V., Miller, R.G. & Kent-Braun, J.A., 1997. Central motor drive is increased during voluntary muscle contractions in multiple sclerosis. *Muscle & Nerve*, 20(10), pp. 1213–1218.

Ng, A.V. et al., 2004. Functional relationships of central and peripheral muscle alterations in multiple sclerosis. *Muscle & Nerve*, 29(6), pp. 843–852.

Nicklin, J., Karni, Y. & Wiles, C.M., 1987. Shoulder abduction fatigability. *Journal of Neurology Neurosurgery & Psychiatry*, 50(4), pp. 423–427.

Nicolle, M.W., 2002. Myasthenia gravis. *The Neurologist*, 8(1), pp. 2–21.

Nielsen, B. & Nielsen, M., 1962. Body temperature during work at different environmental temperatures. *Acta Physiologica*, 56(2), pp. 120–129.

Noseworthy, J.H. et al., 2000. Multiple sclerosis. *New England Journal of Medicine*, 343(13), pp. 938–952.

Nybo, L. & Nielsen, B., 2001. Hyperthermia and central fatigue during prolonged exercise in humans. *Journal of Applied Physiology*, 91(3), pp. 1055–1060.

Paul, R.H., Cohen, R.A. & Gilchrist, J.M., 2002. Ratings of subjective mental fatigue relate to cognitive performance in patients with myasthenia gravis. *Journal of Clinical Neuroscience*, 9(3), pp. 243–246.

Paul, R.H. et al., 2000. Fatigue and its impact on patients with myasthenia gravis. *Muscle & Nerve*, 23(9), pp. 1402–1406.

Petajan, J.H. & White, A.T., 2000. Motor-evoked potentials in response to fatiguing grip exercise in multiple sclerosis patients. *Clinical neurophysiology*, 111(12), pp. 2188–2195.

Petajan, J.H. et al., 1996. Impact of aerobic training on fitness and quality of life in multiple sclerosis. *Annals of Neurology*, 39(4), pp. 432–441.

Ponichtera-Mulcare, J.A., 1993. Exercise and multiple sclerosis. *Medicine and Science in Sports & Exercise*, 25(4), pp. 451–465.

Rampello, A. et al., 2007. Effect of aerobic training on walking capacity and maximal exercise tolerance in patients with multiple sclerosis: a randomized crossover controlled study. *Physical Therapy*, 87(5), pp. 545–555.

Rasminsky, M. & Sears, T.A., 1972. Internodal conduction in undissected demyelinated nerve fibres. *Journal of Physiology*, 227, pp. 323–350.

Rice, C.L., Vollmer, T.L. & Bigland-Ritchie, B., 1992. Neuromuscular responses of patients with multiple sclerosis. *Muscle & Nerve*, 15(10), pp. 1123–1132.

Ringqvist, I., 1971. Muscle strength in Myasthenia gravis: effects of exhaustion and anticholinesterase related to muscle fibre size. *Acta Neurologica Scandinavica*, 47(5), pp. 619–641.

Rutkove, S.B., 2001. Effects of temperature on neuromuscular electrophysiology. *Muscle & Nerve*, 24(7), pp. 867–882.

Saboisky, J. et al., 2003. Exercise heat stress does not reduce central activation to non-exercised human skeletal muscle. *Experimental Physiology*, 88(6), pp. 783–790.

Schauf, C.L. & Davis, F.A., 1974. Impulse conduction in multiple sclerosis: a theoretical basis for modification by temperature and pharmacological agents. *Journal of Neurology Neurosurgery & Psychiatry*, 37(2), pp. 152–161.

Secher, N.H. & Petersen, S., 1984. Fatigue of voluntary contractions in normal and myasthenic human subjects. *Acta Physiologica*, 122(3), pp. 243–248.

Sener, H.O. & Yaman, A., 2008. Effect of high temperature on neuromuscular jitter in myasthenia gravis. *European neurology*, 59(3–4), pp. 179–182.

Sethi, K.D., Rivner, M.H. & Swift, T.R., 1987. Ice pack test for myasthenia gravis. *Neurology*, 37(8), pp. 1383–1383.

Sharma, K.R. et al., 1995. Evidence of an abnormal intramuscular component of fatigue in multiple sclerosis. *Muscle & Nerve*, 18(12), pp. 1403–1411.

Sheean, G.L. et al., 1997. An electrophysiological study of the mechanism of fatigue in multiple sclerosis. *Brain*, 120, pp. 299–315.

Slawta, J.N. et al., 2002. Coronary heart disease risk between active and inactive women with multiple sclerosis. *Medicine and Science in Sports & Exercise*, 34(6), pp. 905–912.

Smith, K.J. & McDonald, W.I., 1999. The pathophysiology of multiple sclerosis: the mechanisms underlying the production of symptoms and the natural history of the disease. *Philosophical Transactions of the Royal Society of London (Biological Sciences)*, 354(1390), pp. 1649–1673.

Symonette, C.J. et al., 2010. Muscle strength and fatigue in patients with generalized myasthenia gravis. *Muscle & Nerve*, 41(3), pp. 362–369.

't Hart, B.A., 2016. Why does multiple sclerosis only affect human primates? *Multiple Sclerosis*, 22(4), pp. 559–563.

Uhthoff, W., 1890. Untersuchungen über bei multiplen Herdsklerose vorkommenden Augenstorungen. *Archiv für Psychiatrie und Nervenkrankheiten*, 21, pp. 55–106.

White, A.T. et al., 2000. Effect of precooling on physical performance in multiple sclerosis. *Multiple Sclerosis*, 6(3), pp. 176–180.

White, L.J. & Dressendorfer, R.H., 2004. Exercise and multiple sclerosis. *Sports Medicine*, 24, pp. 1077–1100.

Index

Milton Keynes UK
Ingram Content Group UK Ltd.
UKHW040106071024
449327UK00019B/849